DEEP NUTRITION

BLENDING CULTURES, BRIDGING TIME

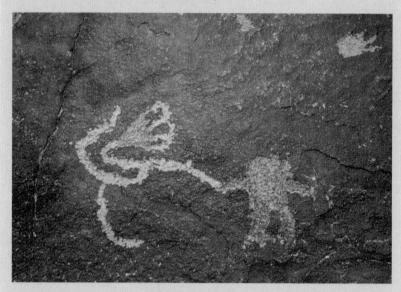

Pteroglyph found on Anasazi Ridge, New Mexico. The childlike glyph on the right is probably Anasazi, agrarians who lived between 400 and 1000 A.D. The left is possibly Numic, hunter gatherers who displaced the Anasazi after 1200 A.D. No one knows for certain what story it tells. What most attracted me to this particular petroglyph, however, is how the meaning of the original has been modified in a wonderful way, by a younger artist who attached his own symbol to it, in much the same way that our own ancient genetic code has been modified over time by everyone who has carried it.

DEEP NUTRITION

Why Your Genes
Need Traditional Food

Catherine Shanahan, M.D.
Luke Shanahan

FLATIRON
BOOKS
NEW YORK

To Buddy

*Of all the souls we have ever met,
he was the most human.*

DEEP NUTRITION. Copyright © 2008, 2016 by Catherine Shanahan and Luke Shanahan. All rights reserved. Printed in the United States of America. For information, address Flatiron Books, 175 Fifth Avenue, New York, N.Y. 10010.

www.flatironbooks.com

Design and production by March Tenth, Inc.

The Library of Congress Cataloging-in-Publication Data is available upon request.

ISBN 978-1-250-11382-5 (hardcover)
ISBN 978-1-250-11383-2 (e-book)

Our books may be purchased in bulk for promotional, educational, or business use. Please contact your local bookseller or the Macmillan Corporate and Premium Sales Department at 1-800-221-7945, extension 5442, or by e-mail at MacmillanSpecialMarkets@macmillan.com.

A substantionally different edition of this book was previously self-published in 2008.

First Flatiron Books Edition: January 2017

10 9 8 7 6 5 4 3 2 1

CONTENTS

AUTHOR'S NOTE

This book is for John Doyle.

Soon after John retired, he and his wife relocated from Ohio to Clearlake, north of Napa County, California. They came to be close to their son, to watch their new grandbaby grow, and to play in a four-season outdoor paradise. But weeks after relocating, John picked up his two-year-old granddaughter and felt a searing pain shooting through his back. What should have been a simple strain that might have resolved itself in a few days simply got worse—to the point that he needed help taking a shower. A stoic man, he endured the pain for two weeks before going to see his doctor. An X-ray showed a funny shadow, and the follow-up MRI identified a benign mass growing around his nerve that his doctors thought might be contributing to the pain. He counted himself lucky that the tumor was caught before it became inoperable. So John and his wife came to the hospital where I worked, in Napa, for what should have been a routine neurosurgical procedure. And that's when his luck ran out.

The routine surgery turned out to be not at all routine. It was complicated by an infection, and the infection was complicated by a blood clot in John's spinal cord that, by the time we met, made it impossible for him to walk or control his bladder and bowel. As his primary care physician, I saw John multiple times a week, and always there was a new problem. It was tragic. To this day, I remember his case in detail; I remember the frustration of dealing with a new medical issue each time he came in for an office visit only to see another problem pop up a few days later. Everything I'd hoped to help people to avoid—by writing books and posting articles on my blog and speaking in public—and all the work I'd done, was to prevent bad things from happening to good people the way they were happening to John. His body was falling apart, and in spite of how easily it all could have been prevented, I'd never had the opportunity for early intervention. John was not my patient until it was already too late.

This book is for John's wife, Margaret. Six months after we met, John Doyle was dead. His infection never cleared and he developed another clot that stopped his heart. After her husband of almost fifty years passed, the RV Margaret and John were going to travel in together became difficult to manage, and aside from her son and grandchild, she didn't know anyone in Clearlake. She relocated to a retirement community in Napa, where I continued to treat her for insomnia, depression, and anxiety. Unlike John, she'd always tried to eat right, so aside from stress-induced conditions, she was in good shape. Unfortunately, their son followed John's eating habits more than Margaret's, giving low priority to healthy eating and, unknowingly, putting his offspring at risk.

This book is for John's young granddaughter, Kayla. Her dad and his girl-friend were dedicated parents, and when baby Kayla developed eczema, her mom's pediatrician advised switching to formula. It didn't help. But by the time they figured that out, her mother's breast milk production had stopped. At age three, Kayla developed a limp that turned out to be the result of a brain tumor. Margaret took her RV back up to Clearlake and parked it in her son's driveway so she could help out. Like so many of my health-conscious patients, she found herself staring down at two generations of failing health, a scenario that too many health practitioners would just chalk up to bad luck.

The story of the Doyle family—a story of life interrupted, of hopes, dreams, and plans taking a sudden, unfortunate turn—is one I see play out in my office all the time. These are stories that could have happier endings.

The narrative of this entire family would have played out differently had they benefited from preventative intervention. But in the current healthcare system, people don't receive the most powerful form of preventative medicine—a comprehensive dietary education. We hear about barriers to healthcare all the time, but that was not John Doyle's problem. He was lucky enough to have had excellent insurance; it covered all his bills and granted him plenty of access to every specialist he needed, whenever he needed it. What John's medical providers couldn't offer him—what few doctors can offer any of their patients—was a crash course in healthy eating. Without this knowledge, he was left vulnerable to a most insidious killer: the standard American diet.

His previous doctors never spoke to him about diet. And why would they? Medical doctors are simply not trained to consider how a person's diet might contribute to medical conditions other than obesity, diabetes, or heart disease. What little we physicians do learn about preventing illness is so useless that few of us even abide by it ourselves. Since there's not much by way of standardized nutrition training, any doctor interested in nutrition must take it upon himself to study on his own. And any physician hoping to fully understand how nutrients and toxins act in the body would need a particularly strong background in biochemistry and cell physiology.

When my own health took a turn for the worse in 2001, I leaned heavily on my undergraduate training at Rutgers University and graduate work at Cornell studying biochemistry and molecular biology as I tried to flush out any possible connection between my health problems and my diet. The deeper I dug, the more critical that training became. The revelations were so profound, I immediately started putting them to use to help my patients.

Like most doctors, I had an average of seven minutes with each of my patients. So although there was no time for a wholesale revision of their dietary program, I could at least leave them with some key advice—like cut out vegetable oils and reduce sugars—that would, more often than not, produce amazing benefits. I'm talking about reversing high triglycerides, hypertension, eczema, recurring infections, migraines, and more.

As much as hospitals and clinics like to talk about wellness and prevention, the truth is, a real discussion about healthy eating cannot take place in a doctor's office. This is why in order to check off the "nutrition-discussion box" they rely on sound-bites, like "eat your colors," which doesn't really mean much, or "everything in moderation," which, in a world where toxins are marketed as health foods, can be harmful advice. Providing real dietary guidance requires far more time with patients than insurance models currently allow. You could fill a book with what needs to be discussed for anyone to adopt a truly healthy diet—which is why, in 2003, I started writing this one.

Five years later, *Deep Nutrition* was complete, and the book started to catch on. People around the world wrote me, sharing stories of how their lives had been changed for the better by implementing its principles. Soon thereafter, the L.A. Lakers took interest. Head trainer Gary Vitti and strength and conditioning coach Tim DiFrancesco felt that good nutrition was being underutilized in the NBA. And so, with me as a member of their training staff, we developed the PRO (Performance Recovery Orthogenesis) Nutrition Program and created a partnership with Whole Foods Markets to ensure that no player, whether on the road or at home, would have to rely on junk food if they didn't want to. Since that time other NBA teams have developed relationships with Whole Foods Markets with excellent results—a trend toward real food in professional sports that is certain to grow.

I don't think of *Deep Nutrition* as a diet book. It's a book that gives you control over your own health destiny. It's an alternative to handing that control over to the financial interests of hospitals and multinational corporations—institutions that see you as little more than an image on an X-ray and will turn a blind eye to lucrative procedures performed without proper medical indication. You don't want to have to depend on anyone else—well-meaning or not—to set your life back on track. And you don't need to.

Deep Nutrition isn't just a diet book. It's an *I'm going to enjoy my retirement* book. It's an *I'm not dependent on medications* book. A *My kids are healthy* book. It's an *I have all the energy I need* book. An *I get to see my granddaughter's graduation* book. An *I can play whatever sport I want* book. An *I can do anything I put my mind to* book. It's first and foremost an *I'm getting to live the life I want* book, because to live the life you want, the life you imagine for yourself, you first need to take control over your health.

You can think of diet as a strategy, a tool—the most powerful of all tools—to accomplish the task of optimizing your health. When my husband, Luke, and I wrote the first edition of *Deep Nutrition*, my intent, as a physician, was to give that tool to as many people as I possibly could. And it brings me such joy and satisfaction that the original edition did help a lot of people. Every time a patient bought dozens of copies to share with their families, I felt grateful. When athletes like Kobe Bryant, Steve Nash, Dwight Howard, and Bryce Salvador started adapting its principles, becoming role models for their fans, and even helping to implement these principles inside the leagues in which they operate, I felt grateful. And when leading health experts, bloggers, physicians, nutritionists, and authors began to incorporate many of our ideas into their own work, I felt grateful. I felt grateful because I knew that each of these people were using the book as a tool to change the course of their own health destinies.

As I had hoped, *Deep Nutrition* changed the conversation.

But it didn't do enough.

Sadly, the general trajectory of America's health has not changed—not even close. Statistics show our country is less healthy than it was in 2008. There are now more people struggling with obesity, more children with autism, more food allergies, more traumatic brain injuries from which athletes and soldiers don't fully recover. There's much more work to be done. And thankfully, there is also now new, powerful scientific data at our disposal to bring the concepts of *Deep Nutrition* up-to-date, and plenty of additional research that reaffirms the basic tenets of the book as well as research demanding an expansion of some of those concepts into new territories.

For those of you who purchased the original edition and have lived in accordance with my advice—those of you who knew in your bones that traditional food using well-sourced produce and humanely raised animal products made intuitive sense—I'm happy to be able to say that all the new science available confirms that you banked on the right ideas. But as the science of nutrition continues to evolve, and the wellness conversation right along with it, there's a lot more to talk about. With this new, updated edition, I hope to bring you four categories of information I believe you'll find useful in your journey towards optimizing your health.

I. This Edition of *Deep Nutrition* Answers Your Questions

In the first edition of *Deep Nutrition* I presented the key ideas I thought were important to anyone wanting the big picture of human health. It was really *my* book. This expanded edition is *your* book.

I have not just updated the science and added new chapters. I've also responded to all the insightful questions, feedback, criticisms, and demands for fuller explanations that I've heard from readers in response to the first edition. Many are built into the expanded chapters. Others, particularly topics that are on everyone's minds right now, such as detoxification, genetically modified organisms (GMOs), animal rights and sustainability, gluten, brain health, and the microbiome, are addressed in a separate Frequently Asked Questions chapter.

While practicing medicine in Kauai, Hawaii, I asked Luke if he could help me write a small pamphlet to explain what I knew to be true about nutrition in simple terms for my patients. Soon, that pamphlet grew into the first edition of *Deep Nutrition*. Never did I anticipate that it would give rise to a community. Some of my readers have taken the ideas presented in the book and added to them, lecturing on nutrition or even writing their own books. Many have started businesses—hip new broth bistros, catering companies—that celebrate the dietary concepts I describe. It's been incredible to hear from this community. Six years after its publication, I still receive daily phone calls, emails, and comments on social media from people whose lives have been changed for the better by implementing the ideas in the book. I've heard hundreds of stories of hope from young families with new children; from adults healing from chronic pain; from people who have recovered from disease, who have experienced physical rejuvenation, or who feel better in their sixties than they ever did in their twenties. Stories like this reassure me that this book is as relevant today as it was when we first wrote it.

Since its publication, I have witnessed hundreds of my clinic patients experience astonishing health reversals after applying the *Deep Nutrition* principles. I have watched happily as they return with lower blood pressures, cholesterol abnormalities eradicated, skin conditions cleared, migraines resolved, moods stabilized, auto-immune diseases—sometimes disabling—drastically improved or in remission. And I have received a flood of testimonials that confirm the body's seemingly miraculous capacity to heal when provided a true, human diet.

Here are just a few of the ways adopting *Deep Nutrition* has changed the lives of its readers:

FOR ADULTS

- Improved mood
- Hunger is curbed and need for snacking disappears
- Stronger joints
- Smoother skin
- Improved fertility
- Fewer infections
- Near elimination of heart attack and stroke risk
- Allergic reactions diminish
- Reduced risk of dementia

FOR CHILDREN

- Improved learning capacity
- Fewer tantrums and behavior problems
- Improved jaw growth and reduced need for orthodontia
- Improved immune system and reduced allergies
- Increases in potential height
- Puberty occurs at the normal age and rate

But the stories that touch me most deeply speak to a kind of *awakening* when it comes to our relationship with food. This is a trend that started long before *Deep Nutrition*, but I feel that I'm augmenting that new awareness when people tell me how our book "completely changed their relationships with food." They rhapsodize passionately about clearing their kitchen cupboards, dusting off their grandmothers' cookbooks, seeking out farmers whose practices include revitalizing overworked soil, and treating their animals with the respect they deserve.

That brings me to something else I'll be discussing in this edition: important lessons to be learned from the vegan/vegetarian community that benefit the animals raised for food, the environment, and of course, our health. While omnivores and vegans necessarily disagree about one of the central ethical questions of our time—*Is it ever okay to eat animals or dairy?*—there is much vegans and conscientious omnivores already agree about, and the sooner those two groups get together and discuss those commonalities, the sooner we can start to make a significant change in human health, and the healthier our planet.

2. This Edition of *Deep Nutrition* Offers a Plan

It's one thing to know what's good for you. But the real work begins when you decide to organize your daily routine around a new way of eating. The number-one request I receive is for more specific, practical instructions on how to implement the *Deep Nutrition* concepts into our lives. So this edition includes an entire section that will guide you, step-by-step, on how to make the switch to the ultimate healthy lifestyle. Much of what is included in this new chapter has come from our readers, who have generously shared not just their success stories, but also the nitty-gritty details of exactly what they did first and how they handled the complexities of building these better habits into the swirl and chaos of daily life. And of course this edition includes what everyone has asked for most of all: meal plans and recipes!

Because I do talk a lot about the value of animal products to our health, it's not always obvious that there's a benefit to be gained by following the *Deep Nutrition* principles even without eating meat. So I've created a plant-strong meal plan to help readers following a vegetarian or vegan lifestyle to optimize their nutrition as well.

3. This Edition of *Deep Nutrition* Includes More Evidence

To those of you who went out and spread the word about *Deep Nutrition* among your family and friends, whether you're a dietician, doctor, nutritionist, or trainer who made it required reading among your clients and patients, or a chef, student, foodie, science enthusiast, or homemaker who simply believes in the message and wants to spread it, I thank you. Your way of thinking is starting to catch on. More people are talking about the harms of sugar—even doctors! More people are refusing to take antibiotics unless they're absolutely necessary. More people are taking the need for sleep seriously. More people are interested in fostering a relationship with beneficial bacteria: taking probiotics, avoiding antibacterial soaps and lotions, even fermenting their own kombucha, kefir, yogurt, sauerkraut, and more. More people are concerned about animal welfare and are willing to pay more for meat if it comes from farmers who are conscientious about being good stewards of the land and taking proper care of their animals.

If you are already on board with all of that, this edition will arm you with the new science that has come to light since 2008. These fascinating new insights—from research in all areas of health—show that you were right to believe in the *Deep Nutrition* message. Like me, you probably believe that if everyone (or at least most people) do not get on board in a big way, then health in the United States, and elsewhere, is certain to decline even further. So it's not just a matter of your personal health improving; it's a matter of whether or not you want to live in a society where our failing health is the only thing people talk about.

The good news for us is, according to all the research in all the health-related fields that has come out since the first edition of *Deep Nutrition* was published, those of us who believe that diet is central to good health are on the right page. And every day researchers around the world release more evidence that a good diet can do more than anything else to improve quality of life. The bad news is that we're still not all in agreement about what a good diet is. And because of the continued misinformation supporting consumption of a continually less nutritious food supply, we now are experiencing the predicted results of worsening health. In fact, in some areas of health, the problems are picking up pace—incidents of food allergies, diabetes, and mental illness have only increased since 2008. This updated edition offers those of you who are on the cutting edge of educating others more ammunition to help you do the good work you do.

4. This Edition of *Deep Nutrition* Presents a More Focused Attack

In 2012, I walked into my office where a fax placed on my desk labeled "FROM CIA PRESIDENT" was marked "URGENT." In this case, the CIA did not refer to the international agency based in McLean, Virginia. It stood for the Culinary Institute of America. The fax was sent in response to an article Luke and I wrote for the *Napa Register* entitled "The Canola Blob." Our article explained that this toxic oil, touted as "heart healthy," had displaced not just butter and cream but also olive, coconut, and peanut oils from the menus of most of the Napa Valley's finest restaurants—including one that was once described as "the best restaurant in America." We intended to sound the alarm that canola—together with other refined, bleached, and deodorized (RBD) vegetable oils—was anything but heart healthy. To the contrary, I warned that canola and other vegetable oils are largely responsible for the majority of fatal heart attacks and disabling strokes, as well as a raft of other familiar diseases, in the United States. We hoped to draw the attention of chefs and start a conversation. So we were actually quite pleased to be issued, from the president of the CIA, a summons to call him "to discuss [our] spreading wrong information."

It turned out the president, Charles Henning, was an affable gentleman who kindly invited us to "break bread" and discuss the source of our difference in opinion. Several days later, Luke and I found ourselves sitting at a table with Mr.

Henning at the open-air restaurant overlooking the rolling green vineyards and stately oaks in the valley below. He had prepared quite a treat for us, including a tasting flight of olive oil paired with chocolates. He was quite passionate about the quality of his olive oils, and spent a few moments detailing the great care taken to preserve the delicate antioxidants responsible for its pale green color and complex flavors. I was genuinely impressed at the breadth of his understanding of biochemistry, so I told him, "Not many people could explain the science of oxidation in such clear detail. But as we're here because of our difference of opinion on canola, I have to ask, If you recognized that care must be taken to protect the nutrients in olive oil, why not consider what the processing does to canola, which is never treated so gently? If canola is so healthy, why aren't we having a canola tasting?"

And that's when I got a taste of the bitter truth. "We have to feed the masses. There's just not enough olive oil for everyone," Mr. Henning told me. So there we had it.

This is tough to admit. In the first edition of *Deep Nutrition*, I made the argument that vegetable oil was toxic and that its consumption was also a leading cause of deadly heart attacks and strokes, among many other things. But for some reason, of all the arguments I made in *Deep Nutrition*, this is the one nobody cared much about.

Well, almost nobody. The L.A. Lakers did. And Mark Sisson did—he's making the only currently available brand of mayonnaise you can find commercially that does not have vegetable oil. Thankfully, most of the people who wrote letters and most of the people I've spoken with have gotten the message. But unlike every other topic discussed in that original text (topics like nutrient density and the reduction of empty carbs, the health benefits of healthy fats and fermented foods to help support a thriving microbiome, the benefits of bone stock, and the value of pasture-raised animals), the vegetable oil argument has yet to really move the needle.

My failure to sound the alarm among chefs is especially upsetting because I put so much faith in chefs. As you will soon discover, I believe that flavor equals nutrition; seeking out and enhancing flavor almost invariably leads to the enhancing of nutrient value. If you understand this concept, then it's no great leap to suggest that chefs are the original nutritionists and that the approach of gifted chefs is the same approach we should take as nutritionists and consumers of nutritional information. The problem is, when it comes to the vegetable oils, many chefs abandon their instincts, opting for the far cheaper vegetable oils because of their flavor neutrality or high smoke point. Some even claim to be looking out for their customers' health or, commonly, for the safety of their peanut-oil-sensitive patrons. In reality, when chefs cook with these oils or drizzle olive oil atop a ramekin of canola and pass it off as pure olive oil, or instruct their staff to keep customers guessing about what oils they're actually eating by answering all oil questions with the innocuous-sounding, "It's a blend," chefs are simply listening to the restaurant owner or, more specifically, to the owner's accountants. But those chefs looking only to the bottom line are selling their customers, as well as their own food establishments, short.

I visited a popular chain restaurant with Los Angeles-based chef and restaurant finance consultant Debbie Lee, and together we looked over a buffet of sustainably sourced ingredients—all ruined by cooking in toxic oil. I asked Chef Debbie what it would cost per dish for a restaurant to use olive oil instead of vegetable oil. She estimated it to be roughly fifty cents per plate. Maybe that sounds like a lot in a restaurant that sells its salads for $2.75, where that extra fifty cents is a big bump, but vegetable oil has slithered its way into the best restaurants in the country. In fact, twenty-six of the twenty-nine five-star hotels on the NBA tour use vegetable oils or blends in place of olive oil for pizza sauces, salad dressings, hollandaise, marinades, mashed potatoes, baked goods—you name it. There's no dish that cutting corners won't ruin. At fifty bucks a plate for some of these high-end dinners, you'd think they could toss in a few pennies for you to enjoy your dinner without a dose of toxicity. When I learned that culinary great and restaurateur Thomas Keller, whose flagship restaurant was minutes from my office, uses vegetable oils in his restaurants (and recommends them in his cookbook recipes), I realized that vegetable oils like canola are not only ruining our health, they're a threat to the entire culinary enterprise.

Maybe because I explained how vegetable oil is bad for so many reasons—from damaging arteries to causing fatty liver and interfering with cell development—I failed to get the message across. Perhaps I should have picked a single target. Maybe it was because I also said high levels of sugar are toxic. Maybe it's because I didn't say that the average health-conscious consumer gets 15–30 percent of their daily calories from this stuff, and the ordinary eater 30 to 60 percent.[1] Maybe these oils are still so ubiquitous because they are tasteless and odorless and it's hard to know when some cost-cutting corporation is sneaking them into your food. Perhaps these oils are still so prevalent just because there's so much else gone wrong with the food we buy—from GMOs to endocrine disrupting pesticides to herbicides to worries over gluten—that the issues with vegetable oils get lost.

So in this updated edition of *Deep Nutrition*, I've added a chapter focusing on the harms of vegetable oils in the brain. Why the brain? First of all, any disease that damages your brain threatens your very identity. There's nothing more devastating than that. Second, because we don't screen for brain problems using objective testing. We rely on our patients to alert us when something is wrong inside their heads. But obviously there's a catch: you may not realize there's something wrong because your brain has stopped working right. Unlike the other vital organs, the brain lacks a sensory system to alert us when it's in pain (headaches are thought to originate in intracranial blood vessels, not the metabolically stressed neurons). And last, because the brain often suffers when vegetable oils damage the other tissues in the body, like the gut, our blood and lymphatic circulations, the immune system, and even our genes. Damage to these systems can generate downstream effects that lead to specific impacts on the brain.

So much data has come in since 2008 that has convinced me these oils are particularly harmful to the brain that I was tempted to write a book on the topic. For example, researchers in Milan have shown one of the harmful compounds in vegetable oil degrades the internal highways of nerve cells called intermediate filaments.[2] Another group at Mt. Sinai fed the metabolites of vegetable oil to mice in varying concentrations, and the mice that ate the most oil developed the equivalent of Alzheimer's at the earliest age.[3] Because of the avalanche of new evidence pointing to vegetable oils as the most powerful brain-killing chemicals, when the opportunity to publish this revised and updated editon of *Deep Nutrition* arose, I knew I needed to add this chapter. The information just can't wait any longer. Because this chapter is so packed with information and has such serious implications regarding the many brain and mood disorders that are now commonplace, I hope you read it particularly closely—in fact, I hope you think of it as a book within a book.

THE NEXT GENERATION

The age of technological health solutions is coming to an end.

Our nation's technophilia started in earnest just after World War II, when advancements in medicine and pharmaceuticals gave rise to the notion that if we ever got sick, modern medicine would come to our rescue, gradually turning more and more of the responsibility for our health over to government, corporations, and other perceived authorities. These same authorities convinced us that women could finally be freed from the confines of the kitchen if only they were willing to abandon traditional ingredients and recipes and place their trust, instead, in industrial products from corporations such as Dupont, which promised "better living through chemistry." This idea caught on so well that now, when the natural requirements for health seem inconvenient, we're conditioned to look to one or another corporation for a shortcut around those requirements.

And how's that working out for us?

A quarter of infections are now resistant to antibiotic therapy, and we've recently discovered each course kills hundreds of species of beneficial bacteria that may never come back to help us fend off the bad bugs again.

Our war on cancer has had minimal effect, if any. In fact, cancer seems to be thriving in the U.S. population. In 1960 a woman's lifetime risk of developing breast cancer was one in twenty-two. Now it's one in eight.[4] And the incidence of childhood cancer has increased nearly 60 percent.[5]

Cardiovascular disease is still the number-one killer of men and women.[6] More Americans than ever are living with seriously impaired mental functioning from Alzheimer's. According to the Alzheimer's Foundation, 44 percent of the population between age seventy-five and eighty-five carries a diagnosis, and are, or will soon be rendered, dependent on others to care for their basic needs.[7] What's the point of spending all this money on living longer when the tarnish of Alzheimer's robs any remaining shine from your golden years, taking from you every memory of who you are?

We're sicker than ever. Healthcare is the number-one driver of the U.S. economy. The pharmaceutical industry now has the spare change to lobby Congress with more dollars than the combined expenditures of oil, gas, and military defense. Keep in mind, this is the very same industry that has failed to stem the tide of obesity, heart disease, diabetes, cancer, Alzheimer's, autism, and the rest.

Technology has failed to keep us healthy. And now millions of people are getting wise to the fact that the only technology that has consistently provided us with healthy children, healthy hearts, and healthy minds is the technology that has been under constant development and quality improvement since life on Earth began: the technology of nature.

The more you plug into this technology of nature, the healthier you will be. This is the bedrock argument of *Deep Nutrition*. And of course the best way to plug in to nature is through well-sourced ingredients whose nutritional value is protected and enhanced using the same culinary techniques that have served us for millennia.

Whether you are one of the people who shared the first edition of this book with friends and family—and if you are, thank you!—or you are about to be introduced to *Deep Nutrition* concepts for the first time, I hope this book can serve as a science-backed articulation of the commonsense beliefs you already feel in your bones: fake foods are bad for us. Food has a powerful influence on your health. Source and tradition really do matter. Given the right diet, the human body has a remarkable ability to provide a lifetime of optimal health.

If you would like to better understand just how deep these truths run and how exactly to harness nature's power to inspire better health, then this book is for you.

INTRODUCTION

This book describes the diet to end all diets.

That's easy to say, of course. All kinds of nutrition books claim to describe the one and only, best-of-all diet—the last one you'll ever need. The truth is, there really are a lot of good diets out there. You're already familiar with some of them: the Okinawan, the Mediterranean, and the French—who, paradoxically, live long, healthy lives though their foods are so heavy and rich.

As a physician, I've often wondered—as have many of my patients—what it is, exactly, that makes all these good diets so special. If the people in Japan, eating lots of fish and fresh vegetables, and the people of the Mediterranean, eating dairy and foods drenched in olive oil, can enjoy superior health, and attribute their good health to the foods they eat, then how is it that—enjoying apparently different foods—they can both lay claim to the number-one, best diet on earth? Could it be that many cultures hold equal claim to a fantastically successful nutritional program? Might it be that people all over the world are doing things right, acquiring the nutrients their bodies need to stay healthy and feel young by eating what appear to be different foods but which are, in reality, nutritionally equivalent?

This book comprehensively describes what I like to call the Human Diet. It is the first to identify and describe the commonalities between all the most successful nutritional programs people the world over have depended on for millennia to protect their health. The Human Diet also encourages the birth of healthy children so that the heritage of optimum health can be gifted to the next generation, and the generations that follow.

We like to talk about leaving a sustainable, healthy environment for our children. The latest science fuses the environmental discussion with the genetic one; when we talk environmental sustainability, we are necessarily talking about our genomic sustainability.

This is also the first book to discuss health across generations. Because of a new science called *epigenetics*, it will no longer make sense to consider our health purely on the personal level. When we think of our health, we think of our own bodies, as in "I feel good," "I like my weight," "I'm doing fine." Epigenetics is teaching us that our genes can be healthy or sick, just like we can. And if our genes are healthy when we have children, that health is imparted to them. If our genes are ailing, then that illness can be inherited as well. Because epigenetics allows us to consider health in the context of a longer timeline, we are now able to understand how what we eat as parents can change everything about our children, even the way they look. We'll talk about how, with the right foods, we can get our genomes into shape to give our kids a fighting chance.

Each chapter is chock full of scientific revelations you can use to take positive action toward better health. If you have digestive system problems, you will learn how to act as a gardener of your intestinal flora to better protect yourself against pathogenic infections. If you're fighting cancer, you'll learn that sugar is cancer's favorite food and how cutting sugar helps you start to starve it out. If you suffer from recurring migraines, frequent fatigue, irritability, or concentration problems, you will learn how eliminating toxic oils and adding more fresh greens into your diet can free you from these syndromes.

One of the most important new concepts of *Deep Nutrition* is the idea that the foods parents eat can change the way their future children look. Actually, it's not entirely new. Most of us are familiar with fetal alcohol syndrome, a developmental impairment characterized by a set of facial abnormalities caused by alcohol consumption during pregnancy. Those very same developmental impairments can be caused by malnutrition during pregnancy or early childhood. I see this every day in my clinic. On the pages here, I'll explain why following the standard dietary recommendations currently promoted by nutritionists and dietitians means running the risk that your child's development will be similarly affected. To protect your children from these potentially life-altering problems, I provide a game plan to help ensure mom's body is adequately fortified with all the nutritional supplies a growing baby requires—something I call the sibling strategy.

There's been a reluctance to equate good looks with good health—even, for that matter, to broach the subject. But with the healthcare infrastructure creaking under the bloat of chronically ill children and adults, it's time to get real. We're not talking about abstract aesthetic concepts of beauty. If you're planning on having children, and you want them to have every opportunity in life, you want them to be healthy *and* physically attractive. How do we know what's attractive? We met with the world's leading expert in the science of beauty to find out for ourselves what, exactly, makes a person pretty or plain. His name is Dr. Stephen Marquardt. He's a highly sought-after plastic surgeon living outside Los Angeles, and his "Marquardt Mask" shows how the perfect human face is the inevitable result of a person's body growing in accordance with the mathematical rules of nature.

You're going to meet another maverick, a man who should be considered the father of modern nutrition. Like Marquardt, a plastic surgeon, this modest dentist refused to accept the idea that it was natural for children's teeth to crowd and shift as haphazardly as tombstones on frost-heaved ground. Teeth should fit, he insisted. He traveled the world to determine if living on traditional foods would ensure the proper growth of children so that their teeth, their eyes, and every organ in their bodies would match one another in perfect proportion, ensuring optimum function and extraordinary health. He discovered that human health depends on traditional foods.   proves that this is so because our genes expect the nutrients traditional foods provide.

The most important single idea you're going to come away with is that there is an underlying order to our health. Sickness isn't random. We get sick when our genes don't get something they expect, one too many times. No matter your age, meeting these genetic expectations will improve your health dramatically. This is why we've devoted the bulk of the plan section of the book to describing what, exactly, your genes expect you to eat: the Four Pillars of the Human Diet. These foods will unlock your genetic potential, literally rebuilding your body one molecule at a time as fast as you can feed it. Of coure, this doesn't all happen overnight. The longer you continue to provide your body rejuvenating nutrition, the more benefits you will enjoy.

The first thing you will notice is more mental energy—usually within the first few days. As I tell my patients who elect to embark on this healing journey, the real you is obscured behind layers of cognitive static. Like a cell phone signal flickering in and out, the communication between regions of your mind is partially blocked. You don't even know who you really are until your mind is fully operational.

But before you can discover that potential, it is essential that you learn to recognize two toxic substances present in our food that are incompatible with normal genetic function: sugars and vegetable oils. These are not just toxic to people who have food sensitivities or certain medical conditions like leaky gut or prediabetes. They're toxic to every living thing. By eliminating vegetable oil and reducing foods that raise blood sugar, you will make caloric space to accommodate the nutrition your body craves.

When you have finished reading this book, you will have completely revised the way you think about food. We're going to put calorie counting and struggling to find the perfect ratio of carbs to protein to fat on the back burner. These exercises don't reveal what really matters about your food. Food is like a language, an unbroken information stream that connects every cell in your body to an aspect of the natural world. The better the source and the more undamaged the message when it arrives to your cells, the better your health will be. If you eat a properly cooked steak from an open-range, grass-fed cow, then you are receiving information not only about the health of that cow's body, but also about the health of the grasses from which she ate, and the soil from which those grasses grew. If you want to know whether or not a steak or a fish or a carrot is good for you, ask yourself what portions of the natural world it represents, and whether or not the bulk of that information remains intact. This requires traveling backward down the food chain, step by step, until you reach the ground or the sea.

In the following chapters, you will learn that the secret to health—the big secret, the one no one's talking about—is that there is no secret. Getting healthy, really healthy, and staying healthy can be easy. Avoiding cancer and dependence on medications, staving off heart disease, keeping a razor-sharp mind well into advanced years, and even having healthy, beautiful children are all aspects of the human experience that can be, and should be, under your control. You can live better, and it doesn't have to be that difficult. You just have to be armed with the right information.

No matter what you already believe about diet, medicine, or health—including the limits of your own health—the book you're about to read will enable you to make better sense of what you already know. To answer what is for many people a nagging question: *Who's right?* What's the simple, complete picture that ties all the best information together, so that I can know, once and for all, which foods my family is supposed to eat and which ones we need to avoid? How can I be sure that what I'm preparing for my children will give them a better chance to grow normally, succeed in school, and live long, happy lives?

What am I supposed to make for dinner?

This book will give you the answer.

PART ONE

The Wisdom of Tradition

WHAT DO THE TOUGHEST MEN IN HISTORY ALL HAVE IN COMMON?

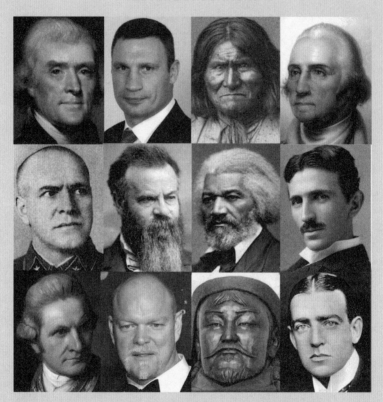

They all ate the same foods. From left to right starting from the top row: Thomas Jefferson, Wladimir Klitschko, Geronimo, George Washington, Georgy Zhukov, John Powell, Frederick Douglass, Nikola Tesla, James Cook, Magnus Samuelson, Genghis Khan, Ernest Shackleton.

Whether battling their way to victory, surviving months of bitter arctic cold, or leading a nation, the greatest men in history were no sissies. They look tough because they are tough. They are men of grit, determination, and extraordinary physiology.

CHAPTER I

Reclaiming Your Health
The Origins of Deep Nutrition

- We are less healthy today than our ancestors, despite boasting a longer lifespan.

- Nutrition science of the 1950s convinced people that the only healthy foods were relatively bland.

- An optimal human diet is full of both nutrition and flavor.

- By disregarding culinary traditions, we've predisposed ourselves to genetic damage.

Ask ten people what the healthiest diet in the world is and you'll get ten different answers. Some people swear by the Okinawa diet. Others prefer the Mediterranean or the French. But have you ever wondered what it is about all these traditional diets that makes the people living on these dietary strategies so healthy? This book will describe the common rules that link all successful diets. These rules constitute the Four Pillars of World Cuisine, which make up the understructure of the Human Diet. Throughout history, people have used them to protect their own health and to grow healthy, beautiful children.

In other words, they used diet to engineer their bodies. Most of us probably have something we'd want to change about the way we look and feel, or a health problem we'd like to be free of. What if you knew how to use food to upgrade your body at the genetic level?

Any improvement you've ever wished for your body or your health would come from optimization of your genetic function. Your genes are special material inside every one of your cells that controls the coordinated activity in that cell and communicates with other genes in other cells throughout your body's many

3

different tissues. They are made of DNA, an ancient and powerful molecule we'll learn more about in the next chapter.

Think about it: What if you could re-engineer your genes to your liking? Want to be like Mike? How about Tiger Woods? Halle Berry? George Clooney? Or maybe you want to change your genes so that you can still be you, only better. Maybe you want just a modest upgrade—a sexier body, better health, greater athleticism, and a better attitude. When you start to consider what you might be willing to pay for all this, you realize that *the greatest gift on Earth is a set of healthy genes.* The lucky few who do inherit pristinely healthy genes are recognized as "genetic lottery winners" and spend their lives enjoying the many benefits of beauty, brains, and brawn. Being a genetic marvel doesn't mean you automatically get everything you want. But if you have the genes and the desire, you can, with intelligent choices and hard work, have the world at your feet.

Back in the mid-1980s, a handful of biotech millionaires thought they had the technology to bring daydreams like these to life. They organized the Human Genome Project, which, we were told, was going to revolutionize how medicine was practiced and how babies were conceived and born.

At the time, conventional medical wisdom held that some of us turn out beautiful and talented while others don't because, at some point, Mother Nature made a mistake or two while reproducing DNA. These mistakes lead to random *mutations* and, obviously, you can't be a genetic marvel if your genes are scabbed with mutations. The biotech whiz kids got the idea that if they could get into our genes and fix the mutations—with genetic vaccines or patches—they could effectively "rig the lottery." On June 26, 2000, they reached the first milestone in this ambitious scheme and announced they'd cracked the code.

"This is the outstanding achievement not only of our lifetime but in terms of human history," declared Dr. Michael Dexter, the project's administrator.[8]

Many were counting on new technology such as this to magically address disease at its source. Investors and geneticists promised the mutations responsible for hypertension, depression, cancer, male pattern baldness—potentially whatever we wanted—would soon be neutralized and corrected. In the weeks that followed, I listened to scientists on talk shows stirring up publicity by claiming the next big thing would be made-to-order babies, fashioned using so-called designer genes. But I was skeptical. Actually, more than skeptical—I knew it to be hype, an indulgence of an historically common delusion that a deeper understanding of a natural phenomenon (like, say, the orbits of the planets) quickly and inevitably leads to our ability to control that phenomenon (to manipulate the orbits of the planets). Add to this the fact that a decade earlier, while attending Cornell University, I had learned from leaders in the field of biochemistry and molecular biology that a layer of biologic complexity existed that would undermine the gene-mappers' bullish predictions. It was an inconvenient reality these scientists kept tucked under their hats.

While the project's supporters described our chromosomes as static chunks of information that could be easily (and safely) manipulated, a new field of science, called *epigenetics*, had already proved this fundamental assumption wrong. Epigenetics helps us understand that the genome is more like a dynamic, living being—growing, learning, and adapting constantly. You may have heard that most disease is due to random mutations, or "bad" genes. But epigenetics tells us otherwise. If you need glasses or get cancer or age faster than you should, you very well may have perfectly normal genes. What's gone wrong is how they function, what scientists call *genetic expression*. Just as we can get sick when we don't take care of ourselves, it turns out, so can our genes.

YOUR DIET CHANGES HOW YOUR GENES WORK

In the old model of genetic medicine, diseases were believed to arise from permanent damage to DNA, called mutations, portions of the genetic code where crucial data has been distorted by a biological typo. Mutations were thought to develop from mistakes DNA makes while generating copies of itself, and therefore, the health of your genes (and Darwinian evolution) was dependent on random rolling of the dice. Mutations were, for many decades, presumed to be the root cause of everything from knock-knees to short stature to high blood pressure and depression. This model of inheritance is the reason doctors tell people with family histories of cancer, diabetes, and so on that they've inherited genetic time bombs ready to go off at any moment. It's also the reason we call the genetic lottery a lottery. The underlying principle is that we have little or no control. But epigenetics has identified a ghost in the machine, giving us a different vision of Mother Nature's most fantastic molecule.

Epigenetic translates to "upon the gene." Epigenetic researchers study how our own genes react to our behavior, and they've found that just about everything we eat, think, breathe, or do can, directly or indirectly, trickle down to touch the gene and affect its performance in some way. These effects are carried forward into the next generation, where they can be magnified. In laboratory experiments researchers have shown that simply by feeding mice with different blends of vitamins, they can change the next generation's adult weight and susceptibility to disease, and these new developments can then be passed on again, to grandchildren.[9]

It's looking as though we've grossly underestimated the dictum "You are what you eat." Not only does what we eat affect us down to the level of our genes, our physiques have been sculpted, in part, by the foods our parents and grand-parents ate (or didn't eat) generations ago.

The body of evidence compiled by thousands of epigenetic researchers working all over the world suggests that the majority of people's medical problems do not come from inherited mutations, as previously thought, but rather from harmful environmental factors that force good genes to behave badly, by switching them on and off at the wrong time. And so, genes that were once healthy can, at any point in our lives, start acting sick.

The environmental factors controlling how well our genes are working will vary from minute to minute, and each one of your cells reacts differently. So you can imagine how complex the system is. It's this complexity that makes it impossible to predict whether a given smoker will develop lung cancer, colon cancer, or no cancer at all. The epigenetic modulation is so elaborate and so dynamic that it's unlikely we'll ever develop a technological fix for most of what ails us. So far, it may sound like epigenetics is all bad news. But ultimately, epigenetics is showing us that the genetic lottery is anything but random. Though some details may forever elude science, the bottom line is clear: *we* control the health of our genes.

The concept of gene health is simple: genes work fine until disturbed. External forces that disturb the normal ebb and flow of genetic function can be broken into two broad categories: toxins and nutrient imbalances. Toxins are harmful compounds we may eat, drink, or breathe into our bodies, or even manufacture internally when we experience undue stress. Nutrient imbalances are usually due to deficiencies, missing vitamins, minerals, fatty acids, or other raw materials required to run our cells. You may not have control over the quality of the air you breathe or be able to quit your job in order to reduce stress. But you do have control over what may be the most powerful class of gene-regulating factors: food.

A HOLISTIC PERSPECTIVE OF FOOD

Believe it or not, designer babies aren't a new idea. People "designed" babies in ancient times. No, they didn't aim for a particular eye or hair color; their goal was more practical—to give birth to healthy, bright, and happy babies. Their tools were not high technology in the typical sense of the word, of course. Their tool was biology, combined with their own common sense, wisdom, and careful observation. Reproduction was not entered into casually, as it often is today, because the production of healthy babies was necessary to the community's long-term survival. Through trial and error people learned that, when certain foods were missing from a couple's diet, their children were born with problems. They learned which foods helped to ease delivery, which encouraged the production of calmer, more intelligent children who grew rapidly and rarely fell sick, and then passed this information on. Without this nurturing wisdom, we—the dominant species on the planet as we are presently defined—never would have made it this far.

Widely scattered evidence indicates that all successful cultures accumulated vast collections of nutritional guidelines anthologized over the course of many generations and placed into a growing body of wisdom. This library of knowledge was not a tertiary aspect of these cultures. It was ensconced safely within the vaults of religious doctrine and ceremony to ensure its unending revival. The following excerpt offers one example of what the locals living in Yukon Territory in Canada knew about scurvy, a disease of vitamin C deficiency, which at the time (in 1930) still killed European explorers to the region.

> When I asked an old Indian . . . why he did not tell the white man
> how [to prevent scurvy], his reply was that the white man knew too
> much to ask the Indian anything. I then asked him if he would tell me.
> He said he would if the chief said he might. He returned in an hour,
> saying that the chief said he could tell me because I was a friend of
> the Indians and had come to tell the Indians not to eat the food in the
> white man's store. . . . He then described how when the Indian kills
> a moose he opens it up and at the back of the moose just above the
> kidney there are what he described as two small balls in the fat [the
> adrenal glands]. These he said the Indian would take and cut up into
> as many pieces as there were little and big Indians in the family and
> each one would eat his piece.[10]

When I first read this passage in a dusty library book from the 1940s called *Nutrition and Physical Degeneration*, it was immediately obvious just how sophisticated the accumulated knowledge once was—far better than my medical school training in nutrition. My textbooks said that vitamin C only comes from fruits and vegetables. In the excerpt, the chief makes specific reference to his appreciation of the interviewer's advice to avoid the food in the trading posts ("white man's store"), demonstrating how, in indigenous culture, advice regarding food and nutrition is held in high esteem, even treated as a commodity that can serve as consideration in a formal exchange. We've become accustomed to using the word *share* these days, as in "Let me *share* a story with you." But this was sharing in the truest sense, as in offering a gift of novel weaponry or a fire-starting device—items not to be given up lightly. In fact, the book's author admitted consistent difficulty extracting nutrition-related information for this very reason. There is an old African saying, "When an elder dies, a library burns to the ground." And so, unfortunately, this particular human instinct—an understandable apprehension of sharing with outsiders—has allowed much of what used to be known to die away.

Today we are raised to think of food as a kind of enriched fuel, a source of calories and a carrier for vitamins, which help prevent disease. In contrast, ancient peoples understood food to be a holy thing, and eating was a sanctified act. Their songs and prayers reflected the belief that in consuming food, each of us comes in contact with the great, interconnected web of life. Epigenetics proves that intuitive idea to be essentially true. Our genes make their day-to-day decisions based on chemical information they receive from the food we eat, information encoded in our food and carried from that food item's original source, a microenvironment of land or sea. In that sense, food is less like a fuel and more like a language conveying information from the outside world. That information programs your genes, for better or for worse. Today's genetic lottery winners are those people who inherited well-programmed, healthy genes by virtue of their ancestors' abilities to properly plug into that chemical information stream. If you want to help your genes get healthy, you need to plug in, too—and this is the book that can help.

For fifteen years, I have studied how food programs genes and how that programming affects physiology. I've learned there is an underlying order to our health. Getting sick isn't random. We get sick because our genes didn't get what they were expecting, one too many times. Most importantly, I've learned that food can tame unruly genetic behavior far more reliably than biotechnology. By simply replenishing your body with the nourishment that facilitates optimal gene expression, it's possible to eliminate genetic malfunction and, with it, pretty much all known disease. No matter what kind of genes you were born with, I know that eating right can help reprogram them, immunizing you against cancer, premature aging, and dementia, enabling you to control your metabolism, your moods, your weight—and much, much more. And if you start planning early enough, and your genetic momentum is strong enough, you can give your children a shot at reaching for the stars.

WHO AM I?

In many ways, it was my own unhealthy genes that inspired me to go to medical school and, later, to write this book. I'd had more than my fair share of problems from the beginning of my sports career. In high school track, I suffered with

Achilles tendonitis, then calcaneal bursitis, then iliotibial band syndrome, and it seemed to me that I was constantly fitting corrective inserts into my shoes or adding new therapeutic exercises to my routine. In college I developed a whole new crop of soft tissue problems, including a case of shin splints so severe it almost cost me my athletic scholarship.

When my shin splints got bad enough that I had to start skipping practice, I paid yet another visit to the team physician. Dr. Scotty, a squat, mustached man with thick black hair and a high-pitched voice, told me that this time he couldn't help me. All I could do was cut back my training and wait. But I was sure there was something else I needed to do. Perhaps I had some kind of dietary deficiency? Applying my newly acquired mastery of Biology 101, I suggested that perhaps my connective tissue cells couldn't make normal tendons. Like many of my own patients today, I pushed Dr. Scotty to get to the bottom of my problem. I even had a plan: simply take some kind of biopsy of the tendon in my leg and compare the material to a healthy tendon. My ideas went nowhere, as I imagine such suggestions often do. Dr. Scotty furrowed his bushy eyebrows and said he'd never heard of any such test. I'd read stories in *Newsweek* and *Time* about the powerful diagnostics being brought to us by molecular biology. In my naiveté, I couldn't believe Dr. Scotty didn't know how to use any of that science to help me. I was so confounded by his unwillingness to consider what seemed to me to be the obvious course of action, and so enamored with the idea of getting to the molecular root of physical problems—and so enthralled by the promise of the whole burgeoning biotech field—that I scrapped my plans to be a chemical engineer and enrolled in every course I could to study genetics. I went to graduate school at Cornell, where I learned about gene regulation and epigenetics from Nobel Prize–winning researchers, then straight to Robert Wood Johnson Medical School in New Jersey, in hopes of putting my knowledge of the fundamentals of genetics to practical use.

I then found out why Dr. Scotty had been dumbfounded by my questions years before. Medical school doesn't teach doctors to address the root of the problem. It teaches doctors to treat the problem. It's a practical science with practical aims. In this way, medicine differs quite drastically from other natural sciences. Take, for instance, physics, which has built a body of deep knowledge by always digging down to get to the roots of a problem. Physicists have now dug so deep that they are grappling with one of the most fundamental questions of all: How did the universe begin? But medicine is different from other sciences because, more than being a science, it is first and foremost a business. This is why, when people taking a heart pill called Loniten started growing unwanted hair on their arms, researchers didn't ask why. Instead, they looked for customers. And Loniten, the heart pill, became Rogaine, the spray for balding men. Medicine is full of examples like this, one of the most lucrative being the discovery of Sildafenil, a medication originally used to treat high blood pressure until it was found to have the happy side effect of prolonging erections and was repackaged as Viagra. Since medicine is a business, medical research must ultimately generate some kind of saleable product. And that is why we still don't know what leads to common problems like shin splints.

I didn't go to medical school to become a businesswoman. My dreams had sprouted from a seed planted in my psyche when I was five, during an incident with a baby robin. Sitting on the street curb in front of my house one spring morning, the plump little fledgling flew down from the maple tree to land on the street in front of me. Looking directly at me, he chirped and flapped his wings as if to say, "Look what I can do!"—and then I saw the front tire of a station wagon roll up behind him. In a blink, the most adorable creature I'd ever seen was smashed into a feather pancake, a lifeless stain on the asphalt. Dead. I was outraged. Overwhelmed with guilt. Whoever was driving that car had no idea of the trauma he'd just inflicted on two young lives. This was my first experience with the finality of death, and it awoke a protective instinct that has driven my career decisions ever since: prevent harm. It was why I'd wanted to be a chemical engineer (to invent nontoxic baby diapers) and why I had gone to medical school. I was all about prevention, and that meant I needed to understand what makes us tick and what makes us sick.

Unfortunately, soon after enrolling in medical school, I found that the gap between my childhood dream and the reality of limited medical knowledge was enormous—so enormous that I concluded it wasn't yet possible to breach. To pursue my dream of preventing harm, the best I could do was practice "preventive medicine," and the best place to do this was within the specialty of primary care. To tell the truth, I kind of forgot about the whole idea of getting to the bottom of what makes people sick, and for many years after graduation I went on with ordinary life. Until something drew me back in.

RESPECTING OUR ANCIENT WISDOM

It was those malfunctioning genes of mine, again. Shortly after moving to Hawaii, I developed another musculoskeletal problem. But this one was different from all the others. This time no doctor, not even five different specialists, could tell me what it was. And it didn't go away. A year after I developed the first unusual stinging pain around my right knee, I could no longer walk more than a few feet without getting feverish. It was unlike anything I'd ever heard of. I'd had exploratory surgery, injections, physical therapy, and I'd even seen a Hawaiian *kahuna*.

But everything I tried seemed to make the problem worse. Just as I was giving up hope, my husband, Luke, came up with an idea: try studying nutrition. As an excellent chef and an aficionado of all things relating to cuisine, he'd been impressed by the variety and flavors he encountered at the local Filipino buffets. Like many professional chefs I've spoken with since, he suspected there might be other opinions out there on what healthy food might actually be. Having fought his own battles against malnutrition while growing up on the wrong side of the tracks in a small town, he recognized that there were nutritional haves and have-nots, just as with everything else. And he suspected that my high-sugar, convenience-food diet put me in the have-not category and might even be impairing my ability to heal.

Sure, I thought, everyone has an opinion. I—on the other hand—went to medical school. *Hel-l-l-lo-o-o* . . . I took a course on *nu-tri-tion*. I learned *bi-o-chem-is-try*. I already knew to eat low-fat, low-cholesterol and count my calories. What more did I need to know? The next day, Luke brought home a book. Had I not been literally immobilized, I may never have bothered opening Andrew Weil's book *Spontaneous Healing* and started reading.

Medical school teaches us to believe that we're living longer now, and so today's diet must beat the diets of the past, hands down. This argument had me so convinced that I never considered questioning the dietary dogma I'd absorbed throughout my schooling. But we need to take into account the fact that today's eighty-year-olds grew up on an entirely different, more natural diet. They were also the first generation to benefit from antibiotics, and many have been kept alive thanks only to technology. Today's generation has yet to prove its longevity, but given that many forty-year-olds already have joint and cardiovascular problems that their parents didn't get until much later in life (as I found in my practice), I don't think we can assume they have the same life expectancy. And the millennium generation's lifespan may be ten to twenty years shorter.[11] I was going to get my first inkling of this reality very soon.

Once I cracked the book open, it didn't take much reading to bump into something I'd never heard of before: omega-3 fatty acids. According to Weil, these are fats we need to eat, just like vitamins. These days, our diets are so deficient that we need to supplement. This blew my mind. First of all, I'd thought fats were bad. Secondly, we were supposed to be eating better today than at any point in human history. Either he was off base, or my medical education had failed to provide some basic information. Like a kid who gets into the bathtub kicking and screaming and then doesn't want to get out, I soon couldn't get enough of these "alternative" books. They gave me valuable new information—and hope that I might walk normally again.

In another publication, I came across an intriguing article entitled "Guts and Grease: The Diet of Native Americans," which suggested that Native Ameri-

cans were healthier than their European counterparts because they ate the entire animal. Not just muscle, but all the "guts and grease."

> According to John (Fire) Lame Deer, the eating of guts had evolved into a contest. [He said] "In the old days we used to eat the guts of the buffalo, making a contest of it, two fellows getting hold of a long piece of intestines from opposite ends, starting chewing toward the middle, seeing who can get there first; that's eating. Those buffalo guts, full of half-fermented, half-digested grass and herbs, you didn't need any pills and vitamins when you swallowed those."[12]

I liked the voice of authority this Native American assumed, as if he were drawing from a secret well of knowledge. I also liked that the article's authors offered healthy people instead of statistics of lab simulations as evidence. At the time, the approach struck me as novel—focusing on health rather than disease. Early European explorers Cabeza de Vaca, Francisco Vaquez de Coronado, and Lewis and Clark described Native Americans as superhuman warriors, able to run down buffalo on foot and, in battle, continue fighting after being shot through with arrows. Photographs taken two hundred years later, in the 1800s, capture the Native American's imposing visage and broad, balanced bone structure. Presenting a people's stamina and strength as evidence of a healthy diet seemed reasonable, and it rang true with my own clinical experience in Hawaii: the healthiest family members are, in many cases, the oldest, raised on foods vastly different from those being fed to their great-grandchildren. I began to doubt my presumption that today's definition of a healthy diet was nutritionally superior to diets of years past.

Still, the dietary program of Native Americans seemed bizarre. Reading the passage about two grown men chewing their way through an animal's unwashed, fat-encased intestine forever changed the way I remember the spaghetti scene from *Lady and the Tramp*. It also brought up some serious questions. For one thing, wouldn't eating buffalo poo make the men ill? And isn't animal fat supposed to be unhealthy? The first issue—eating unwashed intestine—was too much for me to tackle (though later I would). So I sank my teeth into the matter of the health effects of animal fat.

Two things I learned about nutrition in medical school were that saturated fat raises cholesterol levels, and that cholesterol is a known killer. Who was right, the American Medical Association—whose guidelines are used to teach medical students—or John (Fire) Lame Deer?

This was how I began to close the knowledge gap that years ago had derailed me from pursuing further studies of the fundamentals of disease. To determine

HYGIEIA: GODDESS OF NUTRITION
IN THE HIPPOCRATIC OATH

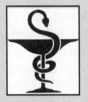 **Hygieia's Bowl.** In Greek mythologic emblems, Hygieia is depicted holding a bowl, from which she feeds the serpent, a symbol of medical learning. In ancient Greece the philosophy of wellness was balanced by two complementary ideas. The female, Hygieia, the goddess of health, personified the first. Hygieia was all about building healthy bodies with sound nutrition from the start—prenatally and throughout the formative years of childhood—and maintaining health for the rest of a person's life. In other words, she embodied the most effective form of preventive medicine there is. When that first line of defense failed, and people succumbed to infections or the inevitable accident, Aesculapius, the god of medicine, acted as a kind of Johnny-on-the-spot. He provided knowledge of healing surgical procedures and therapeutic potions. The Hippocratic oath I took on graduation day invokes the wisdom of Aesculapius, Hygieia, and Panacea, the god of potions or cure-alls. But like hundreds of other fresh-faced M.D.s standing beside me in the lecture hall, hands raised, I had no idea who Hygieia was or what she stood for.

Over the last 3,000 years of civilization, the male aspect of medical science has taken over. Hygieia, which was once a highly scientific and advanced compendium of nutritional information, has been reduced to simplistic notions of cleanliness, like washing your hands and brushing your teeth. It's time to bring Hygieia back.

the best dietary stance, I would look at all the necessary basic science data (on free radicals, fatty acid oxidation, eicosanoid signaling, gene regulation, and the famous Framingham studies), which, fortunately, I had the training to decipher. It took six months of research to get to the bottom of this one nutritional question, but I ultimately came to understand that the nutrition science I'd learned in medical school was full of contradictions and rested on assumptions proved false by researchers in other, related scientific fields. The available evidence failed to support the AMA's position and overwhelmingly sided with that of John (Fire) Lame Deer.

This was a big deal. Contrary to the opinion of medical leaders today, saturated fat and cholesterol appeared to be beneficial nutrients. (Chapter 8 explains how heart disease really develops.) Fifty years of removing foods containing these nutrients from our diets—foods like eggs, fresh cream, and liver—to replace them with low-fat or outright artificial chemicals—like trans-fat-rich margarine (trans-fat is an unnatural fat known to cause health problems)—has starved our genes of the chemical information on which they depend. Simply cutting eggs and sausage (originally made with lactic acid starter culture instead of nitrates, and containing chunks of white cartilage) from our breakfasts to replace them with cold cereals would mean that generations of children have been fed fewer fats, B vitamins, and collagenous proteins than required for optimal growth.

Here's why: the yolk of an egg is full of brain-building fats, including lecithin, phospholipids, and (only if from free-range chickens) essential fatty acids and vitamins A and D. Meanwhile, low-fat diets have been shown to reduce intelligence in animals.[13]

B vitamins play key roles in the development of every organ system, and women with vitamin B deficiencies give birth to children prone to developing weak bones, diabetes, and more.[14, 15] Chunks of cartilage supply us with collagen and glycosaminoglycans, factors that help facilitate the growth of robust connective tissues, which would help to prevent later-life tendon and ligament problems—including shin splints![16]

By righting the wrong assumptions that mushroomed from this one piece of nutritional misinformation, I had already gained a greater understanding of the root causes of disease than I'd thought possible. A single item of medical misinformation—that cholesterol-rich foods are dangerous—had drastically changed our eating habits and with that our access to nutrients. The effect on my personal physiology was to weaken my connective tissues, an epigenetic response that had already managed to change the course of my life in ways that I can't begin to calculate. After reading every old-fashioned cookbook I could get my hands on, and enough biochemistry to understand the essential character of traditional cuisine, I changed everything about the way I eat. For me, eating in closer accordance with historical human nutrition corrected some of my damaged epigenetic programming. I got fewer colds, less heartburn, improved my moods, lost my belly fat, had fewer headaches, and increased my mental energy. And eventually my swollen knee got better.

WHAT OUR ANCESTORS KNEW THAT YOUR DOCTOR DOESN'T

It seems like every day another study comes out showing the benefits of some vitamin, mineral, or antioxidant supplement in the prevention of a given disease. All these studies taken together send the strong message that doctors still underestimate the power of nutrition to fortify and to heal. Of course, people know this intuitively, which is why dietary supplements and nutraceuticals sell so well. Unfortunately, in all this research there is also something that's not talked about very often: artificial vitamins and powdered, encapsulated antioxidant products are not as effective as the real thing—not even close. They can even be harmful. A far better option is to eat more nutritious *food.*

To identify the most nutritious foods, I studied traditions from all over the world. The goal was not to identify the "best" tradition, but to understand what all traditions have in common. I identified four universal elements, each of which represents a distinct set of ingredients along with the cooking (or other preparation technique), that maximize the nutrition delivered to our cells. For the bulk of human history, these techniques and materials have proved indispensable. The reason that so many of us have health problems today is that we no longer eat in accordance with any culinary tradition. In the worst cases of recurring illnesses and chronic diseases that I see, more often than not, the victim's parents and grandparents haven't, either. This means that most Americans are carrying around very sick genes. But by returning to the same four categories of nourishing foods our ancestors ate—the Four Pillars of World Cuisine— our personal genetic health will be regained.

GENETIC HEALTH AND WEALTH

The health of your genes represents a kind of inheritance. Two ways of thinking about this inheritance, *genetic wealth* and *genetic momentum,* help explain why some people can abuse this inheritance and, for a time, get away with it. Just as a lazy student born into a prominent family can be assured he'll get into Yale no matter his grades, healthy genes don't have to be attended to very diligently in order for their owners' bodies to look beautiful. The next generation, however, will pay the price.

We've all seen the twenty-year-old supermodel who abuses her body with cigarettes and Twinkies. For years, her beautiful skeletal architecture will still shine through. Beneath the surface, poor nutrition will deprive those bones of what they need, thinning them prematurely. The connective tissue supporting her skin will begin to break down, stealing away her beauty. Most importantly, deep inside her ovaries, inside each egg, her genes will be affected. Those deleterious genetic alterations mean that her child will have lost *genetic momentum* and will not have the same potential for health or beauty as she did. He or she may benefit from mom's sizable financial portfolio—but junior's genetic wealth will, unfortunately, have been drawn down.

That's a real loss. Over the millennia, our genes developed under the influence of a steady stream of nourishing foods gleaned from the most nutritionally potent corners of the natural world. Today's supermodels have benefited not just from their parents' and grandparents' healthy eating habits, but from hundreds, even thousands, of generations of ancestors who, by eating the right foods, maintained—and even improved upon—the genetic heirloom that would ultimately construct a beautiful face in the womb. All of this accumulated wealth can be disposed of as easily and mindlessly as the twenty-year-old supermodel flicking away a cigarette.

Such squandering of *genetic wealth*—a measure of the intactness of epigenetic programming—has affected many of us. My own father grew up drinking powdered milk and ate margarine on Wonder Bread every day at lunch. My mother spent much of her childhood in postwar Europe, where dairy products were scarce. Because they had inherited genetic wealth from their parents, my parents never had significant soft tissue problems in spite of these shortcomings. But those suboptimal diets did take a toll on their genes. Much of the genetic wealth of my family line had been squandered by the time I was born. Unlike my parents and grandparents, I had to struggle to keep my joints from falling apart.

Fortunately for me, my story is not over—and neither is yours. Thanks to the plasticity of genetic response we can all improve the health of our genes and rebuild our genetic wealth.

Anyone who has chronically neglected a plant and watched its leaves curl and its color fade knows that proper care and feeding can have dramatic, restorative effects. The same applies to our genes—and our epigenetic programming. Not only will you personally benefit from this during your lifetime with improved health, normalization of fat distribution, remission of chronic disease, and resistance to the effects of age, your children will benefit as well. If you think saving money for college or moving to a neighborhood with a good school system is important, then consider the importance of ensuring that your children are as healthy and beautiful as they can be. If you start early enough, the fruits of your efforts will be clearly visible in the bones of your child's face, the face they may one day be presenting to the one person who can give them the opportunity—over all the other candidates—to inaugurate the career of their dreams. It all depends on you—what you eat and how you choose to live. I am not a specialist in stress reduction (though stress reduction is vital), and I won't be talking that much about exercise other than to describe how different types of exercise will help you lose weight and build healthy tissue. However, by virtue of my training and subsequent studies, I am an expert at predicting the physiologic effects of eating different types of food. And my basic philosophy is simple.

DEEP NUTRITION

I subscribe to the school of nutritional thought that counsels us to eat the same foods people ate in the past because, after all, that's how we got here. It's how we're designed to eat. Epigenetics supplies the scientific support for the idea by providing molecular evidence that we are who we are, in large part, because of the foods our ancestors ate. But because healthy genes, like healthy people, can perform well under difficult conditions for a finite amount of time, there is, in effect, a delay in the system. Since nutritional researchers don't ask study participants what their parents ate, the conclusions drawn from those studies are based on incomplete data. A poor diet can seem healthy if studied for a twenty-four-hour period. A slightly better diet can seem successful for months or even years. Only the most complete diets, however, can provide health generation after generation.

Diet books that adopt this long-term philosophy such as *Paleodiet, Evolution Diet,* and *Health Secrets of the Stone Age* have been incredibly successful partly by virtue of the philosophy itself, which has intuitive appeal. Fleshing out the bare bones of the nutritional philosophy with specifics—real ingredients and real recipes—is another matter. Authors of previously published books are still working on the old random mutation model, and so fail to account for how quickly genetic change can occur. In going all the way back to the prehistoric era, they take the idea too far to be practical. Their evidence is so limited it's literally skeletal—gleaned from campfire debris, chips of bone, and the cleanings of mummified stomachs. These books do give us fascinating glimpses of life in the distant past. And I'm impressed by how the authors use modern physiologic science to expand tiny tidbits of data into complete dietary regimes. But each of these books, often citing the same information, leaves us with contradicting advice. Why? The data they have is simply too fragmented, too old, and too short on detail to give us meaningful guidance. How can we reproduce the flavors and nutrients found in our Paleolithic predecessors' dinners when the only instructions they left behind come in the form of such artifacts as "the 125,000-year-old spear crafted from a yew tree found embedded between the ribs of an extinct straight-tusked elephant in Germany" and "cut marks that have been found on the bones of fossilized animals."[17]

The authors do their best to make educated guesses, but clearly a creative mind could follow this ancient trail of evidence to end up wherever they like.

Fortunately, we don't have to rely on prehistory or educated guesses. There is a much richer, living source of information available to us. It's called *cuisine*. Specifically, authentic cuisine. By "authentic," I'm not talking about the Americanized salad-and-seafood translation of Mediterranean or Okinawan or Chinese diets. I'm not talking about modern molecular gastronomy or functional food or fast food. The authentic cuisine I'm referring to is what fondest memories are made of. It's the combination of ingredients and skills that enable families in even the poorest farming communities around the world to create fantastic meals, meals that would be fit for a king and that would satisfy even the snarkiest of New Yorkers—even, say, a food connoisseur whose glance has been known to weaken many a *Top Chef* contender's knees. I am of course referring to former punk-rock-chef-turned-world-trotting-celebrity, Anthony Bourdain.

As evidence that there's plenty of detailed information surviving to inform us exactly how people used to eat (and still should), I submit Bourdain's travel TV show *No Reservations*, which ran from 2005 until 2012. Bourdain served up the colorful, vastly inventive, and diverse world of culinary arts for an hour each week in your living room. Bourdain got right to the heart of his host country's distinct food culture, beginning each show by casting a historical light on the local food. Guided by food-wise natives, he ended up at the right spots to sample food that captured each geographical region's soul. More often than not, these spots were the mom-and-pop holes-in-the-wall where people cook food the way it has been cooked in that country for as long as anyone can remember. Shows like Bourdain's have helped to convince me that, culinarily speaking, growing up in America is growing up in an underdeveloped country.

While Americans have hot dogs and apple pie, Happy Meals, meatloaf, casseroles, and variations on the theme of salad, citizens of other countries seem to have so much more. In one region of China, a visitor could experience pit-roasted boar, rooster, or rabbit, with a side of any number of different kinds of pickles or fermented beans, hand-crafted noodles, or fruiting vegetation of every shape, size, color, and texture. In burgeoning, ultramodern cities, at the base of towering glass buildings around the world, farmers markets still sell the quality, local ingredients pulled from the earth or fished from the rivers and lakes that morning. My point is not to suggest that America isn't a wonderful country with our own rich history of cuisine. My point is that we're out of touch with our roots. That disconnection is the biggest reason why we have bookshelves full of conflicting nutritional advice. It's also why, though many of us still have good genes, we have not maintained them very well. Like plump grapes left to bake on a French hillside, American chromosomes are wilting on the vine. They can be revitalized simply by enjoying the delightful products of traditional cuisine.

The messy amalgamation of vastly different dishes comprising every authentic cuisine can be cleaved into four neat categories, which I call the Four Pillars of World Cuisine. We need to eat them as often as we can, preferably daily. They are:

1. Meat cooked on the bone
2. Organs and offal (what Bourdain calls "the nasty bits")
3. Fresh (raw) plant and animal products
4. Fermented and sprouted foods—better than fresh!

These categories have proved to be essential by virtue of their ubiquitousness. In almost every country other than ours people eat them every day. They've proved to be *successful* by virtue of their practitioners' health and survival. Like cream rising in a glass, these traditions have percolated upward from the past, buoyed by their intrinsic value. They have endured the test of time simply by being delicious and nutritious, and in celebrating them we can reconnect with our roots and with each other, and bring our lives toward their full potential.

TENDING THE SACRED FLAME

Not too long ago (and without understanding genetics, stem cell biology, or biochemistry) cultures everywhere survived based on living in accordance with the cause and effect realities of their daily experience. If someone ate a certain red berry and got sick, berries from that bush would be forbidden. If a mother developed a strong craving for a specific mushroom or kind of seafood or what-have-you during her pregnancy and went on to enjoy a particularly smooth and easy delivery of a healthy baby, then this association would be added to the growing body of collective wisdom. Their successes are now memorialized in our existence and in the healthy genetic material we have managed to retain. Solutions to the all-important omnivore's dilemma—the question of what we *should* be eating—are all around us, encapsulated in traditions still practiced by foodies, culinary artists, devoted grandmothers, and chefs throughout the world, some in your very own neighborhood. Unfortunately, this wisdom has gone unappreciated, thanks to the cholesterol theory of heart disease and other byproducts of what Michael Pollan calls "scientific reductionism" (a decidedly unscientific exercise, as Pollan explains in his popular book, *In Defense of Food*).[18]

Fortunately, those who love—really love—good cooking and good food have kept culinary traditions alive. In doing so, not only have their own families benefited, they also serve as the modern emissaries of our distant relatives, carriers of an ancient secret once intended to be shared only with members of the tribe. Today, we are that tribe. And that message—how to use food to stay healthy and beautiful—is the most precious gift we could possibly receive.

Throughout this book I will highlight the power of food to shape your daily life. In fact, every bite you eat changes your genes a little bit. Just as the genetic lottery follows a set of predictable rules, so do the small changes that occur after every meal. If the machinery of physiologic change is not random, and is instead guided by rules, then who—or what—keeps track of them? In the next chapter, we'll see how the gene responds to nourishment with what can best be described as intelligence, and why this built-in ability makes me certain that many of us have untapped genetic potential waiting to be released.

CHAPTER 2

The Intelligent Gene
Epigenetics and the Language of DNA

- "Good genes" make us healthy, strong, and beautiful and represent a kind of family fortune we call genetic wealth.

- We hear all the time that harmful gene mutations that cause disease are random, but the latest science suggests that's not always true.

- We don't need to wait for technology to synthesize disease-free genes or designer babies.

- Simply by giving our genes the nutrients they've come to expect, we can accomplish a lot, with zero risk.

- Reorienting our financial priorities around healthy eating rebuilds our family's genetic wealth and is the best investment we can make.

I remember getting caught up in the excitement when Halle Berry took the stage at the 2002 Oscars, how she stood before the audience and tearfully thanked God for her blessings. "Thank you. I'm so honored. I'm so honored. And I thank the Academy for choosing me to be the vessel for which His blessing might flow. Thank you." A laudable Hollywood milestone, Berry was the first woman of African-American descent to be awarded the Oscar for a leading role. While so much focus was placed on what made this actor, and that evening, unique in the history of Hollywood movies, I couldn't avoid the nagging feeling that there was something familiar about the woman in her stunning gown, something about her face that reminded me of every other woman who had, over the years, clutched the little golden statue in her hands. What was the link between Ms. Berry and all her Academy-honored sisters like Charlize Theron, Nicole Kidman, Cate Blanchett, Angelina Jolie, Julia

Roberts, Kim Basinger, Jessica Lange, Elizabeth Taylor, Ingrid Bergman, and the rest? Yes, they are all talented masters of their craft. But there was something else about them, something more obvious, maybe so obvious that it was one of those things you just learn to take for granted.

Then it occurred to me: They are *all* breathtakingly gorgeous.

Like Halle Berry, we are all vessels—not necessarily designed to win Oscars—but made to eat, survive, and reproduce genetic material. So if you happen to win an Oscar, you could make history by extending one last note of gratitude to your extraordinary DNA. When your PR agent chastises you the next morning, just explain to her that we are all active participants in one of the oldest and most profound relationships on our planet—between our bodies and our DNA, and the food that connects both to the outside world. Halle Berry's perfectly proportioned, fit, healthy body is evidence of a happy relationship between her genes and the natural environment, one that has remained so for several generations. As this chapter will explain, if you hope to create a more fruitful relationship with your own genes, to get healthier and improve the way you look, you need to learn to work with the intelligence embedded within your DNA.

DNA'S GIANT "BRAIN"

Every cell of your body contains a nucleus, floating within the cytoplasm like the yolk inside an egg. The nucleus holds your chromosomes, forty-six super-coiled molecules, and each one of those contains up to 300 million pairs of genetic letters, called *nucleic acids*. These colorless, gelatinous chemicals (visible to the naked eye only when billions of copies are reproduced artificially in the lab) constitute the genetic materials that make you who you are.

If you stretched out the DNA in one of your cells, its 2.8 billion base pairs would end up totaling nearly three meters long. The DNA from all your cells strung end to end would reach to the moon and back at least 5,000 times.[19] That's a lot of chemical information. But your genes take up only 2 percent of it. The rest of the sequence—the other 98 percent—is what scientists used to call *junk*. Not that they thought this remaining DNA was useless; they just didn't know what it was for. But in the last two decades, scientists have discovered that this material has some amazing abilities.

This line of discovery emerges from a branch of genetics called *epigenetics*. Epigenetic researchers investigate how genes get turned on or off. This is how the body modulates genes in response to the environment, and it is how two twins with identical DNA can develop different traits.

Epigenetic researchers exploring this expansive genetic territory are finding a hidden world of ornate complexity. Unlike genes, which function as a relatively static repository of encoded data, the so-called junk DNA (more properly called non-coding DNA) seems designed for change, both over the short term—within our lifetimes—and over periods of several generations, and longer. It appears that junk DNA assists biology in making key decisions, like turning one stem cell (an undifferentiated cell that can mature into any type of cell) into part of an eye, and another stem cell with identical DNA into, say, part of your liver. These decisions seem to be made based on environmental influences. We know this because when you take a stem cell and place it into an animal's liver, it becomes a liver cell. If you took that same stem cell and placed it into an animal's brain, it would become a nerve cell.[20] Junk DNA does all this by using the chemical information floating around it to determine which genes should get turned on when, and in what quantity.

One of the most fascinating, and unexpected, lessons of the Human Genome Project is the discovery that our genes are very similar to mouse genes, which very much like other mammalian genes, which in turn are surprisingly similar to those of fish. It appears that the proteins humans produce are not particularly unique in the animal kingdom. What makes us uniquely human are the regulatory segments of our genetic material, the same regulatory segments that direct stem cell development during in-utero growth and throughout the rest of our lives. Could it be that the same mechanisms facilitating cell maturation also function over generations, enabling species to evolve? According to Arturas Petronis, head of the Krembil Family Epigenetics Laboratory at the Centre for Addiction and Mental Health in Toronto, "We really need some radical revision of key principles of the traditional genetic research program."[21] Another epigeneticist puts our misapprehension of evolution in perspective: mutation- and selection-driven evolutionary change is just the tip of the iceberg. "The bottom of the iceberg is epigenetics."[22]

The more we study this mysterious 98 percent, the more we find it seems to function as a massively complicated regulatory system that serves to control our cellular activities as if it were a huge, molecular brain. A genetic lottery winner's every cell carries DNA that regulates cell growth and activity better than your average Joe's. Not because they're just dumb-lucky, but because their regulatory DNA—their chromosomal "brain" located in the vast non-coding portions of their chromosomes—functions better. Just like your brain, DNA needs to be able to remember what it's learned to function properly.

One example of what can happen when DNA "forgets" how to operate is cancer. Cancer develops in cells that have misunderstood their role as part of a cooperative enterprise and lost their ability to play nice in the body. The DNA running a cancer cell essentially becomes confused, believing its job is to in-

THE NUCLEUS: WHERE FOOD PROGRAMS GENES

A special chamber in every cell, called the nucleus, houses and protects all your DNA. Inside the nucleus, DNA is divided into chunks called *chromosomes*. Though each would measure several feet when uncoiled, all forty-six chromosomes are packed into just a few microns of space, spooled tightly around tiny structures called *histones*. These spooled threads of genetic information can loosen up to make a given section of DNA available for enzymes to bind to it, thus "turning on," or *enabling expression of*, that particular gene or set of genes. Nutrients from food, such as vitamins and minerals, as well as hormones and proteins your body makes play various roles in regulating this winding and unwinding, called "breathing." The more we learn, the more we understand that our genes have a life of their own. The field of epigenetics is just beginning to scratch the surface of this dynamic gene regulation control system. One thing we do know is that chromosomal data is computed in analog terms rather than digital, enabling our DNA to store and compute far more information than previously imagined.

struct the cell it operates to divide and keep dividing without regard for neighboring cells until the growing mass of clones begins to kill its neighbors. This is an example of how epigenetics can work against us.

One of the *positive* functions of epigenetics is to come up with novel and creative solutions to less-t genes to make intelligent compromises. Take the development of the eye, for example. Nested inside the retina at the back of the eye is the optic disc, which acts as the central focal point for light inputs that represent what eye doctors call central vision. Something as simple as an inadequate supply of vitamin A during early childhood can force the genes to figure out how to build the disc as best it can under suboptimal nutritional circumstances. The result? Instead of a perfectly round disc you get an oval one, which can cause near-sightedness and astigmatism.[23] Not a perfect outcome, of course, but without this ability to compromise, DNA would have to make more drastic decisions, like reabsorbing the malnourished optic disc cells entirely, leaving you blind.

The creativity of this problem-solving "intelligence" does not operate without reference. Each solution is guided by a record of every challenge your DNA, and your ancestors' DNA, has ever faced. In other words, your DNA learns.

HOW CHROMOSOMES LEARN

To understand the genetic brain, how it works, and why it might some-times forget how to function as perfectly as we may wish, let's get a closer look at chromosomes.

Each of your forty-six chromosomes is actually one very long DNA mol-ecule containing up to 300 million pairs of genetic letters, called *nucleic acids*. The genetic alphabet only has four "letters," A,G,T, and C. All of our genetic data is encrypted in the patterns of these four letters. Change a letter and you change the pattern, and with it the meaning. Change the meaning, and you very well may change an organism's growth.

Biologists had long assumed that letter substitution was the only way to generate such physiologic change. Epigenetics has taught us that more often, the reason different individuals develop different physiology stems not from perma-nent letter substitutions but from temporary markers—or *epigenetic tags*—that attach themselves to the double helix or other nuclear material and change how genes are expressed. Some of these markers are in place at birth, but through-out a person's life, many of them detach, while others accumulate. Researchers needed to know what this tagging meant. Was it just a matter of DNA aging, or was something else—something more exciting—going on? If everyone devel-oped the same tags during their lives, then it was simple aging. But if the tagging occurred differentially, then it would follow that different life experiences can lead to different genetic function. It also means that, in a sense, our genes can *learn*.

In 2005, scientists in Spain found a way to solve the mystery. They prepared chromosomes from two sets of identical twins, one set aged three and the other aged fifty. Using fluorescent green and red molecules that bind, respectively, to epigenetically modified and unmodified segments of DNA, they examined the two sets of genes. The children's genes looked very similar, indicating that, as one would expect, twins start life with essentially identical genetic tags. In contrast, the fifty-year-old chromosomes lit up green and red like two Christmas trees with different decorations. Their life experiences had tagged their genes in ways that meant these identical twins were, in terms of their genetic function, no lon-ger identical.[24] This means the tagging is not just due to aging. It is a direct result of how we live our lives. Other studies since have shown that epigenetic tagging occurs in response to chemicals that form as a result of nearly everything we eat, drink, breathe, think, and do.[25] It seems our genes are always listening, always on the ready to respond and change. In photographing the different patterns of red and green on the two fifty-year-old chromosomes, scientists were capturing the two different "personalities" the women's genes had developed.

This differential genetic tagging would help explain why twins with identical DNA might develop completely different medical problems. If one twin smokes, drinks, and eats nothing but junk food while the other takes care of her body, the two sets of DNA are getting entirely different chemical "lessons"—one is getting a balanced education while the other is getting schooled in the dirty streets of chemical chaos.

In a sense, our lifestyles teach our genes how to behave. In choosing between healthy or unhealthy foods and habits, we are programming our genes for either good or bad conduct. Scientists are identifying numerous techniques by which two sets of identical DNA can be coerced into functioning dissimilarly. So far, the processes identified include bookmarking, imprinting, gene silencing, X chromosome inactivation, position effect, reprogramming, transvection, maternal effects, histone modification, and paramutation. Many of these epigenetic regulatory processes involve tagging sections of DNA with markers that govern how often a gene uncoils and unzips. Once exposed, a gene is receptive to enzymes that translate it into protein. If *un*exposed, it remains dormant, and the protein it codes for doesn't get expressed.

If one twin sister drinks a lot of milk and moves to Hawaii (where her skin can make vitamin D in response to the sun) while the other avoids dairy and moves to Minnesota, then one will predictably develop weaker bones than the other and will likely suffer from more hip, spine, and other osteoporosis-related fractures.[26] The epigenetic twin study tells us that it's not only their X-rays that will look different, their genes will, too. Scientists are becoming convinced that failure to attend to the proper care and feeding of our bodies doesn't just affect us, it affects our genes—and that means it may affect our offspring. Research shows that when one sibling has osteoporosis and the other doesn't, you'll find the genes encoding for bone growth in the osteoporotic member have gone to sleep, having been tagged, temporarily, to stay unexposed and dormant.[27] Fortunately, they'll wake up from their slumber if we change our habits. Unfortunately, returning to the example of the twin who smoked, she may have lost too much bone to ever catch up to her milk-drinking, vitamin D-fortified sister. What is worse, any epigenetic markings she developed before conceiving children can be (as we know from studies like the fat-mouse study described below) transmitted to her offspring—so that her avoidance of bone-building nutrients has consequences for them. Her children will inherit relatively sleepy bone-growth genes and be born epigenetically prone to osteoporosis. You could say that when it comes to remembering how to build bone, the epigenetic brain has grown a wee bit forgetful. Marcus Pembry, professor of clinical genetics at the Institute of Child Health in London, believes that "we are all guardians of our genome. The way people live and their lifestyle no longer just affects them, but may have a knockoff effect for their children and grandchildren."[28]

What fascinates me most is the intelligence of the system. It seems our genes have found ways to take notes, to remind themselves what to do with the various nutrients they are fed. Here's how. Let's say a gene for building bone is tagged with two epigenetic markers, one that binds to vitamin D and another that binds to calcium. And let's say that when vitamin D and calcium are both bound to their respective markers at the same time, the gene uncoils and can be expressed. If there is no calcium and no vitamin D, then the gene remains dormant and less bone is built. The epigenetic regulatory tags are effectively serving as a kind of Post-it note: *When there's lots of vitamin D and calcium around, make a bunch of the bone-building protein encoded for right here.* When they do, *voilà!* You're building stronger, longer bones! It's truly an elegant design.

Of course, DNA doesn't "know" what a given gene actually does. It doesn't even know what the various nutrients it contacts are good for. Through mechanisms not fully understood, DNA has been programmed at some point in the past by epigenetic markers that can turn certain DNA portions on or off in response to certain nutrients. The entire programming system is designed for change; these markers can, apparently, fall off or be removed, causing the genetic brain to forget, at least temporarily, previously programmed information.

WHAT MAKES DNA FORGET?

Recent discoveries suggest that, just as with many of us, DNA tends to become a bit forgetful with advancing age.

One of the most well-studied risk factors for having a child with a brain-development disorder is paternal age. While every egg carried in a woman's ovaries was created before she was even born, men continuously produce fresh batches of sperm, beginning at puberty. With the onset of puberty, spermatogonia (precursors of fully functioning sperm) begin dividing about twenty-three times each year. Each division is a critical process as not only do all three billion letters of the DNA code need to be replicated perfectly but so, too, does all the epigenetic bookmarking that will allow that DNA to "remember" which genes to turn on or off in response to nutrient and hormone signals—a set of coordinated functions that is essential for optimal growth and health throughout the future child's life.

While numerous "proofreading" enzymes ensure near-perfect fidelity of DNA replication, this is not the case with epigenetic bookmarking.[29] This suggests environmental circumstances at the time of replication have a relatively much greater impact on epigenetic fidelity than on the rate of genetic (DNA) mutation, a fact borne out in the latest research.[30] In other words, if a man

lacks adequate raw materials for bookmarking, then the bookmarking simply won't go that well during the manufacturing process of that particular batch of sperm. Unfortunately, uncorrected errors tend to accumulate as a man ages. Neurological disorders like autism, bipolar disorder, and schizophrenia have been found to be more common among the children of older men who also have very high rates of abnormal bookmarking.[31]

But it's not only a man's age that can influence genomic memory. It's also how well a man takes care of himself. I believe it's quite possible for older men to significantly increase their odds of having perfectly healthy babies if they support their testicular sperm factories by eating well—a powerful strategy in assuring quality control on the sperm production line.

In 2014, geneticists working in conjunction with Albert Einstein College of Medicine in New York found evidence supporting the idea that low levels of certain nutrients could promote these reproduction errors. Folic acid, B12, and a number of essential amino acids are used for a type of epigenetic bookmarking called methylation; a lack of any one of these vital nutrients would result in undermethylation and critical bookmarks may be omitted. Their research showed bare patches of missing methylation occurring almost exclusively in the out-of-the way places of the gene, where the DNA is tightly coiled and therefore harder for the methylation equipment to reach.[32] If this is really the case, then it would seem that optimizing a man's diet would effectively fortify him against these errors and the diseases they may cause.

GOOD NUTRITION CAN HELP REVERSE
SOME EPIGENETIC MISTAKES

I just showed you evidence supporting the idea that a good diet can help prevent epigenetic mistakes that lead to permanent mutation. But can diet fix past mistakes before they rise to the level of mutation? In other words, can good nutrition enable your genes to return to an earlier, more adaptive strategy, thus averting the possibility that this strategy may be added to the permanent genetic record in the form of a mutation?

The following two studies demonstrate how a strategy involving a predisposition to being overweight can be toggled on or off by modulating nutrition in utero.

A 2010 study looking into how poor maternal nutrition and obesity affects subsequent generations concluded, "Poor in utero nutrition may be a major contributor to the current cycle of obesity."[33] The article shows that children born to overweight mothers are epigenetically programmed to build adipose

tissue in unhealthy amounts. This suggests that millions of malnourished moms are, unbeknownst to them, programming their children for a lifetime of being overweight, and that this predisposition for putting on the pounds can be passed down to that child's children as well.

Did one mom without access to proper nutrition doom all the subsequent generations to be overweight? Here's where the good news comes in. As much as bad nutrition can lead to undesirable traits, good nutrition can compel the epigenetic adaptation system to reprise an earlier strategy appropriate for a more optimal nutrition environment.

Some of the classic epigenetic research suggests that forgotten strategies may be recalled, at least in some circumstances, when genes are given improved nutritional support. And this is why I believe we all have the potential to be—or at least give birth to—genetic lottery winners, because a forgetful genome can potentially be retrained.

This second study shows how optimizing in utero nutrition can have the opposite effect, by convincing the epigenome to abandon the weight-gain strategy and opt for one geared toward optimal body composition. Dr. Randy Jirtle, at Duke University in Durham, North Carolina, studied the effects of nutrient fortification on a breed of mice called *agouti*, known for their yellow color and predisposition for developing severe obesity and subsequent diabetes. Starting with a female agouti raised on ordinary mouse chow, he fed her super-fortified pellets enriched with vitamin B12, folic acid, choline, and betaine and mated her to an agouti male. Instead of exclusively bearing the kind of overweight, unhealthy yellow-coat babies she'd previously given birth to, her new litter now also included a few healthy brown mice that developed normally.[34] You could interpret this study as follows: the agouti breed has regulatory DNA that's essentially been brain damaged by some past traumas in the history of the lineage. As a result, agouti chromosomes, unlike those of other mice, are typically incapable of building healthy, normal offspring. In this study, researchers were able to rehabilitate the agouti's genome by blasting the sleepy genes with enough nutrients to wake them up, reprogramming their genes for better function.

This has enormous implications for us, as researchers are finding abnormal regulatory scars all over our genes. These scars act as records of our ancestors' experiences—their diets, even what the weather was like during their lives. For example, toward the end of World War II, an unusually harsh winter combined with a German-imposed food embargo led to death by starvation of some 30,000 people. Those who survived suffered from a range of developmental and adult disorders, including low birth weight, diabetes, obesity, coronary heart disease, and breast and other cancers. A group of Dutch researchers has associated this exposure with the birth of smaller-than-normal grandchildren.[35]

This finding is remarkable, as it suggests the effects of a pregnant woman's diet can ripple, at the least, into the next two generations. Unlike the agouti mice, which required massive doses of vitamins, these people would possibly respond well to normal or only slightly above normal levels of nutrients as their genes have been affected only for a short while—just a generation or two (unlike the mice)—meaning it might not take quite so much extra nutrition to wake them up.

Some epigenetic reactions are not merely passed on but magnified. In a study of the effects of maternal smoking on a child's risk of developing asthma, doctors at the Keck School of Medicine in Los Angeles discovered that children whose mothers smoked while pregnant were 1.5 times more likely to develop asthma than those born to non-smoking mothers. If grandma smoked, the child was 1.8 times more likely to develop asthma—even if mom never touched a cigarette! Those children whose mothers and grandmothers both smoked while pregnant had their risk elevated by 2.6 times.[36] Why would DNA react this way? If you look for the logic in this decision, you might see it like this: by smoking during pregnancy, you are telling the embryo that the air is full of toxins and that breathing is sometimes dangerous. The developing lungs would do well to be able to react quickly to any inhaled irritants. Asthmatic lungs are over-reactive. They cough and spit at the slightest whiff of foreign aerosols. Still, I believe even a genome as abused as this can be reminded of normal function.

Why do I have so much faith in the restorative power of good epigenetic care? Because contrary to the old ways of thinking, we now know that most diseases are not attributable to permanent mutation but rather to misdirected genetic expression.[37] As we've seen, environmentally derived chemicals mark the long molecule with tags that change its behavior. Such a system, according to the author of the seminal agouti mouse study, Randy Jirtle, seems to exist to provide a "rapid mechanism by which [an organism] can respond to the environment without having to change its hardware."[38] This way, any physiologic tweak or modification can be recalled based on its apparent success or failure. Call it test marketing for a proposed "mutation." That may seem a rather sophisticated operation for a molecule to pull off, but remember we're talking about a molecule that has been in development ever since life on Earth began. With this new understanding of how DNA works, we can now appreciate how easily nutrient deficiencies or exposure to toxins might lead to chronic disease—and how readily these diseases might respond to eliminating toxins and improving nutrition.

At Yale's Center for Excellence in Genomic Science, Dr. Dov S. Greenbaum shares my faith in the intellect behind the design of our genetic apparatus. In describing how junk DNA functions to guide evolution, he writes, "The movement of transposable junk results in a dynamic system of gene activation, which allows for the organism to adapt to its environment."[39] He describes the function very much like Jirtle, adding that this transposition system "allows for the organism to adapt to its environment without redesigning its hardware."[40] To further the analogy, it's conceivable that genetic modifications are introduced under a protocol similar to that used by software designers: test for bugs, then run concurrent with other software on a provisional basis (the beta version of the program), then integrate into the operating system, and finally—when proved to be indispensable—build it into the hardware.

This might have been exactly what happened with the human gene for making vitamin C. After generations of nonuse (due to abundance of vitamin C in our food), the gene would have grown very "sleepy." Eventually, when epigenetic "test marketing" had demonstrated that we could live without being able to make our own vitamin C, a mutation within the gene permanently deactivated it. How, exactly, might this test marketing work? Certain markers increase the error rate during reproduction, and thus a temporary epigenetic change can set up the gene to be permanently altered by a base pair mutation.[41] Genes are like tiny protein-producing machines that create different products. If a factory worker (think epigenetic tagging) shuts off one machine and everything in the cell continues to run smoothly over the ensuing generations, then that particular machine (gene) can be refashioned to produce something else, or turned off altogether. The more we learn about epigenetics, the more it seems that genetic change—both the development of disease and even evolution itself—is as tightly controlled and subject to feedback as every other biologic process from cell development to breathing to reproduction, and, therefore, isn't so random after all.

What helps regulate all these cellular events? Food, mostly. After all, food is the primary way we interact with our environment. But here's what's really remarkable: those tags that get placed on the genes to control how they work and help drive the course of evolution are made out of simple nutrients, like minerals, vitamins, and fatty acids, or are influenced by the presence of these nutrients. In other words, there's essentially no middleman between the food you eat and what your genes are being told to do, enacting changes that can ulti-

GUIDED EVOLUTION?

In 2007, a consortium of geneticists investigating autism boldly announced that the disease was not genetic in the typical sense of the word, meaning that you inherit a gene for autism from one or both of your parents. New gene sequencing technologies had revealed that many children with autism had new gene mutations, never before expressed in their family line.

An article published in the prestigious journal *Proceedings of the National Academy of Sciences* states, "The majority of autisms are a result of de novo mutations, occurring first in the parental germ line."[42] The reasons behind this will be discussed in Chapter 9.

In 2012, a group investigating these new, spontaneous mutations discovered evidence that randomness was not the sole driving force behind them. Their study, published in the journal *Cell*, revealed an unexpected pattern of mutations occurring 100 times more often in specific "hotspots," regions of the human genome where the DNA strand is tightly coiled around organizing proteins called *histones* that function much like spools in a sewing kit, which organize different colors and types of threads.[43]

The consequences of these mutations seem specifically designed to toggle up or down specific character traits. Jonathan Sebat, lead author on the 2012 article, suggests that the hotspots are engineered to "mutate in ways that will influence human traits" by toggling up or down the development of specific behaviors. For example, when a certain gene located at a hotspot on chromosome 7 is duplicated, children develop autism, a developmental delay characterized by near total lack of interest in social interaction. When the same chromosome is deleted, children develop Williams Syndrome, a developmental delay characterized by an exuberant gregariousness, where children talk a lot, and talk with pretty much anyone. The phenomenon wherein specific traits are toggled up and down by variations in gene expression has recently been recognized as a result of the built-in architecture of DNA and dubbed "active adaptive evolution."[44]

As further evidence of an underlying logic driving the development of these new autism-related mutations, it appears that epigenetic factors activate the hotspot, particularly a kind of epigenetic tagging called methylation.[45] In the absence of adequate B vitamins, specific areas of the gene lose these methylation tags, exposing sections of DNA to the factors that generate new mutations. In other words, factors missing from a parent's diet trigger the genome to respond in ways that will hopefully enable the offspring to cope with the new nutritional environment. It doesn't always work out, of course, but that seems to be the intent.

You could almost see it as the attempt to adjust character traits in a way that will engineer different kinds of creative minds, so that hopefully one will give us a new capacity to adapt.

mately become permanent and inheritable. If food can alter genetic information in the space of a single generation, then this powerful and immediate relationship between diet and DNA should place nutritional shifts at center stage in the continuing drama of human evolution.

Evidence for Language in DNA

We have no clear idea how nature keeps track of which programming codes work best for what, or how the many environmental inputs—minerals, vitamins, toxins, and so on—might be translated into a new epigenetic strategy, but some intriguing research offers support to the idea that DNA can indeed take notes.

In 1994, mathematicians observed that junk DNA contained patterns reminiscent of natural language, since it follows, among other things, Zipf's Law (a hierarchical word distribution pattern found in all languages).[46, 47, 48, 49] ·Some geneticists disagree with this assessment, while others think this added layer of complexity might eventually help explain many of DNA's hidden mysteries. But everyone agrees there's plenty of space in junk DNA for all kinds of data storage. Junk DNA is a large enough repository of information to function as a kind of chemical software programmed to, for want of a better term, *recognize* something about the dietary conditions provided it and then include this updated information when it reproduces itself. Some molecular biologists feel that this capability to orchestrate a measured response to environmental change demands that we consider the language encoded in junk DNA as "important for . . . the evolution process" implying the existence of an "independent mechanism for the gradual regulation of gene expression." This suggests that evolution involves more than the previously accepted mechanisms of selection and random mutation. The field of evolutionary study that explores how all three of these mechanisms guide evolution is called *adaptive evolution.*

One example of the logic underlying DNA's behavior can be found by observing the effects of vitamin A deficiency. In the late 1930s, Professor Fred Hale, of the Texas Agricultural Experiment Station at College Station, was able to deprive pigs of vitamin A before conception in such a way that mothers would reliably produce a litter without any eyeballs.[50] When these mothers were fed vitamin A, the next litters developed normal eyeballs, suggesting that eyeball growth was not switched off due to (permanent) mutation, but to a temporary epigenetic modification. Vitamin A is derived from retinoids, which come from plants, which in turn depend on sunlight. So in responding to the absence of vitamin A by turning off the genes to grow eyes, it is as if DNA interpreted the lack of vitamin A as a lack of light, or a lightless environment in which eyes would be of no use. The eyeless pigs had lids, very much like blind cave salamanders. It's possible that these and other blind cave dwellers have undergone a similar epigenetic modification of the genes controlling eye growth in response to low levels of vitamin A in a lightless, plantless cave environment.

Taken together, all epigenetic evidence paints DNA as a far more dynamic and intelligent mechanism of adaptation than has been generally appreciated. In effect, DNA seems capable of collecting information—through the language of food—about changing conditions in the outside world, enacting alteration based on that information, and documenting both the collected data and its response for the benefit of subsequent generations. Junk DNA is full of genetic *treasure*. It may function as a kind of ever-expanding library, complete with its own insightful librarian capable of researching previously written volumes of successful and unsuccessful genetic adaptation strategies. It follows that more complex organisms, with larger cells—whose genomes represent a more complex evolutionary history—would carry relatively more substantial libraries filled with more junk DNA. And we do.[51]

The intelligent librarian stands in direct opposition to the placement of selection and random mutation as the sole mechanisms of genetic change and the development of new species. Given the highly competitive world of survival, it seems obvious that those genetic codes capable of listening to the outside world and using that information to guide decisions would enjoy a marked advantage compared to those stumbling in the dark, completely dependent on luck. This understanding may give rise to an entirely new perspective on how we came to be, placing a new spin on "intelligent design." DNA's ability to respond intelligently to changes in its nutritional environment enables it to take advantage of the shifting cornucopia, exploiting rich nutritional contexts, much the way an interior decorator would make use of a surprise shipment of high-quality silk upholstery fabric. Our genes may help us survive periods of famine and stress by way of experiment, and take advantage of any nutritional glut to experiment further—not blindly, not with random mutations, but with memory and purpose, guided by past experiences encoded within its own structure.

Why does this matter to you?

The chemical intelligence encoded in your DNA and the intelligence of our distant ancestors shared the same ultimate goal: survive. Inside your ancestors' bodies, their genomes shuffled themselves to match nutrient supply with physiologic demands while the people who carried them shared tool-making tips and rumors of food sources which—propelled by this synergy of purpose—would catapult a small group of primates from a nook of the African continent to a state of world domination.

Under the watchful eye of grandmothers and midwives, special foods and preparations proved themselves effective at creating children who could learn faster and grow stronger than the generation before. Children who, naturally, would grow to become parents themselves, able to form their own sets of observations and conclusions about the way the world works and how best to guarantee survival. One of the things that makes human beings (and their ancestors) unique is the sophistication of tool use that enabled consumption of a greater proportion of the edible world than the competition, furthering the agenda of our perpetually reincarnating, self-revising, constantly upgrading, ruthlessly selfish genes. We have managed to shepherd our own genomes through millennia, roaming from one ocean to another, over mountains and across whole continents, and into the modern age.

Those hoping to maintain the product of that achievement—beautiful, healthy human bodies—will want to acquaint themselves with the foods and preparation techniques that allowed us to get this far in the first place. By eating the foods described later in this book, you will be talking directly to your genes. Your foods will tell your epigenome to make your body stronger, more energized, healthier, and more beautiful. And your epigenome will listen.

How smart and responsive is DNA? You could think of it this way. Imagine that when studying a subject for a class, your head never got "too full," and that you could simply add new space for more memories and more knowledge on demand. So that over your lifespan, as you learned more subjects, more languages, read more books, your mind could adapt to accommodate it all. How much stuff would you know? How many problems would you be able to solve better than you can now? Now imagine that you could pass all that learning on to your offspring, so that they started life with all your accumulated wisdom. Maybe not every last detail, but at least the pertinent parts, the details of that multigenerational story that promise to aid in survival and reproduction. And imagine that you, in turn, had inherited your parents' knowledge, and that of their parents, and so on. For thousands of generations since the beginning of your line. Well, that's what DNA is like.

The incredible molecules orchestrating the amazing microcosm of operations inside each and every one of your living cells right now are doing exactly that. Each cell of your body is a vessel carrying a code that has been under constant development since the moment a rudimentary cluster of genetic material ensconced itself within the protection of a lipid coat, defining itself as something different than the primordial sea-world that surrounded it.

Unblocking Your Genetic Potential

Whether you believe in the idea of genetic intelligence or not, the one thing I hope I've made clear in this chapter is that our genes are not written in stone. They are exquisitely sensitive to how we treat them. Like a fine painting passed down through generations, conditions that either harm or preserve are permanently recorded in the provenance of a family's DNA. When the DNA is mistreated, like a Monet painting thrown into the corner of a damp, musty basement, the inheritance loses its value. And the losses may be devastating. Between Halle Berry and the person who carries her luggage, and between all the tall, trim, and beautiful people strutting the red carpets in Hollywood or the tennis courts in the Hamptons and the rest of us who can only watch are untold stories of nutritional starvation, of lost or distorted genetic information. This variability in our ancestors' ability to safeguard their genetic wealth is the reason why today we have so many people wishing for better health, better looks, greater athleticism, and all the manifold benefits of healthy genes.

In Chapter 1, I introduced the idea that the genetic lottery is not random, and in this chapter we saw how genes make what seem to be intelligent decisions guided in part by chemical information in the food we eat. In the coming chapters, we'll see that when we've eaten right—when we've consistently marinated our chromosomes in the chemical soup that enables them to do their utmost best—*Homo sapiens* genes can produce moving sculptures of flesh and blood. This is why beautiful people of every race share the same basic skeletal geometry, and why for the bulk of human history, Hollywood beauties were as plentiful as the stars.

CHAPTER 3

The Greatest Gift

The Creation and Preservation of Genetic Wealth

- Traditional cultures were far more focused on nourishing their children than we are today.

- The knowledge of nutrition and skill at producing healthy food paid off in the form of incredible health and vitality.

- A dentist named Weston Price traveled the world in the 1930s to discover many of these secrets.

- Culinary traditions represent a time capsule of nutritional wisdom.

- Traditional foods are much more diverse and nutrient intense than foods most Americans typically eat.

Egyptologist Mark Lehner walks across what appears to be the smooth surface of a backyard patio until we see that it's actually a giant precision-cut stone in the middle of an abandoned desert quarry. At 137 feet long, it would have been the largest obelisk ever made had it not cracked before being raised from its stone cradle. The obelisk had lain ignored for nearly four thousand years, until archeologists considered just how difficult making it—and then moving it—would be. Over the past few decades, a series of similar discoveries have revealed that ancient civilizations around the world were in possession of technological abilities that far exceed our own. But piecing such history back together again will be challenging. As an article in *Ancient American* theorizing on the possibility that the Incas had found a way to sculpt solid rock using concentrated sunlight explains, the best technology of these cultures was highly prized. "These stonemasons weren't giving away any secrets, or writing them down. Judging by the Freemasons, architects and builders who, some say, trace their lineage back to mystery schools of ancient Egypt, they were a secretive lot."[52]

There is, however, another kind of ancient technology that has had far greater impact on all our lives. The remnants of these great achievements are not waiting to be unearthed. They are walking among us, visible in the form of the high school heartthrob who is also the football star, the eighty-year-old grandmother who also runs marathons, and the celebrities on the covers of *Vogue, Outside,* and *People Magazine.* As you are about to see, nutrition as a tool for optimizing human form and function, and for protecting the integrity of family lineage, was every bit as evolved, refined, and perfected as the tools of mathematics and engineering.

Very much like the jealously guarded trade secrets of ancient stonemasons and civil engineers, the most powerful nutritional secrets, too, were kept close to the chest.[53] If there were as many scientists researching the rituals performed in ancient kitchens as there are researching examples of ancient civil engineering, knowing how to use nutrition to create our own "great works," sculpted in bone and flesh, would be common knowledge. And if women wrote more of our history books, schoolchildren might learn something with more practical application than lists of battles won by various kings. They might learn something along the lines of what a dentist named Weston Price discovered when he traveled the world nearly a century ago, in search of the lost secrets to health.

BODY BY ECOSYSTEM

In the early twentieth century, Westerners were tantalized by the possibility that superhuman races lived just beyond the boundaries of the map. One of the most talked about groups of people were the Hunza, a sometimes-nomadic band of goat and yak herders living in the mountains of what are now Afghanistan and Pakistan. British explorers to these parts claimed to have encountered a rarified land where cancer did not exist, where nobody needed glasses, and where it was commonplace to live beyond a hundred. If these accounts were true, then such people would present Western medicine with a mystery. What was their secret? Pure air? Mineral-rich glacial water? Caloric restriction? True or not, enterprising businessmen soon discovered that the word *Himalayan* was bona fide magic—at least when it was printed on the tonic water bottles they were selling. Amid this circus of conjecture, capitalism, and hucksterism, one extraordinary dentist from Cleveland, Ohio, was determined to inject some much-needed science. This man of introspection and quiet charm invested his own money in an amazing series of journeys, attempting to either verify or impeach these rumors. If people possessing extraordinary fitness were found, he planned to systematically analyze what made them so different from the patients at his dental practice in Ohio.

Price was not exactly the kind of man you'd expect to see rounding mountain trails on a mule. But there he was, a bespectacled, slightly pudgy man of average build pushing sixty. A reserved, meticulous man, his data collection was equally detailed and methodical. His passion for truth was driven by adversity, having lost a son to a dental infection. He became, in his words, distressed by "certain tragic expressions of our modern degeneration, including tooth decay, general physical degeneration, and facial and dental-arch deformities."[54] Price couldn't countenance the idea that human beings should be the only species so riddled with obvious physical defects—like teeth growing every which way inside a person's mouth. After years of studying the source of orthodontic problems in active clinical practice as well as in his lab (animal research was a common practice among the early twentieth-century medical practitioners), he recognized that nutritional deficits could lead to the same kinds of facial deformities in animals that he was seeing in his patients. Contrary to what was believed by many to be true at the time, Price's lab evidence helped convince him that crooked teeth didn't come from "mixing of races," being "of low breeding," bad luck, or the devil. Nutrition science offered a better explanation.

Price's preliminary work in the lab had helped to convince him that human disease arose from the "absence of some essential factors from our modern program." [55] Using the now-dated language of his time, he reasoned that the clearest path to understanding those missing factors would be "to locate immune groups which were found readily as isolated remnants of primitive racial stocks in different parts of the world"—hence the need to travel—and to analyze what they were eating.[56] His plan was simple: count cavities. Count them in mouths of people living all over the globe. Whichever group has the fewest cavities, and the straightest teeth, wins. No fillings or orthodontics allowed. Price was betting that healthy dentition could be used as a proxy for a person's overall health—an assumption that proved correct—and so the number of cavities could be used as an objective, inverse measure of health across people of any racial and cultural background. It was an elegant and efficient plan.

The expeditions involved lugging several 8 x 10 cameras, glass plates, and a full complement of surgical dental equipment. Fortunately, Price had help from a seasoned explorer often featured in *National Geographic*, his nephew Willard DeMille Price, who no doubt greatly enhanced the elder man's ability to return with equipment intact. The resulting tome, *Nutrition and Physical Degeneration*, lays out the products of Price's exhaustive research along with his conclusions. Price was right. Not only were there entire groups of people who enjoyed perfect, cavity-free teeth and spectacular overall health, their finely tuned physiology owed itself to the fact that their traditions enabled them to produce foods with spectacular growth-promoting capacity. Of course, from their perspective, there was nothing extraordinary about their fantastic health. To them, it was only natural.

Price went into his data collection looking for beautiful sets of teeth. But after staring into his subjects' mouths, Price stepped back to notice that something undeniable was staring back at him: robust health and undeniable physical beauty. The perfectly aligned teeth he'd been looking for belonged—with rare, if any, exception—to beautiful people. Beautiful faces with beautiful cheekbones, eyes, noses, lips, and *everything* else—the total package, the physical representation of physiologic harmony.

In each of the eleven countries Price visited, people who had stayed in their villages and continued their native dietary traditions were consistently free of cavities and dental arch deformities. Price couldn't help but notice they also were just plain healthy. So healthy that on his first outing, to Lotchental, a Swiss mountain village isolated by a palisade of towering mountains, he was as awestruck by the townspeople as by the scenery, writing, "As one stands in profound admiration before the stalwart physical development and high moral character of these sturdy mountaineers, he is impressed by the superior types of manhood, womanhood, and childhood that Nature has been able to produce from a suitable diet and a suitable environment."[57] He repeats this theme again and again, as he travels the world. It seems as if Price felt that the beauty and vitality of a given landscape could be conducted into the bodies of those who populated that landscape through the foods they drew from it.

FORM AND FUNCTION: A PACKAGE DEAL

From the beginning of humanity's historic record, one can find numerous references to the idea that physical beauty and health are related. And although social taboo currently proscribes explicitly discussing that relationship, to many it remains patently obvious. True, you may remember your high school football star as less than handsome, riddled with acne, wearing thick glasses and braces, and dependent on pills and an inhaler. But usually our high school heroes receive recognition, admiration, and jealousy as a result of good looks and superior athletic skill. This admiration emerges partly from the fact that we instinctively recognize obvious physical endowments like exceptional stamina and coordination as a byproduct of the ultimate gift—good genes. The genius of Price's work

OLD-FASHIONED BREAKFAST:
FRESH, LOCAL, AND UNPROCESSED

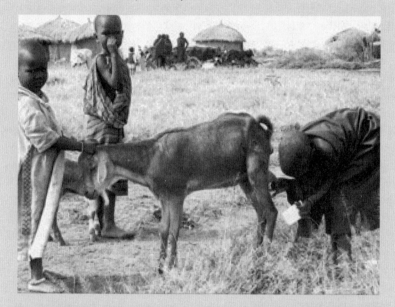

This milk is rich in nutrients bioconcentrated by the goat, which is free to graze on the choicest shoots growing over vast plains of mineral-rich soil. Many small farmers in the United States still raise their animals on pasture, offering the customer a healthy alternative to milk produced by grain-fed animals.

is that he dared to scientifically examine the connection between outwardly visible signs of health and nutrition using the same systematic approach we bring to bear when studying any other biological phenomenon.

The preference for beauty (in our own and other's faces) emerges as a result of the instinctive pattern recognition process that I will describe in detail in Chapter 4. For now, it is crucial to understand that what we consider to be beautiful also serves a survival function. As unfair as it seems, less attractive people have more health problems.[58] All congenital syndromes that distort facial architecture are associated with impairments in physiologic functions like breathing, talking, hearing, walking, and so on. There are hundreds of such syndromes codified so far, recognized on sight by trained pediatricians and resulting in disabilities ranging from poor vision (as in Marfan's Dandy Walker, Cohen and Stickler syndromes—just to name a few) to sinus inflammation and susceptibility to infection (Fragile X, Cornelia De Lange) to hearing loss (chromosomal deletions at 22q11.2, Coffin Lowry) to chewing and swallowing difficulties (Rhett, CHARGE, arthrogryposis).[59] Price recognized that growth anomalies too subtle to warrant characterization as a congenital syndrome are, nevertheless, also associated with functional problems. For example, underdeveloped mandibles don't just look unattractive, they also don't hold teeth very well, which makes it hard to chew and increases the risk of cavities.[60, 61] To our animal minds, these physical traits represent potential liabilities, a weakness in the tribe bordering on contagion. This reaction is deeply ingrained, and it may be why even health professionals are reluctant to investigate the root causes of visible physical anomalies. But Price felt differently. He rejected the age-old notion that the blessings of health and beauty are reserved for those few with the purest souls—the biological equivalent of divine right. His thinking was truly outside the box and even today his research findings are ahead of their time.

If you'd like to get a taste of the kind of vitality Price discovered, what people looked like, and how they lived, do a quick Internet search for indigenous tribes. Start with the San, Maasai, Himba, Kombai, Wodaabe, or Mongolian nomad. Or watch any TV show about tribal life. When you look at the people's faces, notice how particularly well-formed their features are. That is because their diets still connect them to a healthy living environment whose beauty, in a very real sense, expresses itself through their bodies.

One of the first documentary films ever made is called *Grass: A Nation's Battle For Life,* filmed in 1925 by Meriam C. Cooper (who later made *King Kong*). Cooper documents the lifestyle of the Baktiari tribe in the Zardeh Kuh Mountains of what is now Iran. It tracks one leg of the 200-plus-mile journey the tribe made twice a year in the seasonal search of fresh pasture for their goats and pigs. Up and down the rocky mountainsides, old men, pregnant women, and little children herd their stubborn, hungry animals, the leaders breaking through waist-deep snows in bare feet. Five thousand people travel with all their belongings across the 200 high-altitude miles in a little over a month. In distance alone, they covered the equivalent of twenty marathons a year. How did they do it? Genetic wealth. Our twentieth-century Western perspective calls on us to label their lifestyle as subsistence living, since they lacked the accoutrements associated with prosperity. But they didn't carry their gold in leather satchels. Their treasure was safely hidden inside the vaults of their genetic material, and it endowed every member of the tribe with chiseled features, strong joints,

PROFILES IN GENETIC WEALTH

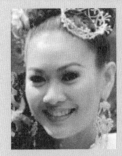 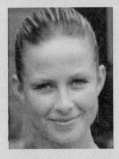 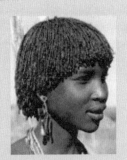

Native Thai (*left*), Danish barmaid (*middle*), Ethiopian woman (*right*). Notice their well-formed features, indicative of ideal geometric facial construction. Whether a people draw nutrition from the family farm, the sea, or the savannah, real food acts as a kind of conduit through which the beauty of the environment can be communicated into our bodies and expressed as human form.

healthy immune systems, and the stamina to achieve athletic feats that few of us would dare attempt. And remember, they did this every season.

HOW THEY WERE BUILT: EXCEEDING THE
RDA BY A FACTOR OF TEN

Contrary to what Westerners tend to assume, indigenous people of the past were not merely scraping by, skinny and starving, desperate to eat whatever scraps they could find. Their lives did revolve primarily around finding food, but they were experts at it, far more capable than we are of making nutrient-rich foods part of daily life. By fortifying the soil, they grew more nutrient-rich plants. By feeding their animals the products of healthy soil, they cultivated healthier, more nutrient-rich animals. And since different nutrients are stored in different parts of the animal, by consuming every edible part of their livestock and the animals they hunted, they enjoyed the full complex of nutritional diversity. They used their own version of biotechnology to create the most nutrient-dense foods possible, foods that functioned to design every sinew and fiber of their bodies.

At eleven locations around the world, Price secured samples of indigenous communities' staple foods for lab analysis. His nutritional survey rivals that of our best nationally sponsored programs in having tested for all four fat-soluble vitamins (A, D, E, and K) and six minerals (calcium, iron, magnesium, phosphorus, copper, and iodine). Here's what he found:

> It is of interest that the diets of the primitive groups . . . have all provided a nutrition containing at least four times these minimum [mineral] requirements; whereas the displacing nutrition of commerce, consisting largely of white-flour products, sugar, polished rice, jams [nutritionally equivalent to fruit juice], canned goods, and vegetable fats, have invariably failed to provide even the minimum requirements. In other words, the foods of the native Eskimos contained 5.4 times as much calcium as the displacing foods of the white man, 5 times as much phosphorus, 1.5 times as much iron, 7.9 times as much magnesium, 1.5 times as much copper, 8.8 times as much iodine, and at least a tenfold increase in fat-soluble activators [Price's term for vitamins].[62]

He continues, listing the findings for each of the other groups he studied. There was a clear pattern: the native diets had ten or more times the fat-soluble vitamins and one-and-a-half to fifty times more minerals than the diets of people in the United States.[63] It is obvious that diets of people living in what doctors at the time would have called "backward" conditions were richer than those living in the technologically "advanced" United States by an order of magnitude. Price's work pulled back the curtain behind which the true glory of humankind's potential now lies obscured. His anecdotes revealed what life could be like across the range of physiologic capacity, from mental balance ("One marvels at their gentleness, refinement, and sweetness of character") to freedom from cancer, a doctor for thirty-six years in Northern Canada who had "never seen a case of malignant disease," and only rarely treated acute surgical problems of the "gallbladder, kidney, stomach, and appendix." And across the age spectrum, from infancy ("We never heard an Eskimo child crying except when hungry, or frightened by the presence of strangers"), to weaning ("Children of Eskimos have no difficulties with the cutting of their teeth") to almost ridiculously easy outdoor birthing where women "would take a shawl and either alone or accompanied by one member of the family retire to the bush and give birth to the baby and return with it to the cabin," to early motherhood, "characterized by an abundance of breastfood which almost always develops normally and is maintained without difficulty for a year," on into midlife ("We neither saw nor heard of a case [of arthritis]") and vitality into older age ("a woman of sixty-two years who carried an enormous load of rye on her back at an altitude of five thousand feet").[64] Though his laboratory was dismantled over fifty years ago, I consider Price's data a more accurate indication of how much nutrition we need than the recommended daily allowance (RDA).

What makes his sixty-plus-year-old data superior to state-of-the-art nutrition science today? Chiefly, the fact that today's state-of-the-art nutrition science leaves much to be desired. While Price's data may be old, he identified the healthiest people he could and then systematically analyzed the nutrient content of their staple foods. But if you ever look into how today's RDAs are set, you'll find a hodgepodge of differing opinions, unstandardized techniques, and poorly thought-out studies. For instance, the RDA of vitamin B6 for infants younger than one year old was set at 0.1 milligram per day based on the average B6 content in the breast milk of only nineteen women. Six of these women did not even themselves consume the RDA of vitamin B6 for their age group, and their breast milk contained only one tenth of the B6 of the women with healthier diets.[65] So you might wonder, then, if a third of the women on which we base our national recommended daily allowances were, by our own definition, undernourished, shouldn't they have been excluded from the study? The fact that they were not suggests to me that the researchers in charge of this study were not interested in what a baby might need to be healthy, but merely in calculating the averages and getting their jobs done. This is just one example of the poor quality research that defines state-of-the-art, modern nutrition science. (It also determines what gets put into infant formula—and what gets left out.)

If you believe Price's data, which I do, then clearly our bodies appear to be accustomed to a far richer stream of nutrients than we manage to sip, chew, swallow, or scarf down in our daily diets. Our need for nutrients is, apparently, quite extraordinary. But what is more extraordinary is the totality to which indigenous cultures, and presumably also our ancestors, involved themselves in the production of these foods. In contrast to our general attitude of nourishment as a necessary evil demanding expediency, traditional life seemed to revolve around collecting and concentrating nutrition. To this end, no methodology—and no recipe—was too bizarre.

I will include here a few examples from Price's book to demonstrate how fully people immersed themselves in the production of food, and a few of the wonderful ingenuities that streamlined this undertaking. In the Scottish Isles, people built their houses using, chiefly, the grass that grew abundantly on the moors. The roofs were loosely woven and chimneyless so that the smoke from their cooking fires would pass directly through the thatch. When the roof was removed and rebuilt in the spring after having been infused with mineral-rich ash all winter, the smoke thatch made fantastic fertilizer for their plant crops, chiefly oats. Their oats, in turn, were superior sources of minerals and were incorporated into many dishes. One of the most important was a fish dish made from baked cod's head (rich in essential fatty acids) that had been stuffed with oatmeal (rich in minerals) and chopped cod livers (rich in vitamins).

On the other side of the world, in Melanesia, the original arrivals to the islands had brought with them a member of the pig family bred for its self-sufficiency at finding forage in the muddy and mountainous landscape. They'd released their hogs into the wild so they could colonize the forests. Soon, the hogs' numbers had grown to the point that one could be hunted down just about anywhere. Every part of the quarry—from snout to tail—would be cooked or smoked or otherwise prepared and eaten. Another Melanesian favorite was the coconut crab, so called because of its ability to sever coconuts from trees with monster claws. To catch the well-armed crabs as they came down from the trees, natives would quickly girdle the tree with grass about fifteen feet from the ground. Upon reaching the grass girdle, the crab—convinced it had reached terra firma—would release its grip, and fall. Stunned, the crab could then be easily gathered. It would be tempting to eat them on the spot. Nevertheless, the crabs were first confined in pens for several days and allowed to gorge on all the coconut they wanted—generally enough to burst their shells. According to Price, "They are then very delicious eating."[66]

Around the world again to Eastern Africa, Price found Maasai life revolved around producing healthy cattle, used primarily for their milk and their blood and only occasionally for their flesh. Maasai men spent nearly a decade learning to tend their animals. This education included everything from identifying the best grazing grounds based on rainfall patterns, to selective breeding, to regularly drawing blood from the jugular vein using a bow and arrow with surgical precision. As the Maasai ate neither fruit nor grain, this milk, either fresh or curdled (and bacteria-enriched), was their dietary staple. Recent studies have shown that Maasai cow milk contains five times the brain-building phospholipids of American milk.[67] In the dry season, when milk yields are low, the Maasai fortify the milk with blood to make another staple drink.

As focused as people once were on the production of healthy food, the chief crop—and the ultimate prize—was the next generation of healthy children. Traditional cultures made a science of it. As we'll see in Chapter 5, step one was planning ahead. Around the world, traditions reflected extensive use of special foods to boost a woman's nutrition before conception, during gestation, for nursing, and for rebuilding before the next pregnancy. Some cultures thought it prudent to fortify the groom's diet in preparation for his wedding ceremony.[68] The

shreds of surviving information suggest such knowledge was quite sophisticated. Blackfoot Nation women utilized the still-unknown nutrient systems found
in the lining of the large intestine of buffalo (and later, cow) to "make the baby
have a nice round head."[69] To ensure easy delivery, many cultures reinforced
preconception and pregnancy diets with fish eggs and organ meats—loaded
with fat-soluble vitamins, B12, and omega-3—as well as special grains carefully
cultivated to be high in important minerals.[70] The Maasai allowed couples to
marry only after spending several months consuming milk from the wet season
when the grass was especially lush and the milk much denser in nutrients.[71] In
Fiji, islanders would hike miles down to the sea to acquire a certain species of
lobster crab that "tribal custom demonstrated [to be] particularly efficient for
producing a highly perfect infant."[72] Elsewhere, fortifying foods didn't just facilitate pregnancy; they made the difference between the baby making it to term or
not. The soil of certain areas around the Nile Delta is notoriously low in iodine,
the lack of which can lead to maternal goiter and infant malformation. Local
tribes knew that burning water hyacinth (rich in iodine) produced ashes capable
of preventing these complications.[73]

These ingrained traditions existed throughout the world and, until recently,
dictated the ebb and flow of daily life. This kind of dedication, study, and wise
use of natural resources is what was required to amass and protect the genetic
wealth that enabled people to survive in a very different, and harsher, wild, wild
world. Of course, these days most of us spend our time fighting traffic, not wild
boar. But the same nutritional input that toughened and fortified the physiologies of these indigenous peoples can still be accessed today for the attainment
of extraordinary health. Were the medical community to bring the same enthusiasm to the engineering and maintenance of healthy bodies as archaeologists
bring to their study of ancient architectural wonders, they would soon call for
a radical revision of what we understand to be a healthy human diet. The construction of a beautiful, sound building is not a matter of chance, but of planning, good materials, and reference to the collected body of relevant science.
Winning the genetic lottery depends upon those very same prerequisites.

Today, at every stage in the process of producing food, we do things differently than our sturdy, self-sufficient ancestors did, wasting opportunities to provide ourselves with essential nutrients at every turn. We fail to fortify and protect the substrate on which the life and health of everything depends: the soil.
We raise animals in unspeakably inhumane and unhealthy conditions, fill their
tissues with toxins, and color the meat to make it appear more appetizing. Being
raised on open pasture is no guarantee that an animal's body, and ultimate sacrifice, will be put to full use; typically, only the muscle is consumed. Much of the
nutrients, bioconcentrated over the animal's life, are thrown to waste. Grains—

ARE WE REALLY LIVING LONGER?

People often say we're living longer than ever. But is that really true? According to an article called "Length of Life in the Ancient World," published in the *Journal of the Royal Society of Medicine* in January 1994, from circa 100 B.C. until 1990, we have managed to tack an additional six years onto the life span. This modest increase is easily attributable not to better nutrition or even better health, but to emergency room care, artificial life support, life-sustaining pharmaceuticals, vaccines, and other technology, not to mention the many leaps in accident prevention. Presuming that it's sensible to gauge health by longevity of lifespan as opposed to longevity of function, the numbers still tell a surprising story. Even though the average life span has increased slightly, according to the United States Census, in the past 200 years the percentage of people living a really long time may actually have gone down:

Percentage of Americans aged 100 in 1830: 0.020
Percentage of Americans aged 100 in 1990: 0.015
Percentage of people living today expected to live to 100: 0.001

even those grown on relatively healthy soil—are too often processed in ways specifically damaging to the most essential, and delicate, nutrients. Once in the kitchen, the consumer takes one last swing at whatever nutrition has survived, through overcooking and the use of cheap, toxic oils. Finally, since we've not been told that certain vitamins and minerals are more bioavailable when combined with acids or fats (see Chapter 7), many of them pass right through us.

Given that we drop the ball at every stage in the process of bringing food to the table, it's not surprising that recent studies show, far from exceeding the RDA as we should be, few of us even meet it. For vitamin A, only 46.7 percent of healthy females meet the RDA,[74] and levels are low in 87 percent of children with asthma.[75] For vitamin D, 55 percent of obese children, 76 percent of minority children, and 36 percent of otherwise healthy, young adults are deficient.[76] For vitamin E, 58 percent of toddlers between one and two years old,[77] 91 percent of preschoolers,[78] and 72.3 percent of healthy females do not consume enough. Zero percent of breastfed infants were found to have achieved the minimum recommended intake of vitamin K.[79] For the B vitamins, only 54.7 percent consumed adequate B2 (riboflavin)[80] for folate, only 2.2 percent of women between the ages of 18 and 35 and 5.2 percent of women aged 36–50 achieved the recommended intake; and for calcium, fewer than 22 percent of African-American adolescent girls consumed the RDA.[81] There are more studies, but you get the idea. Not one study shows 100 percent adequacy of any single nutrient, not to mention adequacy of all measurable nutrients, which would be a better goal. Presumably the vast majority of Americans are deficient in multiple nutrients.

Many of my patients suffer from symptoms that could be attributable to poor nutrition. Problems as common as dry skin, easy bruising, frequent runny noses, yeast infections, and crampy digestive systems are all exacerbated by, if not due entirely to, inadequate nutrition. Unfortunately, testing for vitamin adequacy is not easy. We haven't even defined what "normal" levels are for many nutrients, including essential fatty acids and vitamin K. For those that have been so defined, the normal range may extend all the way down to zero. That's right: you may have none of an essential nutrient in your bloodstream, yet still be considered to have consumed an adequate amount. So why bother testing? And since many vitamins are stored in the liver and other tissues, even if blood levels are adequate, overall body stores may be low. As far as I can tell, the best way to assure nutrient adequacy is not with testing, but with adequate nutrient consumption—itself no simple matter.

Aside from building a time machine and transporting back to the halcyon years of nutritional bounty, in the face of so many barriers to good nutrition, what is an ordinary person to do? Is it remotely possible, in this day and age, to get the nutrients you need without breaking your bank?

Absolutely. You can grow a garden, shop for fruits and vegetables by smell (as opposed to appearance), and buy animal products from farms that raise them humanely—on pasture and outside in the sun. In the coming chapters, I'll go into more detail about special ways to make your food as nutritious as possible. But I can tell you right now, you'll get the most bang for your buck, and the fastest return on investment, if you learn to enjoy something that many kids in many countries aside from this one will fight each other for—the organ meats.

These were the original vitamin supplements, and they comprise key components of almost all truly traditional heritage dishes. They are the missing ingredients whose disappearance from our dinner tables explains many of our health problems, and whose replenishment would go a long way toward improving those dismal nutrition statistics. But like most middle-class Americans, for most of my life I assumed such odd tidbits and wiggly things were best fed to my cats and dogs. I might have thought differently had I been raised some place where traditions of self-sufficiency are still alive and kicking. Some place where children can learn cherished recipes from their parents. Some place where there's plenty of land and open water per capita, where the weather invites people to spend time outdoors with their extended families. Some place like Hawaii.

CROSSING THE CULINARY DIVIDE

The south side of Kauai is known all over the Hawaiian archipelago as Filipino territory; in our old neighborhood about one in three households spoke Illokano. My husband, Luke, a devout meat-eater whose favorite meal is a blood-rare steak, considered himself a serious carnivore until he met these guys. People who catch wild boar with hunting dogs and kill the tusked beasts with knives (not guns, mind you) experience a fuller meaning of the word. There, the majority of households, young and old, could make short work of a large carcass or a sturdy goat leg. When I first moved to Hawaii, given that I am an unworldly American, the culture struck me as slightly terrifying.

Then the inevitable happened: we were invited to a neighborhood buffet for a crash course in local, "any kine" Filipino cuisine. I'd heard about these parties and I knew what kind of stuff awaited us on the rough-hewn picnic table out on the patio behind the sliding glass doors. At the potluck, kids gathered inside to watch and to laugh at the *molikini Ha' Oles* (newly immigrated white folk) trying to cope. Thankfully, a sweet eight-year-old girl took pity on us. Graciously highlighting key ingredients, Kiani guided us through the mystery casseroles, greasy open plates, and bowls of soupy chunks.

First up, *morcon*, a meat, egg, and cheese wrap sliced into neat cross-sections, beautifully setting bright yellow yolk against deep maroon liver. Next, one of those suspiciously chunky soups: tan-colored *paksiw na pata*, pork knuckles and pork meat braised in a mixture of soy sauce, sugar, and vinegar, and flavored with dried lily buds. I couldn't get past the knuckles. More soupy chunks, this time in green and tan, of *balon-balonan*, chicken gizzards softened in vinegar and mixed with water spinach. Beside that, a duo of honeycomb tripe and vegetable stews—*goto* and *callos*. I felt as if I'd wandered into a Klingon delicatessen. But then I noticed, at the far corner of the table, a single lonely looking bowl of sweet potato soup. This I could manage.

Luke was a more enthusiastic guest. The weirder the dish's ingredients, the more he slopped onto his compartmented cardboard plate. This was enormously entertaining to our younger hosts, every scoop generating louder giggling until the adults' attention was drawn to Luke's selections. By the time the table tour was over, he had piled on an unbelievable ten dishes that were now slowly meld-ing into one. Onlookers volunteered approval with a round of claps and cheers.

While Luke transformed the contents of his overflowing plate into a small pile of bones, I began to develop the suspicion that I had been living in a cloistered world. The feeling followed me home, and resurfaced each time I hiked past the goat herds that dot the rolling green hills of Lawai.

I'd worked in Thailand and trekked in Nepal. I'd eaten at hundreds of ethnic restaurants, and in the homes of friends from all over the world. But the potluck meal had really been outside my normal experience of eating. There were things on that table I didn't know you could eat, let alone would want to. At the age of thirty-three, I had learned there's more to meat than meat. While I'd been in my kitchen sprinkling chicken extract powder over rehydrated ramen noodles, just down the road, my Filipino neighbors were stuffing hoofed feet into a boiling cauldron. I wasn't so much horrified as I was envious.

Shortly after this initiation buffet, I fell sick from the infection in my knee and I learned that I'd developed the problem due in large part to nutrient deficiencies. Had I been raised, like my same-aged cohorts in Hawaii, on such wild gastronomic safaris rather than the standard middle-class fare of boneless, skinless white meat, margarine, and frozen vegetables, my life would most certainly have been different.

But there's another piece to this story: I would also very likely look different. The long, slim waist, graceful limbs, perfect vision—and other traits my grandmothers possessed—could have been mine. This may seem like an extraordinary claim. But if you believe what Price discovered, that bad diet can so affect a child's growth that it can manifest in crooked teeth, malocclusions, and jaw anomalies, then it is no great leap to infer that what affects the growth of the bones of the face can affect the growth of all the bones of the skull and of every bone in your body—your entire anatomy.

We all agree it's nice to have straight teeth. But for us to understand how diet affects *all* the proportions of your anatomy someone has to ask a more fundamental question: *How exactly is the human body supposed to be proportioned? What proportions allow for athleticism, ease of movement, and even things like a birth canal wide enough to accommodate the passage of a child?*

In the next chapter we'll see that we already have the answer. Because we all recognize this proportionality instinctively and long ago gave it a name. We call it beauty.

RECIPE FROM *FRENCH COOKING FOR EVERY HOME,*
BY FRANCOIS TANTY, CHEF CUISINE
FOR EMPEROR NAPOLEON III

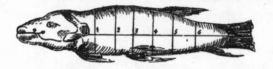

BOILED SALMON OR TROUT.

PREPARATION.—We will tell here how to cook a whole salmon, from about 8 to 10 lbs. and it will be exactly the same with any other fish or part of fish to be cooked "au court bouillon." 1st. Clean and wash your fish, remove the gills and the fins, but preserve the tail, place the fish in a fish kettle (with a grate in the bottom so as not to break it, when you take it from the kettle) with 2 carrots, 1 onion sliced, some thyme and laurel, 6 grains of whole pepper and enough water to cover the fish well. 2d. Let heat and *as soon as it boils* place the fish pan on a corner of the stove and let simmer for about 1 hour without letting boil. 3d. Serve in a long dish on a folded napkin and dispose around the fish or serve apart 2 nice potatoes for each guest, boiled in slightly salted water and carefully carved. Serve the sauce apart. For the sauces see Nos. 151-152-159.

Usually when we buy fish these days it's already filleted and sani-wrapped. But how much closer to the source of your food would you be, and how much more like a top chef would you feel, if you knew how to clean and prepare a beautiful, whole fresh salmon all by yourself?

CHAPTER 4

Dynamic Symmetry
The Beauty-Health Connection

- The way we look speaks volumes about our health because of the fact that form implies function.

- Perhaps because the subject of appearance is so emotionally charged, physicians pretend that disfiguring birth defects and other developmental malformations are unavoidable.

- If doctors and nutritionists were willing to explore the beauty–health connection, every child would have a better chance to grow up healthy.

- A California surgeon created a formula for evaluating the beauty–health connection, based on the same principle of symmetry described by ancient Greeks.

- Athletic bodies and movie-star faces tend to reflect this symmetry, which is, in turn, a reflection of their genetic wealth.

What exactly is beauty? Few people make sense when they talk about it. The subject is either too profound or too emotionally charged to describe objectively. Even talent agents who make their living in the beauty trade characterize it using imprecise euphemisms: a glow, a certain something. Press a publisher, a judge, a casting director, or a news reporter hard enough and you might get them to confess that good looks matter in their fields more than they'd like to admit. On the other hand, feminists like author Camile Paglia have suggested that beauty may all be a big put-on, and that without cover girls, movie stars, and other models saturating the media, we'd be immune to its effects.

Controversial and enigmatic as the subject of beauty may seem, in reality, beauty is simply another natural phenomenon that, like gravity or the speed of

EIGHT HISTORICAL STUDIES OF HUMAN ANATOMY AND ADHERENCE TO PHI PROPORTIONS

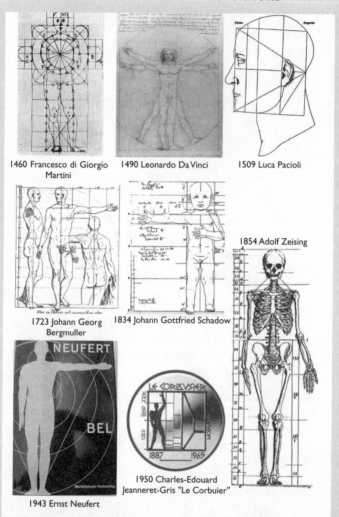

1460 Francesco di Giorgio Martini

1490 Leonardo Da Vinci

1509 Luca Pacioli

1723 Johann Georg Bergmuller

1834 Johann Gottfried Schadow

1854 Adolf Zeising

1943 Ernst Neufert

1950 Charles-Edouard Jeanneret-Gris "Le Corbuier"

Were all these men obsessed with physical beauty? We could say so. But realize that until very recently the concept of beauty, structural integrity, movement, and grace were considered aspects of the same phenomenon. More accurate might be to say they were obsessed with geometric proportion.

light, can be quantified, analyzed, and understood. Though poets and songwriters might object, significant benefits can be derived from deconstructing human beauty using the same tools we would bring to any other scientific question. In fact, beauty can tell us quite a lot about our genetic histories, our bodies, and our health.

This connection is anything but abstract. In ancient times, athletes were considered exemplary demonstrations of the relationship between beauty, strength, and health. Many art historians agree that the Greco-Roman depiction of the idealized male figure is an argument in stone that there is a connection between form and function, symmetry and grace, and that these conjoined qualities are worthy of celebration.[82, 83, 84]

I bear witness to the reality of the beauty-health connection every day in my clinic. And whether they realize it or not, so does every primary care doctor in America: the number-one reason for an office visit is "arthropathies [joint pain] and related disorders"[85] very often attributable to a musculoskeletal imbalance arising from a skeletal asymmetry.[86] The entire field of chiropractic is based on evaluating skeletal alignments—another way of talking about symmetry and balance. Hang around backstage at any professional sporting event where trainers are trying to maintain an athlete's ability to function and you hear words like symmetry, balance, and stability floated around as these professionals discuss how one small asymmetry in physiology or motion has the potential to work its way up the "kinetic chain" leading to secondary imbalances that can disable a player for weeks or months.

Outside the field of medicine, many life-science professionals apply their ability to judge physical attractiveness without hesitation. When a farmer or a racehorse breeder or a rare orchid grower sees obvious disruptions in healthy growth, they naturally consider the nutritional context in which the specimen was raised. If a prize-winning mare gives birth to a foal with abnormally bowed legs, the veterinarian recognizes that something went wrong and, often, asks the logical question, What was the mother eating? But physicians rarely do that, even when life-threatening problems show up right at birth. And we continue to neglect the nutrition-development equation when our patients develop scoliosis, joint malformations, aneurysms, autism, schizophrenia, and so on later in life. If doctors and nutritionists were as willing as other professionals to use their basic senses, every child would have a better chance to grow up healthy.

Our desire for beauty is no simple matter of vanity. The way we look speaks volumes about our health because of the fact that form implies function. Less attractive facial forms are less functional. Children with suboptimal skull structure may need glasses, braces, or oral surgery, whereas children with more ideal architecture won't. [87] This is because suboptimal architecture impairs development of normal geometry, leading to imperfectly formed facial features, be it the eyes or ears or nose or jaw and throat. For example, narrow nasal passages irritate the mucosa, increasing the chances of rhinitis and allergies.[88, 89] When the airway in the back of the throat is improperly formed, a child may suffer from sleep apnea, which starves the brain of the oxygen needed to develop normal intelligence.[90, 91] One of the few instances in which doctors do use visual assessments to screen for health disorders is with a condition known loosely as minor anomalies, also known, much less formally, as the "funny looking kid." It's common enough that it even has an acronym, FLK. This diagnosis is one of the primary reasons for genetic testing. Children with growth anomalies are the group most often found to have genetic diseases and internal organ malformations, and they frequently develop learning disorders, socialization disorders, and cancer.[92] And let's not pretend a person's physical development has no social consequences. Less attractive people rate themselves as less popular,[93] less happy,[94] and less healthy.[95] They are more depressed more often,[96] spend more time in jail,[97] and as adults, they earn less[98] than their more attractive peers.

My personal story feeds right into this discussion. In high school, I competed in cross-country and track at an international level and ultimately earned a four-year college athletic scholarship and an invitation to the Olympic trials for the 1500-meter race. While I suffered more than my fair share of injuries, I always found a way—an orthotic insert or an extra couple of stretching exercises—to keep myself in the competition and remain undefeated. But in college, my body started falling apart faster than it had in high school. The rehab programs and assistive orthotics I'd relied upon could no longer keep me competitive. I soon fell behind the pack. Not long after, I was sidelined. Then redshirted: no more running for an entire season.

If you've ever had the privilege of being involved with competitive sports, you know what happens once you take off that uniform and you're no longer part of the team: you get really introspective. You start asking questions. Why couldn't I have gone further when others did? What's different about me? Did I not bring it in terms of effort or is there something about me physically that just plain doesn't measure up?

It's that last question that haunted me as I began to notice the little differences between my body and the bodies of the girls who went on to national competition. Their waists were longer. Their hips wider and more flexible. They were lithe and supple while my short, blocky waist sat atop the same narrow hips I had when I was twelve, stubbornly refusing to develop.

As a twenty-year-old senior at Rutgers College in New Brunswick, New Jersey, I developed a suspicion, the awakening of perception, that allowed me to begin to see a connection between form, function, and health that I had never fully appreciated before. At that same time, a thousand miles away on the west bank of the widest section of the Mississippi, the man who I would meet five years later and ultimately marry was dealing with his own recurring health issues and asking the very same questions about his own body and how good looks and physical ability and health might all be connected. For both of us, these questions became obsessions that would ultimately collide at the moment we decided to create a simple pamphlet for my patients who wanted a short guide to health and nutrition. A document that ultimately became this book.

We also were equally curious about the inverse circumstance: What happens when everything goes right? In both of our high schools, when Rod Stewart sang, "Some guys have all the luck . . ." we knew who he was talking about: the homecoming king. You may have noticed this in your high school, too. Was he popular? Athletic? Pretty smart? And what about the prom queen? In my high school, she was also the valedictorian and MVP on the soccer team. But why should this be so? What is it about beauty that makes something not only look better but also function better? And what makes us want it so badly?

After years of subsequent research, I discovered that the bulk of evidence suggests that the same conditions that allow our DNA to create health also allow our DNA to grow beautiful people. I call this phenomenon the *package deal effect* because beauty and health are just that—a package deal. The more you have of one, the more you probably have of the other.

And the more you have of each of these qualities, the more other people will be attracted to you. It all boils down to science: when you're attracted to someone else, or when you are decidedly not attracted to another person, you are engaged in a sophisticated scientific enquiry. There's nothing shallow about it; it's as deep as it gets. Like the laws of engineering, chemistry, and physics, the laws of physical attraction emerge from the fabric of the universe and can best be understood using the language of mathematics.

THE MAN WHO DISCOVERED
THE PERFECT FACE

The desire for beauty is so great that some of us take matters into our own hands—or rather, into the hands of a professional—to get a larger helping of its sweet rewards. In 2005 more than 11 million cosmetic procedures were performed in the United States alone. Most procedures involve moving fat, skin, and muscle around the face and body, but an extreme makeover can require breaking and resetting bone. As doctors permanently rearrange our looks, what standards, do you suppose, guide their decisions? The answer is *none*—that is, none aside from their own personal aesthetics and experience. Thankfully, their skills usually leave the patient looking better rather than worse. But their training does not provide them with instructions for rebuilding faces according to any universal standard of ideal facial architecture.

Why not? Simply put, it's complicated. Each person's face has a distinct 3-D geometry that our brains can interpret. We don't know how exactly, and most of us don't need to worry about it. But if plastic surgeons want to build better faces reliably, and if they want to know whether or not they will be repositioning a jaw, a tooth, or an eyebrow in an attractive location that also allows for normal function, they should have at their disposal a blueprint for designing attractive and functional facial geometry. Such was the thinking of a bright, young maxillofacial surgeon at UCLA named Dr. Stephen Marquardt.

This was no ordinary plastic surgeon. This was a man on call for UCLA ER and in charge of reconstructing people's faces after serious vehicular accidents and penetrating trauma. One evening in the late 1970s, Dr. Marquardt couldn't sleep. In two days time he would commence an operation on a woman who'd been in a terrible car accident. It was his job to reconstruct her badly damaged lower face. But one question nagged him all night: How can I be sure she'll be happy with the results? In those days there were relatively few plastic or reconstructive surgeons, even in Los Angeles, and patients would receive their particular surgeon's trademark work—say, Audrey Hepburn's nose—with results so consistent that other surgeons could tell who the patient had seen. Dr. Marquardt realized Hepburn's petite nose, as undeniably cute as it was, might not be the right nose for just anyone. How could a doctor know which nose, or chin, or jaw line is best proportioned for the face of the person on the operating table? Marquardt wondered why there weren't some rules or standards to follow. Would he always have to guess, fingers crossed, or might there be a more dependable approach?

In a search for answers, Dr. Marquardt went to a museum and spent the day examining great works of art. At the end of the day he had a stack of sketches, but no definitive set of rules. He wanted to know what, if any, principle guided the creation of all great works of art. Over the next several months he studied rules of beauty in architecture, art, music, and more. Still, no consistent theme emerged.

Finally, he recognized that he kept running across formulas, like the triangle on the color wheel, and the "rule of threes" as applied in painting, photography, writing, and other art forms. He'd been studying individual subjects to find a common link, and that link was mathematics. At the core of the mathematical principles of beauty lay a set of numbers named after the Italian who first discovered it in the eleventh century—the *Fibonacci Sequence*.

BEAUTY'S SECRET CODE: PHI

You may remember the Fibonacci sequence from The DaVinci Code, in which the cryptologist heroine discovers a series of numbers her grandfather wrote on the floor with invisible ink at the site of his murder: 1, 1, 2, 3, 5, 8, 13, 21. The sequence builds by summing the last two numbers on the end, growing forever. Had the dead man lived to write the next number, he would have written 34— the sum of 13 and 21. If one were looking for a universal code of proportionate growth, this sequence of numbers would be the Holy Grail.

THE GOLDEN RECTANGLE

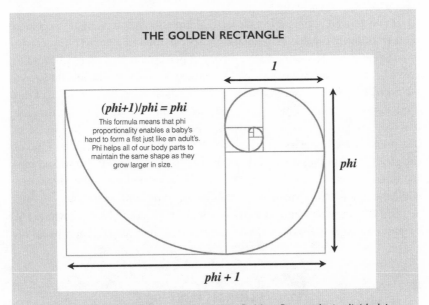

(phi+1)/phi = phi

This formula means that phi proportionality enables a baby's hand to form a fist just like an adult's. Phi helps all of our body parts to maintain the same shape as they grow larger in size.

1

phi

phi + 1

With length phi+1 and height phi, the Golden Rectangle is divided in such a way as to create a square and a smaller rectangle that retains the same proportions as the original. Because of the amazing symmetry of phi, this proportion can be repeated over and over ad infinitum. Drawing a radius equal to the length of the side of the square across each square generated a golden spiral.

As you extend the sequence out to infinity, the ratio of the last two terms converges on an irrational number, approximately 1.618033988. This is the golden ratio, used by the Greeks and Egyptians to design perfectly balanced works of structural art that mystify architects even today. The golden ratio is symbolized by the Greek letter phi: Ö (pronounced fie, rhymes with pie).

The Egyptians and Greeks worshipped phi as a fountainhead of eternal beauty, calling it the *divine ratio*. The Parthenon and other great works of ancient architecture that still stand today do so in part because they were designed around this mathematic principle of ideal proportion, and architects to this day still study them with wonder. The philosopher Socrates saw geometry, in which phi plays a central role in relating various forms, not only as a guiding constant of the natural world but also as a potential source of life itself. Leonardo DaVinci was obsessed with geometric relationships and the structure of the human form; his famous *Vitruvian Man* sketch of a man superimposed on a circle and a square illustrates his own quest for a code of nature that generates living forms.

In his pursuit of the perfect face, Dr. Marquardt discovered that the golden ratio is uniquely capable of generating a special kind of symmetry called *dynamic symmetry*. According to the theory of perception, there are two ways to create harmonic balance within an object or space. One is to divide it into equal parts, creating the symmetry of balance. Biradial symmetry is an example of this kind of symmetry. (See illustrations on pages 61 and 62). The other is a division based on the golden section, creating the perfect form of asymmetry—perfect because the ratio of the lesser part to the greater part is the same as the ratio of the greater part to the whole. (See illustration below.) This is dynamic symmetry. Interestingly, dynamic symmetry characterizes the growth of living matter, while the symmetry of balance characterizes the growth of crystals.

The literature on human beauty is full of references to biradial symmetry, suggesting that if one side perfectly mirrors the other, you've got a beautiful

BEAUTY EMERGES FROM MATH

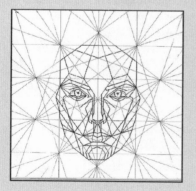

Every line of Marquardt's Mask is geometrically plotted according to the dynamic symmetry of phi. When epigenetic conditions provide for optimal growth, facial features "crystalize" in a pattern that conforms to the mask. This is the female mask. According to Marquardt, the male mask is a variation on the female.

face. But that's a misconception, and here's why: although dynamic symmetry often leads to biradial symmetry, biradial symmetry does not guarantee, or even imply, dynamic symmetry. Put another way, biradial symmetry is a necessary, though not sufficient, characteristic of an attractive human face. As Marquardt explains it: "You can draw Alfred E. Neuman with perfect biradial symmetry but he's not going to turn into Paul Newman." Living, growing beings are dynamic, and that's exactly the kind of symmetry that makes them beautiful.

Dr. Marquardt focused on phi as the essential clue. The divine ratio had to be buried somewhere in the proportions of the perfect human face.

If Hollywood were to set the action to film, they would show a montage of Dr. Marquardt at his desk holding his compass and protractor to a series of cover girls' faces, then a heap of dulled pencils in the foreground as he scratches out another formula involving square roots and algebraic variables. Until finally the moment of epiphany. Cut to Marquardt raising his cipher to the camera: a clear sheet of acetate on which his "Primary Golden Decagon Matrix" is printed in bold, black lines, the angulated mask of a perfect human face.

Marquardt's Mask is a matrix of points, lines, and angles delineating the geometric framework and borders of what Marquardt calls the archetypal face, a plotted graph of the visual ideal our collective unconscious yearns for. Nested within the matrix are forty-two secondary Golden Decagon Matrices, each the same shape as the larger matrix, but smaller by various multiples of phi. These lock on to the primary matrix by at least two vertices.[99] The mask defines the ideal three-dimensional arrangement of every facial feature, from the size of the

BLUEPRINT FOR BEAUTY

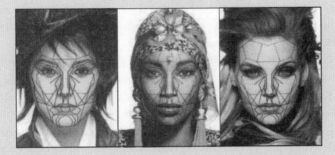

Marquardt's Mask fits neatly over beautiful facial architecture no matter what race.

PRICE MEETS MARQUARDT

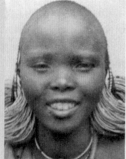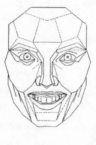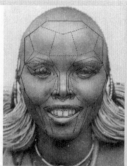

A very high percentage of Maasai and other people Price photographed displayed similar bone structure to this attractive young lady. (Looking into the sun, she is squinting a little bit.)

eyes and their distance from one another to the width of the nose, to the fullness of the upper and lower lip, and so on.

In John Cleese's BBC series *The Human Face*, featuring Marquardt and based largely on his research, the mask transparency is placed atop separate photos of Marilyn Monroe, Halle Berry, and Elizabeth Taylor.[100] Like a glass slipper sliding over Cinderella's foot, the mask fits each face perfectly, revealing the fact that, though each woman could be distinguished through skin tone and hair color, these icons of mega-stardom are all kin of consummate proportion who, by no coincidence, entered the world wearing the same archetypical mask. So much for beauty being in the eye of the beholder. Beautiful people exist not because of luck, but because all DNA is naturally driven to create dynamically symmetric geometry as it's generating tissue growth.

Marquardt's work reveals the specific facial geometry that healthy human DNA creates. His work extends the thinking of a long line of architects and mathematicians who identified phi proportions in the human body: Vitruvius in the first century B.C. (the architect who gave DaVinci the idea for his famous *Vitruvian Man*); Leon Battista Alberti and Francesco di Giorgio Martini in the fifteenth century; Luca Pacioli and Sebastiano Serlio in the sixteenth; Charles-Édouard Jeanneret-Gris, better known as Swiss architect Le Corbusier, in the twentieth. Adolf Zeising could have been speaking for all of them when he pontificated, in 1854, that within the golden ratio "is contained the fundamental principle of all formation striving to beauty and totality in the realm of nature and in the field of the pictorial arts, and that from the very beginning was the highest aim and ideal of all figurations and formal relations, whether cosmic or individualizing, organic or inorganic, acoustic or optical, which had found its most perfect realization however only in the human figure." [101]

Like the Egyptian scientists thousands of years ago who found mathematical order extended throughout their landscape and out into the stars, I believe the same mathematic principles that give order to the universe also govern the growth of every part of every living thing. When that growth proceeds optimally, beautiful and functional biologic structures are the inevitable result. This is not a new idea; it echoes the writings of ancient philosophers from Plato to Pythagoras. What we can now understand that could not have been known in ancient times, however, is precisely how the human brain so easily decides so much math, instantaneously recognizing complex geometric patterns and translating them into an emotion—desire, awe, tranquility, fear.

WHY WE LIKE BEAUTIFUL THINGS: NATURE'S GEOMETRIC LOGIC

Take a walk through a garden, in the woods, or on a beach, and you'll see all kinds of pretty things. If you look a bit closer, you'll notice patterns—curves, whorls, spirals, even repeating numbers. What's behind this? A new discipline, called biomathematics, is all about answering that question. Biomathematicians are confirming that phi and the Fibonacci Sequence are encoded not just in the human face, but in living matter everywhere.

The shape of a pinecone, the segments of insect bodies, the spiral of the nautilus shell, the bones of your fingers, and the relative sizes of your teeth—everything that grows owes its form to the geometry of phi. When a plant shoot puts out a new leaf, it does so in such a way that lower leaves are least obscured, and can still receive sunlight. This is a benefit of a phenomenon called *phyllotaxis*, which describes the spiraling growth of stems, petals, roots, and other plant organs in 90 percent of plants throughout the world.[102] The angle of phyllotaxis is 137.5 degrees, or $1/phi^2$ x 360 degrees. We can see the same pattern of branching, twisting—so-called dendritic growth—when we look at nerve cells in the brain. All these instances of patterned growth are directed not by DNA but by the rules of math and physics which act on living tissue automatically to create pattern. During the course of cellular and tissue growth there comes a point where the flow of genetic information drops away and, like a lunar module floating through space, the organism's growth is now on autopilot. As author, journalist, and TV producer Dr. Simon Singh explains:

> Physics and mathematics are capable of producing intricate patterns
> in non-organic constructions (for example, snowflakes and sand
> dunes). They can offer a range of patterns which will emerge spon-
> taneously, given the correct starting conditions. The theory which
> is currently gaining support says that life operates by using DNA to
> create the right starting conditions, and thereafter physics and maths
> do all the rest.[103]

Biomathematics offers us a fundamentally new perspective of the universe and the living world. It is allowing us to recognize that recurring patterns seen throughout our living landscape are more than just coincidences. They seem to reflect the elemental structure and order of the universe itself.[104, 105]

This organizing force, which helps sculpt a beautiful face, also functions during development of your brain. Within the jelly-like matrix inside our skulls, neurons in the human brain form bifurcating tendrils, called *dendrites* (meaning branches). We call them dendrites because the earliest scientists who peered at neurons under a microscope were reminded of stately, graceful trees. For us to think and learn, these trees must be properly proportioned. This enchanted forest is the hidden landscape where beautiful minds are born.

Why would phyllotactic patterns of growth form inside the dark vaults of our skulls? The most obvious answer is, *Because every healthy part of every living thing follows the same basic formula for growth in order to function.* Just as the golden rectangle delineates phyllotactic growth and helps plants capture more sunlight, the same dynamic symmetry may allow our brains to pack in as many nerve connections per cubic inch as possible, making best use of the limited real estate between our ears. More complex than any computer and more efficient, the network in your brain works because each brain cell is connected to thousands of others. Those connections enable you to recognize faces, flowers, food, and other familiar objects. How? With *pattern*.

Cognition is what mathematicians would call an *emergent property*. Emergence refers to the way complex systems and patterns arise out of a multiplicity of relatively simple interactions. Your thoughts and emotions are, likewise, not based on any individual brain cell's contents, but on the resonance frequencies that arise when millions of interconnected neurons are stimulated.[106, 107] Phi may help our brains work better by using its nimble mathematic flexibility to allow resonance to occur more often. When our nerves are structured so as to contain the maximum internal symmetry, not only can we sustain more complex perceptions, we can better comprehend the relationships between perceptions, memories, thoughts, and other cognitive phenomena. In other words, every specialized sub-portion of our entire brain can function as an interconnected unit, and—*poof!*—consciousness emerges.

The pleasure we derive from looking at attractive people may offer us more insight into how the brain works. If beautiful faces share the same fundamental proportionality as the connections in our brains—phi—then they may trigger a more ordered series of recognizable resonances than faces with less symmetry, which may enable us to recognize the image as a distinctly human face that much faster. The biology of our brains may be such that our brains experience pleasure on having solved the puzzle of sorting out just what it is we're looking at. Every time the brain is presented with an image or sound it is, in essence, being posed a kind of mathematic riddle. The more pleasing the image or harmonious the sound, the fewer the barriers standing between the beholder and the pleasure of the epiphany of a solution. The Fibonacci Sequence may facilitate this process, enabling us to solve these visual or acoustic riddles faster by serving as a template that helps order our minds and orchestrate our thoughts. Not only, then, does phi offer us beauty, it also seems to arrange our nerves in ways that facilitate intelligence.

Instinctive Attraction: The Myth of the Eye of the Beholder

The fact that the architecture of our neural tissue so closely mirrors that of dynamically symmetric, and therefore attractive, objects in the outer world helps to explain how our brains work. It also explains why our brains would prefer images of this same symmetry over others: their familiar geometry resonates instantaneously with our own, making beautiful objects easier to perceive. Suggesting that beauty recognition seems hardwired into our brains, Nancy Etcoff, author of *Survival of the Prettiest,* tells us that "when babies fix their stare at the same faces adults describe as highly attractive, their actions wordlessly argue against the belief that culture must teach us to recognize human beauty."[108]

Consider the complications that would arise if a cheetah sizing up a herd had to be trained to recognize the absence of health, to meticulously weigh the implications of a halting gait or an uneven coat, signs of injury and disease. Without a killer instinct, or an instinctive guide to health, predators would go hungry, social animals would put themselves in contact with disease, and good genes would be diluted with compromised DNA.

This idea, that we humans instinctively recognize the form-function relationship and use the presence or absence of dynamic symmetry to gauge health,

WHY ATTRACTIVE PEOPLE ENTRANCE US

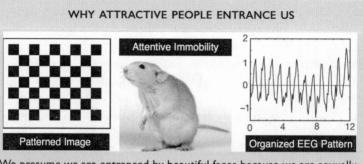

We presume we are entranced by beautiful faces because we are sexually attracted, but it may be that we are attracted to their patterns. When animal researchers show rats checkerboard patterns, the resulting brain waves demonstrate *rhythmic spikes* (upper right panel), which are said to reflect a state of "attentive immobility." While staring at the checkered image, blood flow to the pleasure center of the brain is increased, suggesting the rat enjoys looking at the pattern. Researchers believe this kind of brain activity allows for the "optimization of sensory integration within the corticothalmic neural pathways," which helps the rat "learn" the pattern.

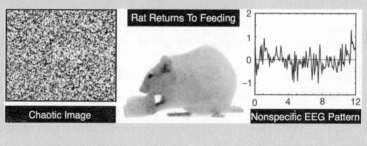

is supported by studies in which people were shown a series of male and female faces, each with varying levels of symmetry, and asked to make judgments about who was healthiest. What emerged was an undeniable positive correlation between the possession of dynamic symmetry and the perception of health.[109] So whether we're a cheetah, a baby, or a doctor, as far as our brains are concerned, dynamic symmetry—and attractiveness—*equals* health.

Of course, the ultimate purpose of this subconscious appreciation of the form–function relationship is the perpetuation of our DNA through the act of reproduction. And when it comes to the mating game, our responses to attractive members of the appropriate sex will typically percolate from their origins

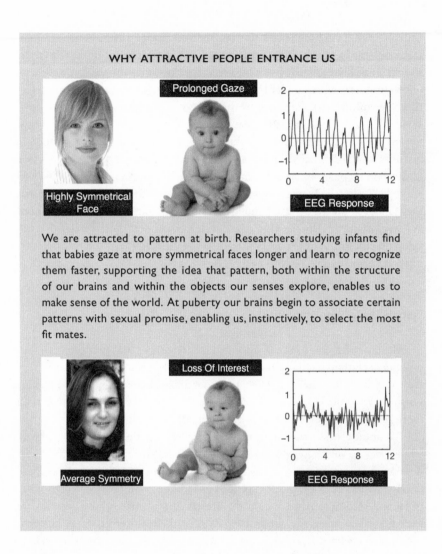

WHY ATTRACTIVE PEOPLE ENTRANCE US

We are attracted to pattern at birth. Researchers studying infants find that babies gaze at more symmetrical faces longer and learn to recognize them faster, supporting the idea that pattern, both within the structure of our brains and within the objects our senses explore, enables us to make sense of the world. At puberty our brains begin to associate certain patterns with sexual promise, enabling us, instinctively, to select the most fit mates.

deep in our psyche to reach the surface, where they can become all-consuming.

The Perfect Mate: In Search of Sexual Dimorphism

When looking for that perfect man or woman, research shows that facial features deviating from Marquardt's geometric blueprint even slightly make a surprisingly large impression—or lack of impression.[110] A set of lips that fall just a millimeter or two short of luscious fullness, or eyes just a fraction of an inch too close together, downgrade a girl from pretty to plain. Take a strong brow and chin and pull them both back a tiny bit, and you change a handsome, dominating man—the kind you might envision as CEO of a company, or captain of the ship in an adventure movie—into a docile-looking office drone. Every curve of our features is sculpted under the influence of nature's tendency toward perfection. Our minds, too, are tuned by the ratio of phi, and so we desire dynamic symmetry, and pursue it with great tenacity. The extreme attraction we have toward sex objects exists because, during puberty, our gray matter is tuned to lust after a well-defined set of sex-specific variations on Marquardt's Mask (see illustration on page 60). These variations on the theme of human attractiveness are collectively called *sexual dimorphism*. While sex-differences in our facial and skeletal development exist in childhood, they become much more pronounced at sexual maturity. The package-deal effect predicts that those bodies that develop the full gamut of sex-specific features are the healthiest, and research correlating female body type with health bears this out.

Female Body Type and Health

Beauty researchers have divided female body types into four categories. In order of declining frequency they are: banana, apple, pear, and hourglass.[111] Several studies performed in 2005 showed that apple-shaped women (with short waists and narrow hips) had almost double the mortality rates of women with more generous curves.[112, 113] Why would that be?

Voluptuousness is an indication of healthy female sexual dimorphism, while a lack of voluptuousness indicates a problem. Normally, the hips and bust develop during puberty as a result of a healthy surge in sex hormones. These developments involve expansion of the pelvic bones along with the deposition of fat and glandular tissue within the breasts. But women whose genetics are such that their spines are abnormally short or their hormonal surge less pronounced—or whose diet is such that it interferes with the body's *response* to hormones—end up with boxier figures. If they're thin, they'll end up as bananas. If they put on weight, it gets distributed in a more masculine pattern—in the belly, on the neck, and around the upper arms—and they'll become apples. Today, after three generations of trans fat consumption (which interferes with hormone expression; see Chapter 7), and with daily infusions of sugar (which interferes with hormone receptivity; see Chapter 9), hourglass figures have become something of a rarity. According to a 2005 study commissioned by Alva products, a manufacturer of designers' mannequins, less than 10 percent of women today develop the voluptuous curves universally recognized as the defining features of a healthy and attractive female figure.[114]

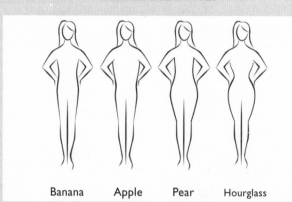

FEMALE BODY TYPES

Banana Apple Pear Hourglass

The hourglass represents normal female sexual development, while the banana develops when sex-hormone receptivity is blunted. While the apple and pear can be found among women with normal body weights, the apple most commonly develops when women with banana-shaped bodies put on weight, and the pear when women with hourglass-shaped bodies put on weight.

In a world of apples, pears, and bananas, writer Nancy Etcoff has suggested that the most beautiful among us are "genetic freaks."[115] It's not an insult: she is merely referencing the statistical improbability of someone growing up to look like, to use her example, Cindy Crawford. But the suggestion seems to capture Etcoff's general thesis accurately: when a stunningly beautiful person is born, it's largely the result of (genetic) chance. These select few, the thinking goes, played the genetic lottery and won big. But I couldn't disagree more. Why would biology program us to be hot for "genetic freaks"? It seems to me far more probable that we are attracted to beautiful bodies because they advertise superlative health. In keeping with this idea, researchers studying the effect of these four female body types on life span find that women with the most attractive of the four body types, the hourglass, not only live the longest, they also live better. Statistics consistently show that having a longer, slimmer waist and more womanly hips correlates with reduced diagnoses of infertility,[116] osteoporosis,[117] cancer,[118] cognitive problems,[119] abdominal aneurysms,[120] diabetes and its complications,[121] and more.

Why Aren't All Bodies Perfect?

So far I've shown you a good deal of evidence that beauty is not incidental, not an accident of fate. It is the default position, the inevitable product of
natural, *unimpeded* growth whose progress conforms to rules of mathematic
proportion. Just as the laws of physics dictate that six-sided crystals inevitably
result when clouds of water vapor form in freezing air, generations of optimal
nutrition prime human chromosomal material for optimal growth. If optimal
nutrition continues throughout childhood development, the laws of biology dictate the final result: a beautiful, healthy person. But if beauty emerges naturally
from well-ordered growth, then why aren't all of us beautiful?

In October 2006, at a meeting in his Huntington Beach, California, home,
I asked Dr. Marquardt his opinion. His answer was, "We are." When I said I
was surprised to hear this from a person who makes his living correcting facial anomalies, he elaborated: "If you put the mask over the population, you'll
see that many people are not that far off from a perfect fit, though we wouldn't
regard them as highly attractive." The variability we do have, he believes, stems
from the fact that "we've evolved past the point of efficiency." In other words,
societal safety nets allow people who aren't perfectly healthy or functional to
reproduce, whereas, in the past, they would simply have died off.

Marquardt's pragmatic explanation sheds some light on the origins of our
current, historically unprecedented level of attractiveness variability. If we examine human history and focus only on access to nutrients, we would find that
with civilization and sedentism (not migrating) came food shortages and disease. But sedentism was also less physically demanding than the wandering,
hunter- or herder-gatherer lifestyle, and so it acted as a kind of safety net. Living
in settled, relatively crowded cities began to chip away at our genetic programming, leading to the rise of disease while simultaneously enabling people with
damaged genes, who might otherwise have died, to survive and give birth to less
healthy children with less dynamic symmetry. Bit by bit, the genetic wealth created by thousands of years of successful survival in the wild was squandered as
poverty or plague denied genes the nutrients they needed. During each period
of nutritional deprivation valuable epigenetic programming was lost.

As time has passed, we have required more and more safety nets and invented correctives like glasses, braces, and thousands of medications. Some
would argue this physiologic fall from grace has not yet proved to be maladaptive for people living in modern industrialized societies, as we are still
successfully reproducing. But that might be changing. Like many doctors in
this country, I'm seeing more young couples frustrated by infertility. How

widespread this problem will become remains to be seen.

I'm certainly not suggesting that only supermodels should have babies. And since I have argued that the genes of all people of every race and every walk of life carry the potential of extraordinary beauty and health, the implications of this chapter run about as far from the specter of eugenics as you can get. What I am saying is that—in the same way that I tell women trying to get pregnant to stop smoking and drinking, take their folic acid, and avoid medications known to cause birth defects—there are nutritional choices you can make to help ensure that your baby will be born healthy and beautiful if that is what you desire. Of course, parents can choose to smoke and drink and ignore their doctor's advice. But I think every one of us deserves the best, latest, most complete information with which to make choices.

In the previous chapters, I've argued that the human genome's adaptability, its intelligence, is so vast that we are only now beginning to unravel its mysteries. What we do know is that its ability to create the perfect human body and maintain health is, as with any master craftsman, limited by the materials it has to work with. In this chapter we learned how powerfully anatomy shapes our destiny. In the last chapter we learned how our ancestors' focus on nutrition paid off in healthy babies and long-lived adults who were vital until the very end.

AN AVERAGE FACE

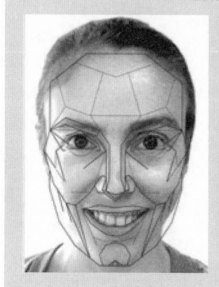

Marquardt tweaked the formula to get the mask to fit my face. If facial growth is disrupted, horizontal (X) and vertical (Y) planes grow disproportionately and perfect dynamic symmetry is lost. According to Marquardt, narrow faces are common, suggesting that when nutritional conditions are suboptimal, the coordination of growth planes is uncoupled, and the X plane shrinks. But if conditions are bad enough, the growth coordination within a plane begins to fall apart. That's why, even with the mask adjustment, my jaw is still too narrow to fit.

So what happens when we forsake those traditions?

Not surprisingly, having been fabricated without all the normal ingredients, people today are developing "old age" diseases in early or midlife as well as other health problems previous generations never even heard of. (*Harrison's Principles of Internal Medicine* from 1990 doesn't even list attention deficit disorder or fibromyalgia in the index, and I didn't hear much about either in medical school. Now, both are common.) If the genetic intelligence needs more nutrients than it's currently getting, and if Price was right, and perfect faces grow where good nutrition flows, you'd expect to see facial form progressively diverging from Dr. Marquardt's definition of the ideal. I think that's exactly what's happening. In the next chapter, you'll read evidence that not only does facial degeneration predictably develop from poor nutrition, the effects are so immediate that you can see it happening within the space of a single generation.

CHAPTER 5

Letting Your Body Create
a Perfect Baby
The Sibling Strategy

■ Mom's nutritional status before and during pregnancy influences how much facial and body symmetry her child develops.

■ In the context of modern diet, birth order correlates with two distinct symmetry shifts away from ideal.

■ Studies show that most women are nutritionally deficient during childbearing years.

■ Eating sweets and fried foods during pregnancy is likely to be as detrimental as smoking and drinking, if not moreso.

■ All evidence suggests that optimizing nutrition represents a powerful strategy for creating healthy, beautiful babies.

Almost nothing gives a woman more pride and confidence than the birth of her first child. After one successful pregnancy, there is an understandable expectation that a second pregnancy will go even more smoothly. And perhaps it will, at least for mom; more distensible pelvic tissues do facilitate an easier second labor.[122] But unless the mother gives herself ample time (generally at least three years) and nutrients for her body to fully replenish itself, child number two may not be as healthy as his older sibling. And so, while big brother goes off to football practice, or big sister gets a modeling job, the second sibling will be spending time in the offices of the local optometrists and orthodontists. It's not that they got the "unlucky" genes. The problem is that, compared to their older sibling, they grew in a relatively undernourished environment in utero.

TIMING IS EVERYTHING

Why does being born second sometimes mean a child's body is second rate? For one thing, most American women have no idea how badly they're eating. One study shows that overall, 74 percent of women "are falling short on nutrients from their diet." [123] And I think even that number is optimistic (see the statistics in Chapter 3 and more below). If most mothers-to-be aren't even taking in enough nutrients for themselves, how can we expect them to properly provide for a growing baby, not to mention one right after the other? But the biggest reason there's often such a difference between number one and number two in cases of rapid-fire conception has to do with how the placenta works.

Even minor nutritional deficiencies can hamper baby's growth. So to better protect baby, nature has provided a built-in safety mechanism, allocating as many resources to the placenta as it can get away with, even if it means putting mom's health at some risk. The baby-protection mechanism is so powerful that even on an all-McDonald's diet, a woman can expect to produce a baby with ten fingers and ten toes. Dr. John Durnin, of Glasgow University, describes the mechanism vividly: "The fetus is well protected against maternal malnutrition—that indeed it behaves like a parasite oblivious to the health of its host." [124] If mom's diet is deficient in calcium, it will be robbed from her bones. If deficient in brain-building fats—as horrible as this sounds—the fats that make up the mother's own brain will be sought out and extracted. [125] Pregnancy drains a woman's body of a wide variety of vitamins, minerals, and other raw materials, and breastfeeding demands more still. As you might expect, the demands of producing a baby draw down maternal stores of a spectrum of nutrients, including iron, folate, calcium, potassium, vitamin D, vitamin A and carotenoids, magnesium, iodine, omega-3, phosphorus, zinc, DHA and other essential fatty acids, B12 and selenium. [126] To the placenta, mom's central nervous system, for instance, is simply a warehouse full of the kinds of fat needed to build baby's central nervous system. Studies show that maternal brains can actually shrink, primarily in the hippocampal and temporal lobe areas, which control short-term memory and emotion. [127] These brain regions are not responsible for basic functioning, like breathing or blood-pressure regulation, and so are relatively expendable. This marvelous nutrient-scavenging ability of a human placenta means that even in conditions of insufficient maternal nutrition the first child may come out relatively intact. Meanwhile, mom's body may be depleted to the point that before and after pictures reveal her spine to have curved, her lips thinned, and she may have trouble remembering and learning new things, or feel anxious and depressed—as in postpartum depression.

NUMBER ONE SON—WHY SO LUCKY?

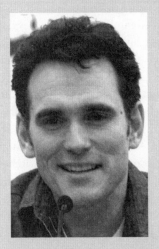 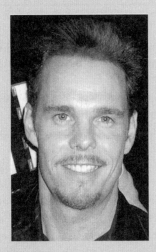

On the left is Matt Dillon, who has been starring in movies since his teens. On the right, the incredibly talented Kevin Dillon, eighteen months his junior. Both men were forty-three when photographed. Why does Kevin look older, and why has he rarely been cast as a romatic lead? The answer: The Sibling Symmetry Shift.

It may sound harsh, but it's just the "selfish" gene at work. Successful genes behave like greedy pirates, commandeering maternal nutrient stores for the benefit of their own optimal replication. However, any child conceived in too short a time for those storehouses to be refilled will be at significant disadvantage. In such depleted conditions, were baby to extract from mother all the nutrients its genes would like it to have, this would put mom's life at significant risk. Following the utilitarian calculus of genetic survival, biology pragmatically chooses not to kill the mother while a baby is gestating and opts, instead, for a compromise. This second baby will be constructed as well as possible in the depleted conditions in order that mom may pull through. Tragically, this exposes the child to a variety of health problems, which can become increasingly noticeable, and even debilitating, as they grow older.

Here's something else to consider. Sugar and vegetable oils act like chemical static that blocks the signals our bodies need to run our metabolisms smoothly.[128] Most women's diets today are high in sugar and vegetable oils, adding to the growth disturbances already caused by missing nutrients. Not only does sugar and vegetable oil consumption disrupt maternal metabolism and lead to gestational diabetes, pre-eclampsia, and other complications of pregnancy, the sugar and vegetable oils streaming through a developing baby's blood block signals in the womb, disrupting the sequence of highly sensitive, interdependent developmental events that contribute to the miracle of a healthy birth.[129, 130]

The consequences of not getting enough nutrients and the introduction of toxins are primarily brought to bear through changes in the infant's epigenome. As we saw in Chapter 2, the epigenome consists of the set of molecules that attach themselves to DNA and other nuclear materials that control when a given gene is turned on or off. These genetic switches inform every aspect of our physiologic function. Diseases previously assumed to be due to permanent mutation—from cancer, to diabetes, to asthma, and even obesity—most often actually result from mistimed genetic expression. And since the proper timing of gene expression requires specific nutrients in specific concentrations, if a second sibling gestates in a lessor nutritional environment than the first, their epigenetic expression will be suboptimal, and growth and development will be impaired. We know, for example, that low birth weight, often due to mom's smoking or high blood pressure (both associated with poor nutrition), puts children at risk for low bone mass and relative obesity for the rest of their lives.[131] Abnormal epigenetic responses due to nutrient deficiency may explain why children of subsequent births are at higher risk for disease, from cancer[132] to diabetes[133] to low IQ and birth defects.[134]

Our skeletal development depends on normal genetic expression, too. Because normal facial growth demands large quantities of vitamins and minerals, and short inter-pregnancy intervals make it unlikely that mom's body would have been given adequate time to replenish all the vitamins and minerals the first baby used up,[135, 136] children born in close succession might reasonably be expected to look different. Previous studies have shown that births less than eighteen months apart increase child mortality and, in some cases, stunt growth.[137, 138] One group of authors' speculation that "a shorter period between births may reduce the ability of the mother to replenish her reserves adequately for this purpose"[139] supports the idea that mom's nutritional health plays an under-appreciated role in baby's ultimate health. But I could find no studies addressing the potentially life-changing influences of birth order on facial development. So I designed one myself.

How Birth Order Affects Our Looks

I began by looking to the stars—TV and movie stars, that is. A glitterati's face is loaded with instances of that special kind of symmetry discussed in the last chapter, called dynamic symmetry, which we recognize by instinct. The actor with "screen appeal," the actress with "that certain something," the up-and-coming journalist groomed for the anchor seat because of her "fresh" face, the photogenic author with the winsome smile—what we're really talking about here is geometry. Our brains are exquisitely sensitive pattern detectors, capable of assessing the architecture of a human face with NASA-like precision. And as NASA was reminded with Hubble, a hair's breadth can make all the difference. Deviations of just a millimeter from the ideal create features that fail to align perfectly with Marquardt's Mask, and we can take all this information in instantaneously. We prefer to fix our gaze on faces with broad foreheads balanced by strong jaws, prominent brows above deep-set eyes framed with nice, high cheekbones—those are the characteristics that tend to bend the angles of the human face toward a more perfect proportionality. As you might have guessed, models and movie stars from Greta Garbo to Angelina Jolie have a habit of hoarding more than their share of dynamic symmetry. And often they are the first born of their family.

In contrast, their younger siblings' faces are often noticeably less symmetrical. Most are characterized by a narrowing of the mid-portion of the face, rounded, indistinct features including noses, cheekbones, and brows, and a weakening of the chin and jaw. Are A-list movie stars always the oldest child in the family? Certainly not, since we're talking about nutrition and nutrition is something that many women can, and often do, take conscious action to improve. But proper nutritional refortification requires time, and I believe this is why those who had older siblings typically had three or more years spaced between them. (Every rule has its exception and Tom Cruise is a notable example.)

Of course, superstar looks are rare (in the modernized world), and the chance for any family to produce even one child of stellar beauty is small. The statistical improbability of one stunner following on the heels of another would predict, with rare exception, any consecutive child to be less attractive than the first regardless of how effectively mom can replenish her nutritional warehouse with baby-building supplies. This would explain a fair, though miserly, rationing of young stars and starlets throughout the general population, but it would fail to account for the fact that the most attractive, most successful siblings are most often the oldest or, in families of three or more, one of the first two. It seemed to me that better nutrition was the simplest, most likely explanation for first-born children with favorable looks, and that a relative short supply of nutrients for

DIFFERENT GEOMETRY

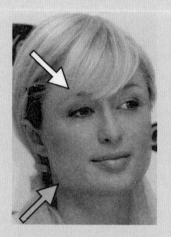 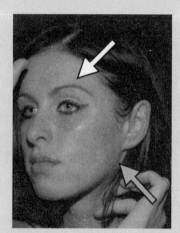

Paris Hilton (*left*, born 1982) and Nicky Hilton (*right*, born 1983). Both girls are lovely, however one's fame far outshines the other's. Arrows shown indicate two of the features that differentiate these attractive women. Gray arrows indicate the corner of the mandible (lower jawbone) called the gonion. Paris has a nearly 90-degree angle within the bone structure of her mandible, while Nicky's is more oblique and her gonion is located much closer to her ear, indicating a smaller, relatively underdeveloped jawbone. White arrows indicate the inflection point of the eyebrow. Paris's eyebrow is angulated, while Nicky's eyebrow is simply curved, indicating less angular orbital bones. Subtle nutritional deficiencies create subtle growth imperfections of the underlying bone. You can find similar tendencies of facial narrowing and midface underdevelopment (termed *retrusion*) in younger siblings of many celebrity families including Beyoncé and Solange Knowles, Penelope and Monica Cruz, Kourtney, Kim, and Khloe Kardashian, Zooey and Emily Deschanel, Vanessa and Stella Hudgens, Nicole and Antonia Kidman.

subsequent siblings was potentially impairing their growth. But before exploring that further, I first wanted to see if the second sibling phenomenon could be found not just among the supermodels of society but also among the rest of us in the general population.

So I expanded my research. With the generous help of office mates, patients who supplied stacks of high school yearbooks from 1969 to 2006, and graduate students from the University of Hawaii, I compiled nearly four hundred groups of siblings, over a thousand faces, cutting and pasting their senior photos (to control for age), organizing them in family groups—some large, some small. To be included in the study, families needed to have at least two siblings born within two years of each other. Just as with the celebrity siblings, among those pictured in the yearbooks, family beauty generally faded according to the same pattern. From oldest to youngest, the jaw grew narrower and receded, the cheekbones flattened out, and the eyes were less deeply set. The closer in age the siblings, the more striking the changes. Unfortunately, birth spacing alone does not prevent this effect. With anything short of an optimal dietary context, if mom's body is asked to produce large numbers of children, then each subsequent baby uses up more of her reserves so that, even with three to four years between births, her body continues to lose nutritional ground. This can magnify the effects of developmental inequalities down the line.

What all these subtle—and sometimes not-so-subtle—rearrangements of the facial features amount to is a loss of dynamic symmetry which, for reasons that have as much to do with health and function as they do with looks, is unlikely to be associated with improvement in quality of life. This may make it seem as though first-born babies have all the advantages. But when we're talking about a baby growing inside mom on a less-than-ideal diet, going first to get a better shot at being more dynamically symmetrical can actually come at a price.

THE SIBLING SYMMETRY SHIFT

In the last chapter, I discussed two distinct kinds of symmetry, biradial (left to right) and dynamic (based on phi proportions).

My examination of the high-school seniors' faces uncovered two unexpected patterns. First, though the first-born exhibited dynamic symmetry, they had less biradial symmetry, which is to say the right half of the face was not a perfect mirror image of the left. Second, the second-born siblings seemed to exhibit the effects of heightened hormonal receptivity.

The first-born might have one eye bigger than the other, or a slightly rotated jaw that ever so subtly torques their smile. One half of the face might be slightly larger than the other. After this discovery I started checking my patients with Temporomandibular Joint Pain (TMJ, or jaw joint pain) for this asymmetry and found it, most often in those with the most long-standing symptoms. At least in my small sample size of several dozen, these patients were usually the first-born children.

As it turns out, the medical literature is peppered with reports of biradial asymmetries occurring more often in first-born children: leg length discrepancy,[140] congenital hip dysplasia,[141] scoliosis,[142] plagiocephaly (flattening on one side of the skull),[143] facial asymmetry including flattening of one cheek with prominence of the other,[144] and left-right asymmetries of the jaw.[145, 146] The authors of such articles generally suggest a link between these disruptions in biradial symmetry and "uterine crowding"—a simple lack of adequate space.[147]

As I see it, we are witnessing two distinct patterns of symmetry disruption, one occurring in first-born children attributable to insufficient uterine expansion, and the other occurring in subsequent children attributable to inadequate nutrition. The problem of inadequate space correlates with a loss of biradial (left-right) symmetry, while the problem of inadequate nutrition correlates with a loss of dynamic symmetry (parts losing their ideal relative proportion).

We've already discussed a potential explanation for relative nutritional deficits in later-born children being simple resource depletion and an inadequate period of time to allow the replenishing of mom's nutritional reservoir. What could be the cause of inadequate uterine growth? This, I believe, has to do with hormones.

The more extreme version of a lack of uterine space is called *intra-uterine growth retardation*, and refers to a fetus that has failed to achieve its genetically determined growth potential. It affects between 5 and 10 percent of pregnancies, most commonly in smokers.[148] Affected newborns suffer lung problems, potentially serious bleeding, and a host of other life-threatening issues. Long-term consequences include cerebral palsy, developmental delay, and behavioral dysfunction.[149] Researchers are recognizing the role of chemical interference from oxidation in disrupting the normal responsiveness of the uterus to hormones like estrogen, progesterone, and more.[150, 151] As we'll see in later chapters, two foods that most powerfully promote oxidative stress are vegetable oils and sugar. In other words, too much vegetable oil and sugar in mom's diet create chemical interference, delaying signal transmission between mom's body and her own uterus. This type of symmetry shift is most pronounced in the first pregnancy due to the fact that, by the second pregnancy, the uterus has been prepped by the first, which is why the second delivery typically goes faster.

It's important to keep in mind that very few of us are perfectly biradially symmetrical, and that minor differences in leg length, for example, should not be considered a matter of great concern. It is only when the asymmetry is pronounced that it is likely to lead to significant musculoskeletal issues down the road.

There is however one situation in which the human body is pushed to such extremes, and the loads that are communicated through the kinetic chain gen-

BIRADIAL SYMMETRY CAN BE A PAIN
IN THE NECK

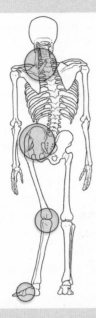

If your skeleton lacks biradial symmetry, your left and right halves are not equal. This is the skeleton of a person with left leg longer than right. Compensations cause abnormal stresses and can predispose a person to developing chronic overuse injuries.

Thoracic and cervical spine: compensatory curve tilts the left shoulder blade and to keep the arm in a position of function the rhomboid minor and levator scapular muscles are chronically activated, predisposing to upper back and neck pain as well as muscle tension headaches.

Lumbar spine: slight curve increases risk of disc herniations and spinal stenosis.

Pelvis: tilted and rotated (left innominate bone anterior) increases risk of sacroiliac joint pain and gluteus maximus muscle strain.

Knee: knock kneed, increases risk of medial joint capsule and ligament strain.

Foot: dropped arch, increases risk of plantar fascitis.

Asymmetry leads to compensation throughout the skeleton. When the skeleton is just standing there, you can imagine the forces of gravity causing pain. Now imagine the skeleton doing something really athletic. You don't have to a be a world-class trainer to imagine this degree of symmetry could cause a person pain. The kinds of discrepancies people like Tim DiFrancesco are looking for are of course far more subtle—partly because if they weren't, the athlete would not likely have made it to elite sports.

erate such powerful forces that, over time, even relatively nominal asymmetries can potentially pose a problem. Here, I'm talking about serious athletes, both professional and amateur. Because these subtle asymmetries can leave an athlete susceptible to repetitive motion injuries or changes in gait and movement, athletic trainer Timothy DiFrancesco of the L.A. Lakers includes symmetry analysis when sizing up a potential recruit: "Performance specialists in the NBA and elsewhere are always looking for the most valid and reliable ways to assess musculoskeletal asymmetry levels. This helps give critical insight into injury susceptibility and an athlete's ability to withstand the rigors of the sport."

I'd like to introduce one additional twist on the Sibling Symmetry Shift. I discovered that some second-born females have fuller lips and more sexually appropriate chins and eyebrows than their older siblings—a woman's chin being a little more pointed and less squared than a man's, and a woman's eyebrows being more arched while a man's are lower and straighter. The pointier female chin and gracefully curved eyebrows are examples of *sexual dimorphism*, the differential development between males and females (introduced in Chapter 4). Human males, in addition to strong, squared chins, tend to have broad shoulders, while women, along with more petite and rounded chins, have slender shoulders, narrow rib cages, wider hips, and fatty breast tissue. So what would explain these second-born girls with the more attractive, sex-specific features?

A woman's body undergoes a miraculous change soon after conception. Under the influence of a new physiologic directive, the functioning of every organ is altered by waves of hormones, all generated by the tiny collection of rapidly dividing cells. Many of these changes are permanent. Of course, no organ is affected more obviously than the uterus. But a modern diet interferes with hormonal signaling, as we'll see later, so the uterus, in particular, can't perform quite so well, at least not at first. Blunted uterine (and placental) estrogen signals could explain why estrogen's effects on a *first* baby girl often appear diminished. A subdued response to estrogen can lead to relatively masculine features: slightly too prominent brow and chin, aggressive-looking eyebrows, and lips not quite filled out. She may be handsome, but she won't turn heads. With mom's uterine infrastructure already built out by the *second* pregnancy, the same level of estrogen produces a more potent response. Incidentally, if the second sibling were a boy, the burst of estrogen receptivity might still create a feminizing effect, sharpening the center of the chin, arching the eyebrows, rounding the forehead, and plumping the lips.

So what does this mean? For one thing, although the development of a beautiful, healthy baby is—as we are so fond of saying—miraculous, it is not a mystery. This spectacular orchestration of events is as dependent upon a strict total adherence to a program of good nutrition as it is vulnerable to its breach. Studying siblings enables us to see *why* we aren't all perfect, and allows us to witness how nutrient deficits change a child's growth in ways that are both predictable and easy to measure.

I call it the Sibling Symmetry Shift because the subtle effects of maternal malnutrition on a child's growth are most readily discernable in the faces of children born in a short time period after an older sibling who, presumably, shares similar genes and thus serves as a kind of control. But as I just described, *no child, not even an only child, is immune from symmetry shifts because the underlying problem is not birth order; it's malnutrition.* While a first baby grows in mother's womb, static interference from dietary sugar and vegetable oils too often disrupts hormonal communication between placenta, uterus, and ovaries, delaying uterine development and reducing physical space for the baby while tending to blunt the child's potential for sexual dimorphism. In a woman's subsequent children, the cellular circuits necessary to coordinate the various baby-making stations (uterus, placenta, etc.) have already been optimized, enabling faster uterine responses (such as quicker growth and speedier deliveries), which permits greater biradial symmetry, and primes the baby's potential for sexual differentiation. But in the context of a modern diet, the cost of going second (particularly with close birth intervals) is often relative maternal nutrient deficiencies that result in relatively less material to build bone, nerve, and so on, thinning and flattening facial features to create a worn-down look.

In Chapter 3, we saw that the vast majority of Americans—and I mean just about everyone—aren't merely malnourished, but severely malnourished. Which should make you wonder: *Doesn't that mean we're* all *suffering from some degree of symmetry shifts?* Most of us are, which is why there seems to be so few genetic lottery winners walking around. And what explains them? How did they, raised by parents who, presumably, followed the same advice my parents did, and ate the same steady diet of frozen, canned, and vitamin-poor fruits and vegetables, mystery meat from poisoned animals, grains grown on mineral-depleted soils, margarine, and everything else that makes our modern diet unhealthy, curry Mother Nature's favor? *They* didn't. Their great-great-grandparents did, by eating such nutrient-rich diets that they imparted the family epigenome with *genetic momentum*, the ability of genes to perform well with suboptimal nutrient inputs for a finite amount of time. And their placentas did, by sending an especially urgent message to mother's bones, brain, skin, muscles, glands, and organs, to release every available raw material for the benefit of the baby. In these one-in-a-million cases, the fetal genome operating in mom's belly can do what it's been doing for a hundred thousand years: create the miracle of a perfectly symmetrical *Homo sapien* baby.

I should be clear that my investigation into the relationships between symmetry shifts and birth order and timing barely scratches the surface. I certainly don't mean to suggest, by introducing my observations, that we can find this pattern in every family without exception. Rather, I'm describing a tendency that I think bears consideration. Nor do I mean to suggest that parents are to blame when congenital malformations affect their children. My hope is that this kind of information will help us do away with the idea that baby-making is simply too formidable or mysterious a task to try to optimize and that we might as well just throw our hands in the air and attribute life-changing symmetry shifts to factors entirely beyond our control.

I believe that we can offer moms solid information to more effectively incentivize their adherence to a healthy diet. What moms need, what they want, is a strategy. A strategy that can help ensure that when their bodies are called upon to engage in the serious project of creating a healthy baby they are nutritionally prepared to allow all those interacting growth-directing systems to join in a coordinated effort. And the proliferation of mommy chat rooms and advice-sharing platforms proves that millions of mothers-to-be are already well aware of the profound impact of nutrition and hungry for the best advice. Given the increase in birth defects, autism, child asthma, child depression, child cancer, and so on that I've observed in the decades since my graduation, years ago I began to suspect that the current strategy—the one recommended by the experts moms most often listen to—has proven to be an epic failure. Nevertheless, I'd sorely underestimated the barriers to disseminating better, more effective child-health–fortifying information by way of the medical establishment.

HOW CONVENTIONAL MEDICINE
LETS MOTHERS DOWN

Doctors get their information from researchers. Researchers can only do research when they can get grant funding. These days, grants come from industry or special interest groups, and tend to support *either* the use of expensive medications and technology *or* a demand for more medical coverage for one of many special interest groups. Few physicians are naive to these realities. But I hadn't fully appreciated the extent to which research must fall into one of these two categories to be funded until I met with researchers at UCLA and UCSF to discuss the possibility that there might be an obvious, though currently overlooked, relationship between modern food and disease.

The trip was a real eye-opener. These researchers held fast to the idea that their primary directive was improving human health. But it soon became clear that their more immediate goal, by virtue of the realities of economics, was the acquisition of grant funds, necessitating a never-ending sequence of compromises between the exigencies of financing and the integrity of the science. I learned from an epidemiologist that various agricultural interests funded most of his research in nutrition, and out of financial necessity, he was directed toward the promotion of the largest crops: fruits.[152] As an epidemiologist, he was unaware that excess fruit consumption leads to health problems due to the high sugar-to-nutrient ratio in fruit. And he was surprised when a colleague pointed out that she'd found, after advising her patients to eat the recommended three to six servings of fruit a day, that doing so raised their triglycerides to unhealthy levels.[153] Hoping to drive home the point that our bodies demand more nutrition than we can get from fruits, vegetables, grains, and low-fat meat, and hoping to stir up interest in doing more research on nutrition and optimal fetal and facial development, I described the results of a pertinent study. It showed that one in three pregnant women consuming what mainstream research suggests would be a healthy diet nevertheless gave birth to babies with dangerously low levels of vitamin A in their blood.[154] Vitamin A deficiency is associated with eye, skeleton, and organ defects. The epidemiologist was fascinated but admitted that his reliance on funding from fruit growers bound him to continue producing more and more research just like he'd already produced—showing that fruits are "good for us." I learned that neither he nor anyone else at UCLA would likely be able to pursue this new nutritional issue or anything similar because there was no giant industry to support it.

Ironically, another researcher at UCLA was examining the so-called *Hispanic paradox*, a term referring to the mysterious finding that recent immigrants from Latin American countries (with a more intimate connection to the products of a traditional diet) have healthier babies than their Caucasian counterparts. Might the mystery be explained by the fact that our Mexican, South American, and other Latin-nation friends are still benefiting from their healthier, homeland diet? The physician I spoke to said that while my argument was plausible, he had not considered the possibility. However, he considered it unlikely that superior Hispanic nutrition was the reason for superior Hispanic maternal-child health. His idea was that Hispanics enjoy a greater network of social supports (in spite of the fact that many have immigrated to this country from thousands of miles away, which fractures families). And he felt that somehow social supports translated into fewer premature births and birth defects. In his publications, he points out that networks of social support are reinforced by community medical clinics. Where did his money come from? State-funded grants for medical clinics serving Hispanic immigrants. I left UCLA impressed by the spirit of optimism but demoralized by the misdirection of its pursuits and the sheer volume of intellectual and financial capital expended on generating the logical contortions necessary to earn funding from various state and industrial entities.

Hoping to find greener pastures elsewhere, I traveled north to speak to a perinatology expert at UCSF. There, I was thrilled to meet with an M.D./Ph.D. with a special interest in prenatal health. We discussed the pattern of facial changes I saw in younger siblings and their implications for improving maternal nutrition. Once again, I was taken aback. The well-respected researcher agreed that there was a relationship between nutrient depletion and skeletal development, but she was unconvinced that the *pattern* of skeletal changes could be due to anything other than chance. In her view, which reflected the general attitude I found at UCSF, it was unlikely that children born in the United States, let alone in the relatively affluent Bay Area, could be exposed to any significant levels of deficiency. Why not? "Because," she explained, "pretty much every pregnant woman is given a prenatal vitamin."

And that's true. Obstetricians and primary care doctors like me routinely write prescriptions for prenatal vitamins to help reduce a woman's risk of pre-eclampsia (an immune system disease causing mother's body to partially reject the baby and give birth prematurely) and to decrease the child's risk of low birth weight and neural tube defects like spina bifida. However, a large study completed in the United States showed that pregnant women using their prenatal pills still develop "combination deficits" of niacin, thiamin, and vitamins A, B6, and B12 that persist throughout each of the three trimesters.[155] Other studies show that prenatal vitamin pills don't solve many nutritional problems. The following are just a few examples:

- **Vitamin D Deficiency:** In studies in which over 90 percent of participants took prenatal vitamins, 56 percent of white babies and 46 percent of black babies were vitamin D insufficient. Insufficiency in early life increases the risk of schizophrenia, diabetes, and skeletal disease.[156]

- **Long Chain Essential Fatty Acids:** As of the date of this writing, there is no recommendation about how much of these to consume, and most people who don't supplement get almost none. But supplementing with cod liver oil during pregnancy has protective and lasting effects on the baby's intelligence.[157]

- **Choline:** Gestational deficiency of choline is associated with lifelong learning deficits.[158] One survey showed 86 percent of college-age women were lacking adequate dietary choline.[159] Choline is not part of any prenatal vitamin supplement commonly marketed in the United States.

While the prenatal pill partially addresses the issue of nutrient deficiency, it does nothing to address the overconsumption of sugar and vegetable oil, both of which interfere with signal transmission required for normal growth and development.

The sad truth is that many, if not most, of the best minds in the research business are satisfied with the status quo. There appears to be very little sense of urgency in the prevention of unnecessary suffering from physiologic default

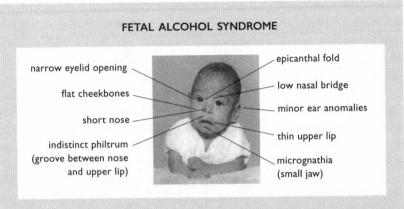

FETAL ALCOHOL SYNDROME

narrow eyelid opening

flat cheekbones

short nose

indistinct philtrum
(groove between nose
and upper lip)

epicanthal fold

low nasal bridge

minor ear anomalies

thin upper lip

micrognathia
(small jaw)

This picture shows the characteristics of FAS. As with The Second Sibling Symmetry Shift, we find tall, narrow skulls, minor ear anomalies, small jaws, thinned lips, and flattened cheekbones. Alcohol's toxic effects occur largely due to cellular membrane damage. Sugar and toxic fats also damage cell membranes (see chapters 8 and 9). Either mechanism would be expected to block signal transmission and thus impair growth.

or disease, and little humility brought to the reality that, in the battle against common childhood and adult diseases, medical research has by any objective account failed miserably. We are told to accept the idea that facial deformities—even relatively minor changes like those I study—occur randomly, all products of the whimsical nature of the "genetic lottery." There was a time when the facial deformities now known to be associated with Fetal Alcohol Syndrome (FAS) were written off as unpreventable.[160] Doctors went on telling their pregnant patients to drink to settle their nerves. And there was a time when the spinal cord and brain malformations we now prescribe prenatal pills to prevent were believed to occur by chance. That changed in 1991, when *The Lancet* published an article entitled, "Prevention of Neural Tube Defects."[161] Provided with un-ambiguous evidence that folic acid deficiency played a role and that better nu-trition could prevent problems like spina bifida, physicians ultimately adopted measures of prevention. We are all served by science's affinity for explanations to natural phenomena. Without it, we are guided only by magical thinking and su-perstition. The witches of Salem weren't possessed; they were poisoned.[162] Hur-ricanes aren't retribution for sinful behavior; they are explicable meteorological phenomena. Likewise, physiologic deficiencies occur for a reason and most can be easily prevented.

I'm sorry to say that such professional complacency is increasingly common in medicine. Although we tell pregnant patients to quit smoking and drinking and to take their prenatal pills, and we screen for certain diseases, the list of childhood epidemics keeps stacking up. That's a tragedy. But for the most part, we physicians simply go about our business assuming someone else will some-day do something about it.

This apathy toward prenatal care has affected the way the general public thinks, as well. I brought up the prenatal pill earlier, so let's look at that as one example. A woman recently came to see me already seven weeks pregnant with her third baby in less than three years. Most women have no idea that the prenatal vitamin pill works best when taken *before* conception because it helps to boost a woman's vitamin levels to prepare for the first ten weeks of pregnancy, the time when the most fundamental decisions about how to shape the baby's body are made. After that window of opportunity has shut, though it can still improve birth weight, the vitamin pill can do little to prevent most major birth defects.[163] This mother's third child will be at high risk not just for disfiguring facial changes but also for skeletal and organ defects which will likely turn him or her into another chronic disease statistic before graduating high school. Still, this is likely the first time you've heard this bit of information about prenatal vitamins, which tells us something about the dissemination of critical child development information in our country. (It might help if we called it a "pre-conception" pill.)

The young mother-to-be certainly had heard nothing of it, but it's not her fault. Our society does not encourage strategizing to optimize a child's health. The medical community is missing the opportunity to prepare mothers' bodies with solid nutrition, giving their babies' genes the materials they need to compose their physiologic masterpiece. Of course, that would involve more than taking a pill. It would require improving the nutrient content of mothers' food.

Synthetic vitamin pills are, of course, a step up from no nutrition at all, but they are a sorry replacement for real food. First, they're not the same as what nature makes. Many vitamins exist in nature as entire families of related molecules, only a few of which can be recreated in a factory. For example, there may be over 100 isomers of vitamin E, but only about 16 are put into tablets.[164] Second, the processing of synthetic vitamins necessarily involves the creation of incidental molecular byproducts, the effects of which are largely unknown. About half of the content of vitamin E tablets are isomers that don't exist in nature, which might explain why some studies show that taking synthetic vitamin E pills increases mortality. Third, without the proper carrier nutrients in the right balance, many vitamins are not absorbed. Fourth, many vitamins work synergistically with other nutrients in ways we don't fully understand. Fifth, who knows what else is in that pill? The entire supplement industry is essentially unregulated, and supplements have been found to be contaminated with toxic compounds including lead or dangerously high levels of copper.[165] But again, there is some benefit to taking certain supplements, especially in pregnancy, because the food supply is so bereft of nutrients when compared with foods from only seventy years ago.[166, 167, 168]

A real danger of the prenatal pill is its psychological effect, how it implies to mothers that the nutrition issue has been addressed and safely removed from their "to do" list. This prenatal vitamin pill, part of "advanced" prenatal care, is widely believed—by health professionals and patients alike—to make up for the fact that today's modern diet is so wantonly lacking. The general idea is that, whatever our mom-on-the-go can't provide to her baby through whatever she's eating, the prenatal vitamin pill can, thus implicitly giving her permission to continue with the standard diet and expose her body to foods that could not be better engineered to deprive a growing child. In my practice, I give all pregnant women who see me a prescription for a prenatal multivitamin, but I make sure they know that it's no magic bullet. If they want to have a healthy, beautiful baby, they have to learn how to eat (see Part Three: Living the Deep Nutrition Way).

Studies like those cited here, showing how poorly nourished we actually are, have presumably been conducted so that perinatologists and other specialists can familiarize themselves with, and begin to address, childhood disease and physiologic deficiencies that result from malnutrition. However, taking action based on what a given study recommends would require personal initiative on the part of individual healthcare providers. But as corporate culture goes, so goes medical culture. We live in the age of consensus and groupthink, where otherwise curious and capable professionals avoid being singled out by huddling in the center of the herd. The herd, in turn, waits for an authority figure to lead the way. So if there is no authority figure acknowledging the importance of a given article's findings, nothing happens. It's as though it were never written.

Long before any of today's ivory towers had been built, and long before a diploma was proof of wisdom, people were making their own observations and drawing conclusions, acting on those conclusions, and passing that wisdom down to their children. Much of that accumulated knowledge pertained either directly or indirectly to the production of healthy babies, yet only a few scattered snippets still remain. These whispers from the past help explain how people used to avoid issues of Sibling Symmetry Shifts and the resulting health problems. And they can still help anyone hoping to become a parent, providing a framework for taking action to better ensure good fertility, a smooth pregnancy, and a healthy, beautiful child.

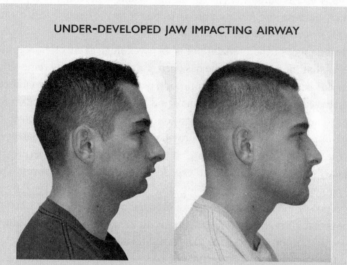

UNDER-DEVELOPED JAW IMPACTING AIRWAY

If I were to tell you that these two young men were twins and that, throughout their school years, one was relentlessly bullied while the other was his protector, which of the two would you peg as the victim and which as his defender? Studies show that the overwhelming majority of us make the very same kinds of character assessments based on facial structure that you probably made just now. In reality, these are before and after photos of one man who underwent surgery to restore his underdeveloped maxila and mandible to more optimal geometry. I include them here because renowned behavioral scientists, most notably Elaine Hatfield and Susan Sprecher, have shown how a lifetime of receiving such judgments begins with one's parents and continues to influence face-to-face interactions every day of our lives. Though subtle, the cumulative effects shape our self-image and ambitions in ways that either impair or facilitate professional accomplishments. Parents who take diet seriously should take pride in their efforts to provide their children with the best chance of success in our highly competitive world.

THE TRADITIONAL STRATEGY
FOR A HEALTHY PREGNANCY

A group of social workers studying access to healthcare in Africa in the 1970s were surprised to discover resistance to the building of more hospitals and clinics from—of all people—local village grandmothers. It's not that these women didn't care about health or feared new technology. They felt that the influx of Western ideas had already caused harm to their children and grandchildren. The new order smacked of an insidious form of imperialism. So when these independently minded African women were politely asked to relinquish their roles as protectors of the community genome, they bridled at the idea. As one member of the Batetela tribe in the Upper Congo River region explained it:

> Today we don't make any decisions about spacing the births of our children. . . . Our ancestors had stronger children because they were not born too close together. Today parents no longer worry about their children getting sick. They think that they can always buy medicine and then the child will get well. This is why couples no longer separate their beds after the birth of a child, as they used to do in the time of our ancestors.[169]

When social workers examined how these traditions eroded, they uncovered an explanation not entirely irrelevant to us: Westerners, including mine owners, state officials, missionaries, and doctors working with these groups, judged the traditional practice of spacing childbirth to be at odds with their long-term goals of expansion and did not support its continuation.[170] "Intimate Colonialism: The Imperial Production of Reproduction in Uganda, 1907–1925" suggests rather provocatively that when companies need workers, they care more about sheer numbers than the quality of workers' lives or their longevity.[171] Such concerns become irrelevant given a large enough pool of potential workers to draw from. And so the systematic spacing of children that was once an "important feature of the control of excellence of child life"[172] is tossed aside as an anachronism, a fractured artifact of female empowerment. But it is not just a women's issue, and it extends beyond the political. We all gain from children's good health, which requires giving mom's body at least three—preferably four—years to refortify her tissues with a generous supply of nutrients.

Nearly a century ago, Mahatma Ghandi preached self-sufficiency as a prerequisite of self-government, reminding his countrymen that "to forget how to dig the earth and to tend the soil is to forget ourselves."[173] Franklin Delano Roosevelt later echoed this principle, saying, "A nation that destroys its soil destroys itself."[174] Two of the most important resources we have are the land that provides

us with food and the farmers who work it on our behalf. If the idea of refortify-
ing a mother's body between births and doing the same with soil between crop
cycles strikes you as related concepts, you're right. Just as we are all custodians
of the genome, traditional farmers are the frontline custodians of the land, going
to great lengths to replenish the ground between crops and to replace all the
minerals required for healthy growth of the plants—even to the point of layering recycled outhouse waste over the ground to recapture nutrients that would
otherwise become depleted. The modern technique is to replace only a few of
the many nutrients crops draw from the ground each year. As a result, our food
supply is of much lower quality now than it was before industrial farming, which
in turn makes fortifying mom's body a tougher task.

While the fact that we still produce bumper crops year after year makes
for good press, in reality the nutrient content of American-grown plants and
animals is far worse than it was during the dustbowls of the 1930s. Farmers call
this the *dilution effect*—more pounds of produce from the same soil means less
nutrition per pound of produce produced. One report showed that packs of sliced
green beans have only 11 percent of the vitamin C claimed on the package.[175]
Another report comparing mineral levels of twenty-seven fruits and vegetables
from 1930 and 1980 found modern produce to be depleted by an average of 20
percent, with calcium dropping 46 percent, magnesium 23 percent, iron 27 percent, and zinc 59 percent.[176] Meat and dairy, which ultimately depend on healthy
soil, have declined commensurately in quality between 1930 and 2002, with iron
content in meat falling an average of 47 percent, 60 percent in milk, and lesser
declines in calcium, copper, and magnesium.[177, 178] When plants and animals are
reared on mineral-deficient soil, not only are they missing nutrients, they're not
as healthy. And their cells are, in turn, less able to manufacture the vitamins and
other nutrients that would benefit us. If we could somehow view these grocery
staples as they now exist nutritionally, they would look like ghostly afterimages
of their former selves, semi-transparent shapes of apples, cucumbers, the various cuts of beef. Of course, in real life it all looks relatively fresh and appetizing.
It had better: most are grown and engineered with eye appeal in mind. These
pretty displays hide the fact that it is more difficult to purchase nutritionally rich
foods today than any time in recent history.

Without healthy soil to nourish them, plants are unable to use the energy
from the sun to manufacture optimal levels of vitamins. Without vitamin- and
mineral-rich plants for animals to eat, they can't add the next layer of chemical/
nutritional complexity *we have evolved to depend on*. We are here today because
our ancestors taught their children how to garden, hunt, and prepare their food
so that they could one day raise healthy children of their own. Their hard work
and due diligence in building and maintaining a healthy environment to support a healthy human genome can, however, only take us so far. We are coasting

along on the nutritional momentum left over from millennia of enacted nutritional and environmental wisdom. If our food is composed of far fewer nutrients than it was four generations ago, it's a fair bet that our physiologies—our connective and nervous tissues, our immune systems, etc.—have taken a hit. What about our genes? Might they be affected as well? What might be the expected effect of generations of nutritional neglect on our own children?

That depends, in large part, on the choices each of us makes. But there is little doubt that physicians like me are going to be very, very busy.

THE OMEGA GENERATION

When I was living and working in Hawaii, four generations sometimes came in to my clinic for an office visit all at once, giving me a front-row view of the impact of modern food. Quite often, this is what I saw: great-grandma, born on her family's farm and well into her eighties, still had clear vision and her own set of teeth. Her weathered skin sat atop features that looked as though they were chiseled from granite. More often than not, she was the healthiest of the bunch and had a thin medical chart to prove it. The youngest child, on the other hand, often presented symptoms of the whole set of modern diseases: attention deficit, asthma, skin disorders, and recurrent ear infections. Like many of today's generation, one or more of his organs wasn't put together quite right. Maybe there was a hole in his heart, or maybe he needed surgery to reposition the muscles around an eye. While the exact effects may be hard to predict, what is predictable, given the dwindling dietary nutrients and proliferation of toxic materials, is some kind of physiologic decline.

Within a given family, the earlier the abandonment of traditional foods for a diet of convenience, the more easily perceptible the decline. I'm thinking of one little boy in particular, the great-grandchild of one of Hawaii's many wealthy missionary families who developed an ear infection during his visit to Kauai from another island. This little boy bore none of his great-grandmother's striking facial geometry. His jaw was narrow, his nose blunted and thin, his eyes set too close, and his cheekbones were withdrawn behind plateaus of body fat. The lack of supporting bone under his eyes made his skin sag into bags, giving him a weary look. His ears were twisted, tilted, and protruded, and his ear canals were abnormally curved, predisposing him to recurring external ear infections.

Narrow face, thin bones, flattened features—sound familiar? This is a dynamic symmetry shift. The nature and degree was something I'd expect to see if he were child number three or four of siblings born in quick succession. But the young man sitting on my exam table was only the couple's second child, and though mom had given herself a full four years between the two, it hadn't

THE REASON MEN SHOULD TAKE PREPARATION FOR PREGNANCY AS SERIOUSLY AS WOMEN

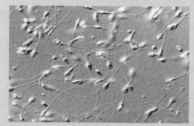 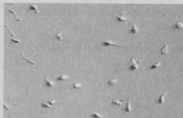

Healthy, high motility *(left)* versus less healthy, low motility sperm *(right)*. Think of the project of making a healthy baby as a competition—because it is. This is a snapshot of what that competition looks like moments after the starting pistol goes off. Already, a survival of the fittest contest has been set in motion, and one winner from each of these two contests will be selected for advancement. Once they enter the world the two finalists will be pitted against all other surviving finalists in the lifelong battle for resources and opportunity.

protected his health. He was the fourth-generation product of a century of nutritional neglect and the consequential epigenetic damage. The last century has derailed our entire culture from the traditions that sustained us, so he is far from alone in enduring visible epigenetic damage. And the consequences impact more than a child's skeletal system; his entire genome is at risk. I believe this is why, according to a landmark 2003 Center for Disease Control (CDC) report, this child, like all others born in 2000, had a one-in-three chance of developing diabetes, a condition that reduces life expectancy by between ten and twenty years.[179] What is going unreported is the fact that it isn't just diabetes on the warpath. Every year, growing battalions of familiar diseases are cutting a wider and wider swath of destruction through the normal experiences of childhood.[180]

Whereas in previous centuries part of a parent's responsibility was to work hard to prevent their children from getting sick, today so many of us are sick ourselves that we've grown to accept disease as one of life's inevitables—even for our children. Today's kids aren't healthy. But rather than make such a sweeping and terrifying declaration, we avert our eyes from the growing mound of evidence, fill the next set of prescriptions, and expand our definition of normal childhood health to encompass all manner of medical intervention. This latest generation of children has accumulated the epigenetic damage of at least the three previous generations due to lack of adequate nutrition along with the overconsumption of sugar and new artificial fats found in vegetable oils. The family

SIX WAYS NUTRITION CAN OPTIMIZE
YOUR CHILD'S GROWTH

1. **Height.** Pour more milk. A meta analysis concluded that for each additional 100 milliliters of milk (roughly 3.3 ounces) consumed daily, children grew an extra 0.2 centimeters (roughly 1/8 inch) per year.[181] Children in the study were aged two to twenty and the study duration ranged from a few months to two years. The study's authors noted that the growth effect was especially powerful in teens. It is not known if higher and sustained milk supplementation would have additive effects. But if avid milk drinker and NBA player Jeremy Lin is any example, at six-foot-three with five-foot-six parents, then perhaps it may.

2. **Vision.** Look for lots of variety. In a study of children between ages seven and ten, children who developed nearsightedness compared to children who did not consumed significantly less of a wide variety of nutrients: protein, fat, cholesterol, vitamin B1, vitamin B2, vitamin C, phosphorus, and iron.[182] Of note, although the myopic children ate roughly 300 fewer calories, there was no difference between the two groups in several anatomic metrics: height, weight, or head circumference. This suggests that while normal height, weight, and head circumference are indications of sufficient nutritional intake they are not definitive indicators of optimal nutrition. It also suggests that the children with normal vision may have been more physically active.

3. **Cognitive development.** Skip starchy snacks. Nutrients shown to correlate most strongly with high IQ include vitamin E, omega-3, and iodine. Studies have shown that the higher a child's vitamin E, the better their language and social skills.[183] Similarly, the higher a newborn's omega-3 (as measured in maternal umbilical cord blood) the higher that child's IQ later in childhood.[184] Additionally, cognition has been shown to be impaired by a "snacky pattern" of eating high-carb foods "characterized by foods that require minimum preparation such as potatoes and other starchy roots, salty snacks, sugar, preserves, and confectionery."[185] Presumably this effect is mediated through reduced nutrition-to-calorie ratio.

4. **Life span.** Beget big babies. Larger children, born to non-diabetic moms, have greater muscle mass, a higher resistance to diabetes and obesity, and longer telomeres (the part of the DNA that determines how many more divisions a cell can undergo, thus influencing cellular lifespan)—all known to be associated with longer life expectancy.[186, 187]

How to grow a big baby without developing gestational diabetes? Aside from being tall and well fed during your own childhood, we don't know much about specific interventions to produce bigger babies. But we do know something about how to avoid having a too-small baby: don't smoke, don't conceive while you're undernourished or underweight, and don't restrict protein (i.e. if you're vegan, you may need to supplement).

5. Immune system. Maximize microbes and micronutrients. Researchers at UC Davis found that individuals with subtle deficiencies of various micronutrients are more prone to develop a variety of common day-to-day infections and are more likely to have more severe infections with prolonged convalescence.[188] Allergies, asthma, and auto-immune illnesses are more prevalent in children with reduced microbial gut flora diversity. Experts recommend breast feeding to optimize early gut flora development and are considering recommending soil-based probiotics.[189, 190] Including fermented foods in a child's diet and encouraging outdoor play would be my preferred methods of introducing immune-boosting probiotics.

6. Puberty. Avoid insulin resistance. Junk food consumption and being overweight are both associated with insulin resistance. Insulin resistance impacts boys and girls in different ways. For girls, it causes precocious puberty, so common today that we find breast development, typical of eleven-year-olds a generation ago, often occurring in seven-year-olds and, rarely, in three-year-olds.[191] Aside from its detrimental psychological effects, precocious puberty typically reduces the child's adult height. In boys, insulin resistance reduces testosterone levels. Low testosterone during puberty is associated with decreased development of muscle mass, impaired growth of the penis and testicles, reduced deepening of the voice, development of breast tissue, and lack of normal male hair growth.[192]

genome has been getting battered relentlessly for almost a century—even during key, delicate periods of replication. The physiologic result of these accumulated genetic insults? Distorted cartilage, bone, brain, and other organ growth. Many physicians have noted an apparent increase in young couples complaining of problems with fertility which, given the implications of epigenetic science, should come as no surprise. Children born today, I'm afraid, may be so genomically compromised that, for many, reproduction will not be possible even with the benefit of high-tech medical prodding. This is why I call these children the Omega generation, referring to the last letter in the Greek alphabet.

Born by cesarean section (often necessitated by maternal pelvic bone abnormalities), briefly breast-fed (if at all), weaned on foods with extended shelf lives—the human equivalent of pet foods—these Omega generation children see the doctor often and, whether first-born or not, will likely suffer from both biradial and dynamic symmetry shifts. In the same way we talk about bracing for the aging baby boomers' medical needs, we had better reinforce the levees of our medical system for the next rising tide: medicine-dependent youth. These children will age faster, suffer emotional problems, and develop never-before-seen diseases. In my experience as a doctor, parents have an intuitive sense that their children are already dealing with more health problems than they ever did, and they worry about their future, for good reason. But no parent is helpless. If you have children, or are planning to, I can think of at least one child who can do something to avoid all this illness and start getting healthy—yours.

RESTORING YOUR FAMILY'S GENETIC WEALTH

If having an Omega generation baby sounds terrifying, you can do something about it. You can get off the sugar and vegetable oils that would block your child's genetic potential. That means cutting out processed food, fast food, junk food, and soda. And you should give yourself at least three, preferably four, years between pregnancies and make every effort to fortify your body with vitamin-rich foods (or if you can't, at least use prenatal vitamins) *before* conception. Those who want to do everything possible to have a healthy baby will find additional instruction throughout this book. But this discussion opens up a new question: *If I do everything right, how beautiful and healthy can I expect my child to be?*

My first answer to that question is that, of course, *all* children are beautiful. But if you're asking if your child will have *extraordinary* health, excel scholastically and in sports, and be so physically striking as to elicit the envy of peers, then the answer is, *It depends.* It depends on how much *genetic wealth* you gave him. Which, in turn, depends on what you inherited from your parents.

Genetics is all about information. Your genetic wealth is a function of how much of the information in your genes has been damaged or remains intact, and how well the supportive epigenetic machinery is able to express the surviving data contained in your genetic code. To gauge the present condition of your genetic data, you can begin by asking your parents and grandparents what they ate when they were little. Find out if you were breastfed. Were they? Learn whatever you can about who was born when (including birth spacing). Dig up as many family pictures as you can find to look for the telltale signs of Second Sibling

Syndrome. The more you know about your family history, and the more objectively you measure your health and appearance along with that of your partner,
the more clues you will have to assess your genetic, and epigenetic, health.

Let's give it a try. Let's attempt to gauge a person's genetic momentum using
Claudia Schiffer as our case subject. Though both her parents were tall and reasonably attractive, you wouldn't guess they could produce the superstar beauty
they did. Their genetic equation was complicated by the fact that her father and
mother were born during the Depression and raised under the conditions of
post-war food shortages. Claudia's secret weapon of genetic wealth may be that
her great-great-grandmother grew up in the most wholesome and remote of
farming communities in Austria, a town near Elbigenalp, which changed very
little in the thousands of years before Claudia's grandmother's birth.[193]

This close relation to someone living in a successful, stable, indigenous society is truly a rare gift. Adding to this, Claudia's father's family was affluent,
meaning that (during their formative years) he and his parents presumably had

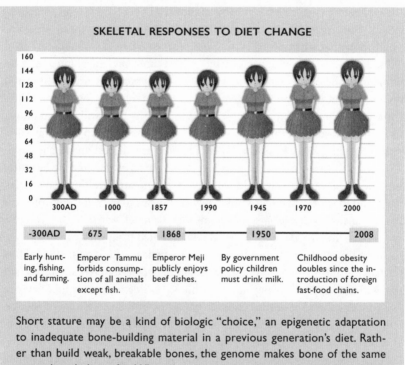

SKELETAL RESPONSES TO DIET CHANGE

300AD	1000	1857	1990	1945	1970	2000

-300AD —	675	1868	1950	2008

Early hunt-ing, fishing, and farming.	Emperor Tammu forbids consump-tion of all animals except fish.	Emperor Meji publicly enjoys beef dishes.	By government policy children must drink milk.	Childhood obesity doubles since the in-troduction of foreign fast-food chains.

Short stature may be a kind of biologic "choice," an epigenetic adaptation
to inadequate bone-building material in a previous generation's diet. Rather than build weak, breakable bones, the genome makes bone of the same
strength, only less of it. When the nutrient supply increases, the genes respond again, taking advantage of the extra material to build a bigger frame.

access to the best foods of the early twentieth century. Put the two together, and keep the good food coming, and—*voilà*—a genome operating under moderate duress for a spell is effectively rehabilitated.

Let's look at a broader example of genetic rehabilitation, this time dealing with height. Height is one of the most desirable proportions for a man. Aside from the obvious social and mating advantages, the professional advantages gained with every additional inch of height are well documented. Studies show that tall men take home higher salaries, obtain leadership positions more often, and have more sex.[194]

Hawaiian archeological evidence shows that for hundreds of years a man's stature helped to secure him a better official position in the class hierarchy. Our language—"big shoes to fill," "big man on campus," "someone you can look up to"—reflects society's universal preference for the tall. The positive perception of the taller among us often extends to women, as well. I am not suggesting that taller people are better, only that height affords certain physical and social advantages. With that in mind, can relatively diminutive parents who want those advantages for their children have a baby who might someday walk tall and rise above the fray to stand head and shoulders above the rest?

Absolutely! This potential is encoded in our genetic memory. We've all heard that we used to be a lot shorter, how few of us could fit into one of those little suits of armor worn by medieval knights. But around the world, accumulating evidence suggests that thousands of years prior, our Paleolithic predecessors were at least as tall, if not taller, than most of us are today.[195] Even in the early Middle Ages, 1,000 years ago, European men were nearly as tall as they are now. What caused the temporary skeletal shrinkage? As the population grew, crowding reduced access to nutrients until stature reached an all-time low in the early 1700s.[196] Improvements in agricultural technology, most notably the series of inventions attributed to lawyer-turned-farmer Jethro Tull, revolutionized the process of tilling soil, vastly increasing productivity.[197] By the late 1700s, having recovered some of its former nutritional inputs, the European genome rebounded—and with it the average European's height. But it would probably have dipped again, so that a tall man today might measure just over five feet, were it not for the early twentieth-century invention of refrigeration. The ability to freeze food meant that fishermen could travel as far as they needed and fill their hulls to brimming. Refrigeration also meant that even during winter, wealthy countries could reach down to the tropics for summer fruits and vegetables, making it profitable for millions of acres of rain forests around the globe to be converted over to crop production. For the past 100 years, industrialized nations have had consistent access to enough nutrition to achieve our Paleolithically pre-programmed height. Of course, height doesn't equal health. But generally speaking, when a genome has access to a *surplus* of complex nutrition, it is far better positioned—and may be said to have a built-in preference—for the production of offspring with more robust, larger frames.

The Sibling Strategy

So what is the strategy I recommend? As we've seen, optimizing a child's growth involves optimizing nutrition in order to best assure the development of biradial and dynamic symmetry, as well as prime the child's body for normal hormone responses in utero.

To optimize nutrition, we need to start eating the Human Diet, as outlined in Chapter 13. To facilitate normal in-utero hormone responses, we need to avoid the dietary substances that can interfere with hormone function, namely toxins. Later, we'll learn more about how sugar and vegetable oils, the two most common toxins in the modern diet, prevent you from being as healthy and beautiful as you deserve to be, and how avoiding them can improve your own and your children's health both immediately and in the long run.

Ideally, you will give yourself at least three months prior to conception to detox and refortify your system but I would recommend six to twelve months if you are prediabetic or overweight because both these conditions can involve profound metabolic and hormonal dysfunction and imbalance. If you are worried about your biologic clock, consider that by improving your nutrition you will not only facilitate faster conception when the time comes, you will also improve pituitary function, essentially reversing time in your baby-making systems.

Avoiding toxins seems like a pretty sound idea. But how, exactly, to do that? It gets confusing because a product can call itself healthy when there's not enough nourishment in it to keep a rat alive. I'm not kidding. According to industry insider Paul Stitt, author of *Fighting the Food Giants*, a popular cereal company did a study in the 1940s that showed its puffed rice product killed rats faster than a starvation diet of water and minerals.[198] Similar puffed and processed whole grain products are still sitting on store shelves today, sold under every major brand label. In fact, even store-bought granola, loaded with unhealthy oils and sugar, makes for an unhealthy way to start your day. Much better alternatives can be found in the fresh food departments, as we'll see. To understand the depth to which our food supply is saturated with products that keep us barely alive, I'll take us back in time to understand where and when things started to go wrong with the way we think about food.

PART TWO

The Dangers of the Modern Diet

CHAPTER 6

The Great Nutrition Migration
From the Culinary Garden of Eden to Outer Space

■ Talking about what constitutes nutritious food as if we're chemists has turned our focus on chemicals and away from what really matters: ingredient source and cooking tradition.

■ Most foods in the grocery are not much different from pet foods.

■ To avoid getting lost in conflicting nutritional paradigms, think like a chef.

■ According to skeletal records, access to greater quantities of animal products historically produces bigger, tougher bodies.

■ Access to nature is the real source of genetic wealth.

> But if thought corrupts language, language can
> also corrupt thought.   —*George Orwell*

In 1987, my friend Eduardo, an antiquities conservator for the Getty Museum in Los Angeles, was called to Laetoli in Northern Tanzania to restore fossilized footprints left by a wandering family of hominids some 3.5 million years ago. Befriended by local tribesmen, Eduardo soon found himself immersed in a world both unimaginably vibrant and deeply spiritual. By day, Eduardo used hypodermic needles to inject poison into tiny plant shoots that threatened to break apart the footprints left by our *Australopithecus afarensis* ancestors. By night, he shared food—on one memorable occasion, the still-beating heart of a goat—with Tanzanian herder-gatherers, known as Maasai, whose culinary rituals had remained largely unchanged for thousands of years.

Hearing Eduardo describe his time with the Maasai, I was reminded of the kind of awe with which Weston Price described the cultures he visited and the people he studied. Eduardo was most impressed by the tribal chief, who, while rumored to have been over seventy years old, was still an impressive physical specimen, standing over six-foot-five, completely free of wrinkles, and still able to keep the peace among his several wives. It seems that few people who journey to visit the Maasai have returned home without feeling profoundly changed. Jen Bagget, a travel writer, describes her visit to Tanzania as if she'd discovered Shangri-La. "With distinctively tall and willowy frames and striking facial features, the Maasai are easily the most beautiful people we've seen in the world. We were instantly captured by their friendly dispositions, open manner, and natural elegance." [199]

The Maasai represent one of the rare surviving intact and functional indigenous cultures. These societies are, in essence, windows into our past. Reading accounts of travelers who've spent time among people like the Maasai, one could get the impression that—as far as human health is concerned—*once upon a time* really existed. In the good old days, people enjoyed an almost idyllic physiologic prosperity. This prosperity was earned, in large part, by the maintenance of an intimate relationship between the people and the land, their animals, and the edible plants that rounded out their diets. As a result of this intimacy, they talked about food differently than we do. To us food is primarily a fuel, a source of energy, and sometimes a source of guilty pleasure. To people who remain connected to their culinary origins, food is so much more. It is part of their religion and identity. And its value is reinforced with story.

> In the beginning, Ngai [the Maasai word for God, which also means
> *sky*] was one with the earth. But one day the earth and sky separated,
> so that Ngai was no longer among men. His cattle, though, needed the
> material sustenance of grass from the earth, so to prevent them dying
> Ngai sent down the cattle to the Maasai. . . . No Maasai was willing to
> break the ground, even to bury the dead within it, for soil was sacred
> on account of its producing grass which fed the cattle which belonged
> to God. [200]

In a few sentences, this story articulates the cattle's central position in Maasai life and the necessary injunction against harming the land. As startled as Eduardo was when invited to take his share of a still-beating goat heart, he might have been more unnerved had they started talking about the total number of calories in their meal, the percentage of their daily intake of protein, carbs, and fat, and the benefits of eating fiber. Such reductionist terminology would have been out of step with the way the Maasai see the world. If they did start talking that way, as a physician, I'd be concerned. Because, no matter where you live, talking about—and then envisioning—food in such arbitrary categories is bad for your health.

Of course, here in the United States, we talk about food that way all the time. These days, very few of us participate in any deeply rooted culinary traditions, let alone share mythical stories connecting the food we eat to the environment it came from. Like everything else, "foodspeak" has to meet the requirements of a sound bite culture and is limited to grunting imperatives such as "eat your veggies," "watch your carbs," and "avoid saturated fat." Having lost the old ways of talking about food, we've also lost the physiologic prosperity that once endowed us with the gift of perfectly proportionate growth. George Orwell warned that the acceptance of newspeak is no small matter; it can ultimately convince us to trade liberty for totalitarianism.[201] So what have we lost by accepting the reductionists' foodspeak?

DRIVEN FROM THE GARDEN:
A RECORD IN THE BONES

Along the western coast of South America, the powerful Humboldt current sweeps north from near the South Pole until its frigid water is blocked by a coastline of sandy plains descending from the high peaks of Peru's Cordillera Mountains. The resulting upswelling current helps to produce several months a year of rain-rich clouds and, in terms of sustaining sea life, is one of the richest currents in the sea. This food-producing confluence of geographic and oceanographic elements helped give rise to the great civilizations of Peru, whose ancient cities are thought to have supported up to a million people.

In the mid-1930s, Weston Price, interested in the effects of nutrition on jaw structure, was drawn to the area by mummies—some fifteen million of which had been buried in mounds and preserved by the succession of seasonal rains on the dry sand. Grave robbers had previously unearthed many of them, so upon his arrival it appeared as though the objects of his intended study had come to greet him. "As far as the eye could see the white bleaching bones, particularly the skulls, dotted the landscape."[202] Price was interested in those skulls because, at that time in America, 25 to 75 percent of the population had some deformity of the dental bones or arches, and he suspected that rate of malformation was an historic anomaly.[203] His visit proved to be illuminating. In a study of 1,276 ancient bones, he "did not find a single skull with a significant deformity of the dental arches."[204] What's most striking about Price's visit to Peru is that when he left the desert mummies to study modern city dwellers, he found the people's structural symmetry and balanced growth patterns had melted away, replaced by what he described as "a sad wreckage in physique and often character."[205]

The Peruvians had changed. Using anthropologic methodology (studying skull structure), Price showed that when a farming population adapts a city lifestyle, this shift can affect bone structure. But how? What was the root of the problem?

Price's discovery was not entirely new. Physical anthropologists have long recognized the diversity of human cranial development, and the anthropologic literature is full of discoveries that link skeletal modifications to dietary changes. For example, when Native Americans migrated down the coast from Alaska to California and the consumption of animal products dropped, the average women's bone size shrank by 9 percent and the men's 13 percent within just a few generations. Meanwhile, brain size dropped 5 and 10 percent respectively.[206] Elsewhere, in South Africa, two distinct episodes of skeletal shrinkage occurred, one 4,000 years ago, the other 2,000. The first coincided with population pressures and the second with the use of pottery, indicating an increased dependence on farming. In the intervening years, absent of farming artifacts, the skeletal size (including the skull and brain space) appears to have recovered.[207] And in the southernmost Andes Mountains, precisely where plants were first domesticated in South America, the fossil record again reveals "farmers hav[ing] a smaller craniofacial size than hunter-gatherers."[208]

Not only is it a consistent finding in the anthropologic record that modifications in diet coincide with modifications in human growth, but there seems to be a general downward trend in size. That is, as groups of modern humans move from hunter-gatherer to agricultural-based lifestyles, their bodies shrink. Why would that be? Bioanthropologists, who consider nutrition in their studies, suggest that "our hunter-gatherer forbearers may have enjoyed such variety of viands [foods] that they fared better nutritionally than any of their descendants who settled down to invent agriculture."[209]

The development of farming has long been thought to represent one of humanity's greatest achievements, the cardinal technologic leap that would set us on course to living easier and healthier lives with every passing century. But this assumption has been challenged lately by both skeletal and living anthropologic evidence. It appears that the hunter-gatherer and herder-gatherer (like the Maasai), who lived in greatest harmony with natural cycles, may have enjoyed an easier lifestyle than all but a few of the wealthiest families today. In fact, Marshal Sahlins, an anthropologist at the University of Chicago, calls hunter-gatherer-style communities (of old) the "original affluent society."[210] In his treatise on hunter-gatherer life, he paints an Arcadian image:

> A woman gathers in one day enough food to feed her family for three days, and spends the rest of her time resting in camp, doing embroidery, visiting other camps, or entertaining visitors from other camps. For each day at

home, kitchen routines, such as cooking, nut cracking, collecting firewood, and fetching water, occupy one to three hours of her time. This rhythm of steady work and steady leisure is maintained throughout the year.[211]

Embroidery? Entertaining visitors? Visiting your neighbors and trading gossip over tea? Though it might sound like something out of *Martha Stewart Living*, this is a fieldworker's description of an average day in the early twentieth-century life of the Hadza, a nomadic band of hunter-gatherers who have lived in the Central Rift Valley of East Africa for perhaps 100,000 years. Many other accounts corroborate the fact that the ecology in certain locations once provided more than enough bounty for the hunter-gatherer to simply sit back and enjoy, at least on the average day.

Hunting and gathering requires a lot of moving around, wandering from place to place chasing seasonal abundance. Farming, on the other hand, enabled us to stay put. Along the banks of the world's mightiest rivers, on some of the world's most fertile soils, societies grew larger and more stratified, developed more tools and technology, and embarked upon ambitious engineering projects like the pyramids. But there was a tradeoff. All the while, agriculturalists struggled to provide the level of nutrition to which their hunter-gatherer genes had grown accustomed. Over generations, this drop-off in nutrition would impair growth so that stature would diminish relative to that of their hunter-gatherer counterparts. You could say that, for the sake of developing agrarian civilizations, these societies chose to swap some of their vitality, toughness, and robusticity for aqueducts, large buildings, and other public works. Of course, if any group of people were to break away from city life and return to nomadic hunting or herding and gathering, they would (as with the migrating Native American tribes mentioned above) reclaim the physique they'd given up; their bodies would grow larger, and their skulls tougher and more robust.

This ability to adjust stature to better match a given nutritional context lends more support to the idea of an intelligent, responsive genome (as the operating mechanism) than to the suggestion that physiologic change depends solely on random mutation. If evolutionary change were dependent on random mutation, then it would be exceedingly unlikely that responses to nutritional change would be so consistent and quick to appear. If, however, an intelligent genome had recorded in its epigenomic library which physiologic adjustments were most appropriate in any given nutritional context, then the epigenomic librarian (see Chapter 2) could simply read the instructions on what to do next. And this is why we see that "throughout the course of human evolution, features of robusticity like supraorbital and occipital tori [boney ridges] have been acquired, lost, or changed in different groups."[212]

If you want to be poetic about it, you could say that the shifting and morphing skeletal and facial features represent the genomic artist at work. Each set of subtle skull feature modifications that have distinguished all the equally beautiful nationalities of human beings is a painted portrait, each one created using different nutritional pigments in varying proportion and displayed on the canvas of world geography. In this way, the intelligence in our genes has generated numerous variations on the theme of human attractiveness. The striking cheekbone, the slender waist and graceful legs, the delicate female chin, and the powerful brow of a dominant male face—all these universally desired features are tweaked a tiny bit to generate the continuum of anatomical variation that is *Homo sapiens*.

But if you look at these anatomical variations the way Dr. Marquardt does and focus on the basic blueprint of our skeletal plan rather than the embellishments, you'll see that in reality very little has changed over time. Though our statures and the prominence of individual facial features may vary, thanks to the genetically programmed growth preference for phi-proportionality, everything fits neatly together. Every part has maintained its functional relationship to every other part. Everything works. This is true of people living everywhere around the world. Or rather it *was* true. Very recently, something changed.

Which brings us back to Price, and those perfect skulls he found scattered on the Peruvian sand. On Price's visit, he recognized that a precipitous drop in proportionality of Peruvian skulls had taken place in contemporary history. There was a key difference in the dentition of ancient and modern Peruvians (and up to 75 percent of the American population) that indicated a process entirely distinct from the nuanced skeletal variations present throughout evolutionary time. That difference: a loss of proportion. Why is that so significant? As we've seen in the preceding chapters, health and beauty are all about proportion. *Dis*proportionality impairs the body's ability to function.

In Chapter 4, we saw that a perfect face—and the bones beneath it—is one that has grown in accordance with a mathematic formula called phi, which defines healthy growth in numerous species of plant and animal life. Dr. Marquardt, the plastic surgeon who discovered how phi-based growth occurs in the human species and created a mask to illustrate it, has shown us that balanced growth occurs in three dimensions, the X, Y, and Z facial planes. When that balanced phi-proportionality is lost, the resulting growth distortions lead to problems. In my own face, the loss of phi-proportionality in the horizontal (or X) dimension narrowed my skull so that my wisdom teeth didn't fit into my head and had to be pulled, and my disproportionately sized eye sockets distorted the shape of my eyeball, forcing my lens to focus light to a point in front of (rather than on) my retinas, blurring my vision. A face that is more severely narrowed than mine may pinch the airway, causing sinus problems. When skull narrowing affects the Z-plane (visible in profile), it may foreshorten the palate, increasing the likelihood of sleep apnea, a condition in which a person's own soft tissues collapse inward and periodically suffocate them, causing fatigue, memory problems, and heart disease.

Phi seems to be the universal template nature uses to ensure that optimal proportionality drives development, even under conditions of varying nutritional inputs. Over the past century or two, however, the typical human diet has diverged so far from anything before that our growth patterns can no longer adhere to the template. The switch from hunting and gathering to farming was accompanied by nutritional sacrifice, yes. But it did not block the ability of the phi-template to continue generating perfect proportionality. Why not? As I've suggested, modern historians have vastly under-appreciated the value of traditional nutritional knowledge. I believe it was this wisdom that enabled people who'd made the shift from hunter-gatherer life to settled life to continue to make (mostly) sound decisions about what kinds of foods they needed to feed their children and expectant parents in order to ensure optimal health. Though history's most celebrated inventions—like trigonometry, plumbing, and the plow—helped give rise to the visible artifacts of civilization, none of this could have been possible had we been severely undernourished. The extraction of adequate nutrition from grains, as on the Scottish Isles, for instance, required advanced biologic technology of soil fortification, fermentation, and other strategies. These vastly undervalued strategies enabled growing populations to maintain nutrition adequate for healthy growth even after leaving the relative bounty of their hunter-gatherer pasts behind. And they did this using the Four Pillars of World Cuisine.

The skeletal record evidences the success of traditional dietary regimes around the world—which universally include all four of the Pillars. If we were to create a visual timeline of the entire human story from nearly 500,000 years ago until today by lining up human skulls on one long table, we would find that, as *Homo sapiens* progressed, migrating across continents and oceans—some finding tiny, isolated islands to call home—all the while changing size and varying features, some skulls, like Paleolithic *Homo sapiens*, would be heavy and robust and others, like recently discovered *Homo floresiensis*, diminutive. But with every skull in our lineup, we'd see teeth well aligned and free of caries,[213] square jaws, and phi-proportionate construction in the X, Y, and Z facial planes.[214] This math is what gives rise to deep and wide eye sockets, powerful male brow ridges and delicate female chins, broadly arched zygoma (cheekbones), and all the other features anthropologists use to define a skull as belonging to a former *Homo sapiens*. These features would be clearly visible in every skull on our table. Until, that is, we walk to the end of the table where the lineup is still being built. In the skulls from the past 100 years or so, we'd see an abrupt change.[215]

Human skulls have recorded within their features every switch from hunter-gatherer to farming lifestyles and every migration from place to place. But our healthy and proportionate bodies had been maintained and protected as if under the aegis of a kind of nutritional Garden of Eden. So what happened to those skulls at the rightmost end of the aforementioned human-timeline table, the ones with the disfigured dentition and disrupted proportion? An examining anthropologist might conclude that we'd left the Garden for good, completely abandoning the diets that had protected us throughout history, and made a pilgrimage to the nutritional equivalent of a barren and inhospitable country. But what no anthropologist could discover by sorting through the bones is *why?* What nutritional sin had we committed?

The answer to that riddle can be found in the pages of a cookbook written over 100 years ago. You see, in order for a burgeoning food industry to convince people to make this journey—this exodus from nature—and to give up traditions with thousands of years of success, it needed to change the way people talk about food.

YOU SAY POTATO . . .

Have you ever heard someone say, "I've been trying to cut out carbs"? Or a TV chef say, "Now, all this dish needs is a protein"? Carbs? A protein? These are biochemical terms. When did we start talking about our foods like chemists? The answer is, not coincidentally, right around the time of the Industrial Revolution.

The Fanny Farmer 1896 Cook Book introduced this new food terminology to a large audience: "Food is classified as follows: Organic or Inorganic," with organic being composed of the following: "1. Proteid (nitrogenous or albuminous); 2. Carbohydrates (sugar and starch); 3. Fats and oils."[216] This new, simplified breakdown of food immediately began influencing our approach to food and diet, and not in a good way. What was once understood holistically—rabbit, potatoes, or hand-pressed oil of *known* origin—would now be seen as so much protein, carbohydrate, and fat. Don't get me wrong. Francis Farmer's cookbook is considered a classic, and deservedly so. But the classification of complex organic systems based only on their more readily isolatable chemical components makes about as much sense as describing the Taj Mahal as so many tons of rock. In terms of isolatable components, a bottle of Romanee-Conti isn't all that different from box wine, but the winemakers of Burgundy would likely argue that there's more to wine than its basic components.

Though you can boil, extract, and refine living tissue to isolate the protein, carb, or fat, you do so only at the cost of everything else that held the cells and organs together. Yanking certain components from living systems—as we do to make flour, sugar, protein slurries, and 90 percent of what's now for sale in the store—and expecting them to approximate their original nutritional value is like removing someone's brain from their body and expecting them to respond to questions. That is not science; it is science fiction. So is the idea that heavily processed food can be healthy.

So where does this terminology, this way of talking about food, get us? It gets us away from talking about the most important aspect of any food, its source. And that, by the way, is exactly how the mass producers of cheaply manufactured processed food products would have it. Now, we can say things like, "Sweet potatoes are really nutritious!" without stopping to consider that some sweet potatoes—those grown in sterile, toxic soil—are nutritionally bereft. We can toss another package of farmed salmon into our shopping cart thinking that it's essentially the same, nutritionally, as wild. And we can buy beef from cows raised on petrochemical-soaked corn, in deplorably crowded conditions, and tell ourselves that, as long as it's tender, it's every bit as good for us as the flesh from happy, roaming, grass-fed animals. Once they've got us believing such absurdities or, worse yet, buying our food reflexively as a thoughtless habit, they can get us to buy just about anything. Why, with a little marketing and the right package, they might even get us to eat dog food.

THE DOG FOOD AISLE

Take a look at the back of a bag of dog or cat food, and here are the ingredients you'll see: corn meal, soy meal, (occasionally) wheat, partially hydrogenated soy or corn or other vegetable oil, meat and protein meal, and a few synthetic vitamins. But guess what? The animal pushing the shopping cart is buying foods with the same list of ingredients for himself. The main differences between donuts, breads, and Cheerios are the quantities of hydrogenated oil and sugar. Cheerios, in turn, are nearly identical to Ramen noodles. Throw on a little salt, and you've got snack chips. Add tomato flakes and bump up the protein powder and—*bam!*—it's Hamburger Helper with noodles. Add a pinch of meat byproducts, take away some tomato powder, and we're in the pet food aisle again, holding a twenty-pound bag of grade A Puppy Chow.

We already know why manufacturers make food this way: it's cheap and convenient to reformulate the basic ingredients of protein, starch, and fat (there are those words again!) into a variety of shapes and textures, coat them in sugars and artificial flavor enhancers, and ship them just about anywhere. That's why they make it. But why would we eat it? Same reason: it's cheap and convenient. These days, a busy parent can buy a frozen lasagna dinner heavy enough to feed a family of five for about what it would cost to make from scratch. It comes in its own disposable aluminum pan, so—no fuss, no muss—the dinner riddle is solved. Like other foods in the supermarket, it keeps forever (or at least a really long time) in the freezer, so if we don't eat it tonight, it'll be ready when we want it. And thanks to the fact that these convenience foods contain protein, fat, and carbohydrates, plus some synthetic vitamins, we can survive on them—at least for a certain amount of time. But that doesn't mean these foods aren't changing us. They are.

As I described earlier, whenever our ancestors moved from one place to another, their diets changed and, in turn, so did their physiologies. And, as you'll recall, each time they relocated from one natural locale to another, though that relocation influenced their stature and relative prominence of certain facial features, their skeletons generally remained perfect examples of function and proportionality. They didn't think of food in terms of carbs and protein and fat. They thought more in terms of good soil, healthy animal, freshly picked. And for this reason, their traditional cultural practices, and the foods they took into their bodies, kept them firmly tethered to the natural world. In other words, they stayed *connected*.

For eons, human beings maintained that connection, thanks to the guidance of their cultural wisdom. But they couldn't have known all the possible consequences of cutting those natural ties. How could they? Until recently, the people of this planet benefited from a relatively stable climate without knowing how easily it could be thrown into chaos; we never had to think about it until it all started breaking down. Indeed, we might have remained blind to the underlying cause had it not been for a handful of prescient climatologists and geologists who, at great professional cost, made certain their warnings were heard. As a result, most of us are fairly well versed in the concepts of climate regulation and instability.

We know, for example, that the Industrial Revolution and subsequent commercial growth created massive carbon dioxide pollution, which magnified the greenhouse effect and is now making global climate warmer. What we don't yet appreciate is the extent to which the Industrial Revolution polluted the food we eat, leading to so many changes in our health and physiologies that it has altered the way we look. Over the past 100 years, we have completed the single most comprehensive dietary shift in the history of our race. This shift, a major dietary migration over vast nutritional territory, has gone on largely unnoticed—even by the medical community—for the following reasons:

- The shift didn't involve moving from one geographic point to another; only our food has changed.

- Except for the very well-off and the recently urbanized, few of us in America have been exposed to the products of culinary tradition and therefore don't know what we're missing.

- Since the migration from real to fake food has occurred over five generations, even our parents were likely born into an environment bereft of culinary tradition.

- Cheap and convenient products catch on quick, and we tend not to ask where they were made or what they were made of, so the easier and cheaper our food gets, the less we think about it.

- The merging of business and science into one corporate body means that medical science can no longer countenance advice incompatible with the interests of commerce.

- A constant stream of new technologic fixes continues to buttress our collapsing physiologic infrastructure, which has so far masked what would otherwise be obvious maladaptive consequences of that collapse.

This last point is the most significant. If needing glasses killed us, we would no doubt pay keen attention to factors that render a child nearsighted. If having oral cavities killed us, we would steer clear of the things known to rot teeth as if our lives depended on it. If there were deadly consequences from inattention to nutritional detail, our nutrition science would be so advanced that it would be, dare I say, effective at preventing disease and capable of promoting health. In the past, when the knowledge of building healthy bodies with nutrition was, in fact, a matter of life and death, it was so highly valued that Dr. Price found many indigenous people reluctant to "disclose

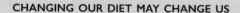

CHANGING OUR DIET MAY CHANGE US

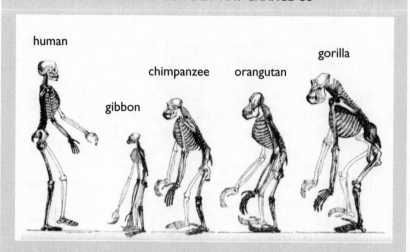

Big brains require brain-building fats like cholesterol, lecithin, choline, saturated fat, and long-chain polyunsaturated fats. These compounds are found in highest concentration in organ meats, cold-water fish, and fish eggs. Today these rich foods are primarily consumed by the wealthy, in high-end restaurants where foie gras, fresh oysters, lobsters, crab, and caviar are staple items. Our hominid ancestors consumed them in greater quantity than other primates.

secrets of their race."[217] As Price discovered, "The need for this [reluctance] is comparable to the need for secrecy regarding modern war devices."[218] We don't think that way anymore. And it's ironic that the kinds of technological advancements that allowed for the mass production of nutritionally wanting processed foods are now necessary to address the physiologic consequences of their consumption.

That's an irony I'd just as soon watch play out from a safe distance. And I'm not alone. *How do I put this delicately?* If you think the wealthy—members of the upper social class—would even *touch* the foods most Americans eat daily, the foods relentlessly touted as healthy, you'd be mistaken. No, the most privileged among us eat very much the way their great-great-great-grandparents did. If we could fly past the iron gates guarding the White House and peer through the dining room windows to see what the guests were eating at President Obama's second inaugural lunch, we'd see this:

FIRST COURSE
Lobster Tails with New England Clam Chowder Cream Sauce

MAIN COURSE
Hickory-Grilled Bison [presumably pasture-raised] *Tenderloin with Wild
Huckleberry Veal Demi-glace Reduction, Baby Golden Beets and Green Beans,
and Strawberry Preserves and Red Cabbage*

THIRD COURSE
Sour Cream Ice Cream and Artisan Cheeses[219]

Those dining on these sinfully rich foods represent the same government whose food pyramid forbids us regular folk from eating anything of the kind. And since we're all supposed to be watching our sodium, we'd hardly risk touching our lips to something as salty as demi-glace or artisan cheeses. Have these culinary daredevils lost their minds, wandering so far outside the protective dietary shadow cast by the food pyramid? Or are their chefs the instigators, luring these susceptible victims over the cliff with the aroma of lobster and cream sauce? Whether through daring, by calculated intention, or by virtue of the same felicitous winds of fate that have caressed other aspects of their lives, one thing is sure: by maintaining their diet of real, traditional foods, the well-heeled have managed to ensconce their genomes inside the walls of a nutritional fortress and defend their physiologic dynasties against the hoi polloi—the swelling masses of the sick and enfeebled.

Given that the privileged can, and frequently do, eat the way we all used to, and given that this shift in eating habits first occurred over a century ago and that the effects of continued nutrient deprivation are magnified with each generation, the widening gap between nutritional-physiologic classes should place the other issues of class differential well into the background. A hundred years ago, two nutritional roads diverged in an evolutionary wood. The less well-off took the one never before traveled, and—judging by the health statistics—that has made all the difference.

It is as if, at the beginning of the twentieth century, ordinary working families were rounded up and ordered to start packing their bags, leave their farms and fertile soil behind, and take their assigned seats in an enormous space cruiser headed for Mars. Most of us would not undertake such a journey without resistance, because we know instinctively that the consequences for our health, and for the health of our children, might prove catastrophic. That is a good instinct, and even though our great-great-great-grandparents may not have known to follow it at the time, that instinct remains alive in every one of their descendants, and it will help get us back to Earth.

LIFE IN OUTER SPACE

In the Florence, Italy, episode of Phil Rosenthal's most excellent PBS series *I'll Have What Phil's Having,* Phil is accompanied by celebrity chef Fabio Picchi and his elderly but remarkably spry mother to visit her rooftop garden. Taking in the 360-degree view of Florence, he is offered, for his pleasure, a small tomato rubbed with the oil of a freshly picked basil leaf. Upon tasting it Phil says with his trademark wide-eyed enthusiasm, *"In Los Angeles it doesn't taste like this!"* Given his reaction, it seemed as though he were tasting a tomato for the first time—and we're talking about one of the superstars of sit-com, creator of *Everyone Loves Raymond,* who could have any ingredient of his choosing flown in first class from anywhere in the world.

Watching the host's eyes roll back with pleasure, his mouth dripping with the juices, I thought to myself, *I'd like to have what Phil's having.* That tomato was the very essence of the word *fresh.* And it made me wonder: if world-traveling bon vivant Phil Rosenthal can be surprised by how much flavor he's still missing out on, then what does that say about the eating experience of the average American on a limited budget? Sadly, I take Phil Rosenthal's experience, and experiences I have had eating vegetables picked fresh from my childhood garden, and rich, creamy milk straight from the collection bucket on a farm in New Zealand, and the ocean-briney opihi scraped just minutes before from the side of a rock of the Southern shore of Kauai, as reminders that, without our noticing, freshness and real flavor have been gradually removed from our eating experiences.

No wonder children and adults alike have been driven away from bland, relatively tasteless vegetables and toward the "super-awesome-mega-intense" options available in fast-food restaurants and the sacks of snack chips stashed away in their cars. But it's not just the sensory experience of real food that our bodies crave. Although food scientists have figured out how to recreate intensity of taste, if not the subtle nuances of real food, they cannot duplicate what Mother Nature does best: create foods that are equally rich in flavor *and nutrition.*

I submit that as our acquaintance with the experiences of real food have been denied us for so long and to such an extreme that the food conglomerates have nudged us, en masse, inch-by-inch, so far from nature that it is as if—with regard to foods produced for shelf life, in depleted soil, in limited space, and marketed as "healthy"—the majority of Americans today have been pushed off the planet and exiled to life in outer space.

Consider this: if we lived confined in some kind of giant penal colony on Mars, what would our diets be like? Would they really be so different from our own modern diets?

Most Martian foods would need to have long shelf lives. Since the shuttle only comes a few times a year, the shipments must be able to last for months. You'll find most space-foods loaded with shelf-stable ingredients such as sugar, flour, protein isolates and hydrolysates, and vegetable oil. ("Sports" and "nutrition" bars contain almost nothing else.) Though these products have been refined and stripped of living, reactive components, many contain toxic preservatives to make them last even longer, including BHT and BHA (the same chemical compounds, incidentally, used by plastic and tire manufacturers).[220] Since vegetable oil is particularly unappealing to micro-organisms (for reasons described in Chapter 8), you will find it incorporated into numerous products and nearly impossible to avoid while living on a Martian diet.

Space food's not big on flavor. The sterile environment can support the growth of a few assorted veggies, including iceberg lettuce and hydroponically grown tomatoes. The occasional shipments of carrots, bell peppers, broccoli, potatoes, apples, and a few more fruits and vegetables offer the splashes of color that help convince inmates they're getting real food, in spite of what their taste buds tell them. To make matters worse, significant nutrient decay occurs during extended transport so that many "fresh" fruits and vegetables actually contain little more nutrition than their canned or frozen counterparts.[221, 222] Fruits and vegetables shipped from Earth are picked unripe, and as a result, they contain significantly lower levels of vitamins (less than half in some cases) than any physiologically mature product.[223] Research suggests such mass-produced products might taste bland because they provide us little more than water and cellulose, some having just one tenth the vitamins or antioxidants of their organically raised cousins.[224]

Space is at a premium on this penal colony, so animals grown for human consumption there are denied access to pasture, sunlight, and room to run. There is no ocean, so fish—genetically engineered for prodigious growth—are farm raised on high-calorie pellets. Chickens, fish, cattle, and hogs are reared in dimly lit containers, fed a mash of corn or soy, and their more perishable fleshy parts (organs) and bones are baked into animal feed or discarded.

The manufacturers on Earth know that the well-educated prisoner is willing to spend his commissary allowance on products labeled "organic." Producers of these products must slightly reduce chemical inputs during production to comply with the labeling rules. Shipments include a small portion of their volume as organic cereals, milk substitutes, meat and cheese substitutes, and desserts, to help these prisoners feel their foods are significantly superior. Other health-conscious inmates—sensing the inadequacy of their diets—follow the lead of U.S. astronauts and take synthetic vitamins, lots of them, unaware that the vitamins manufactured in factories typically fail to approximate the real thing.

You get the idea. It is no great exaggeration to suggest that as far as our bodies are concerned, most of us might as well be living in outer space. Compared to the Maasai, who still root their genes deep within the same nourishing fruits of the earth as their ancestors did 40,000 years ago, our genes are flailing in empty air. The milk the Maasai enjoy today is much the same as it was thousands of years ago when artists drew pictures of people with their cattle on the walls of caves in the Gilf Kabir in Northern Africa (see illustration opposite the title page of this book). More to the point, it carries the same information to their cells. The gray-white substance pumped from our sad cows? Not so much.

Fortunately, you don't need to join a nomadic tribe in the desert to start eating better. All you need to do is follow the recipes laid out in any truly traditional cookbook. In Chapter 10, I will discuss in detail the foundational elements of the *Deep Nutrition* philosophy so that you can pick the best recipes from those available in your favorite cookbooks and on the Internet.

But before we get into which foods you should seek out, I would like to talk to you about two ingredients so harmful and so intrinsic to the modern American diet that with the single act of identifying these troublemakers, you put yourself miles ahead of the game.

THE *KAPU* LIST

Most people are aware of the harmful effects of chemical residues left over from industrial farming and of the preservatives and other agents that have harmful physiologic effects. And those of us who care about our health do what we can to avoid them. These two ingredients are different. Not only does each one seem perfectly engineered to prevent our cells from functioning the way they should, they often appear as a tag-team duo, showing up in the same foods together. I'm talking about vegetable oils and sugar.

I'm not saying that all the pollutants and toxins so often talked about aren't hurting our health. They are. But because vegetable oil and sugar are so nasty and their use in processed foods so ubiquitous that they have *replaced* nutrient-rich ingredients we would otherwise eat, I place vegetable oil and sugar before all others, on the very top of my *don't eat* list.

When traditional people wanted to send the message that certain foods were dangerous (or, in some cases, too special for non-royal persons), they'd place them on a do-not-eat list. In Hawaii, these foods were *kapu*, or forbidden. If they noticed that a food led to deleterious effects in newborns, then they would be *kapu* for expectant moms. Every indigenous society honored such a list; to ignore it could spell disaster for mother or child. Coming up, we'll see why vegetable oil and sugar are the real culprits for diseases most doctors blame on chance, or—even more absurdly—on the consumption of *natural* fats. Once you learn what they do inside your body, I hope you'll put them both on the top of your family's *kapu* list.

CHAPTER 7

Good Fats and Bad

How the Cholesterol Theory Created a Sickness Epidemic

- If we ever want to settle the good-fat/bad-fat debate, we need to listen to the lipid scientists.

- Lipid scientists have been trying to tell us for decades that saturated fat and cholesterol are not the problem.

- Oxidized polyunsaturated fat (PUFA) is dangerous because it is chemically unstable.

- Eliminating toxic fats can make you virtually heart-attack proof.

- Your lipoprotein particle size is the best gauge of your risk of heart attack.

When I was fresh out of medical school, if you had asked me what causes heart disease, I would have answered, "Fat and cholesterol, of course." I felt confident in this advice not only because it was what I had been taught, but because it seemed to make intuitive sense; I could picture fat accumulating inside a person's artery, gradually choking it closed like cooking grease in a pipe. Moreover, the American Medical Association, the American Heart Association, the American Diabetes Association, the American Cancer Society, the American College of Cardiologists, and other organizations endorsed this cholesterol theory of heart disease.

But as I started practicing medicine, one thing about this theory nagged me: Why, if cholesterol is so deadly, were so many of my oldest patients enjoying excellent health after a lifetime of consuming butter, eggs, and red meat?

Not long ago, physicians and scientists at the center of establishment medicine started asking similar questions in light of increasing evidence that the cholesterol issue warranted revisiting. In 2001, a few nutrition scientists at the Harvard School of Public Health went so far as to suggest that "the low-fat campaign has been based on little scientific evidence and may have caused unintended health consequences."[225] Further, they contended that the low-fat, anti-cholesterol campaign might not only be a flop as far as fighting obesity and diabetes were concerned, it could be making both epidemics worse.

Thanks to Michael Pollan and authors of several recent books, who cite this article and others like it, the reading public has witnessed cracks forming in the foundation of modern nutritional thought.[226, 227, 228] As more researchers discover all manner of evidence that animal fat has health-promoting effects (such data has now been published in dozens of academic journals), the pressure is building toward a sea of change in organized medicine.[229] Until that change comes, however, your doctor is unlikely to contradict the official guidelines. Only when current guidelines change to reflect better science will the average doctor's advice on nutrition cease to put patients at risk for those "unintended health consequences."

By the end of this chapter, you may be convinced that there is little reason to fear cholesterol. My hope is that, at the very least, you will recognize that the cholesterol theory of heart disease is far from unassailable and that when your doctor admonishes you to "get your numbers down," you need not accept this advice without objection.

The other thing I want you to understand is that a necessary outgrowth of the indictment of cholesterol is a rejection of the traditional, natural fats that have sustained humankind for thousands of generations. It's a little like the idea Nestle successfully used in the 1940s to sell infant formula to my grandmother and many other women, claiming it was "more perfect than breastmilk."[230] Those who mean to replace natural, traditional foods with modern-day food-like products in the name of health are championing the position that nature doesn't know best; a corporation does. This is an extraordinary claim requiring extraordinary evidence—a burden they have failed to meet.

So why do we fall for it?

To understand how easy it is to sell us completely bogus ideas, to get us begging for products that we barely know anything about, we will begin with the most successful sales pitch in the history of medicine, delivered by a man regarded by many as the hero of modern nutritional thought.

THE MAN WHO BROUGHT US THE LOW-FAT CAMPAIGN

It's 1958. A fit and handsome Ancel Keys stands before a laboratory chalkboard on a CBS documentary entitled *The Search* to warn us of "the new American plague."[231] Onscreen, we see a row of ten little wooden men standing on Keys's desk. He flicks five of them with his finger, knocking them over as he speaks. "The chief killer of Americans is cardiovascular disease. . . . It strikes without warning. Of ten men we can expect five to get it." From that moment forward, America would turn to Keys for advice on preventing heart disease.

The camera reveals Keys in front of a small but attentive group of men dressed in white coats, staged to make it appear as though he were delivering a speech to a cadre of enraptured physicians. Though he never claims outright to be a heart specialist, he wears a doctor's jacket and talks confidently about heart health, looking every bit the part of the reassuring physician as he soberly enunciates just the right words for maximum impact. Delivered with a newscaster's sense of gravitas and the suave confidence of *Madmen's* ad exec character Don Draper, Keys's charisma catapulted him to the front page of *Time* magazine. But unlike Draper, who sold household products using catchy slogans delivered by attractive spokespeople, Keys sold *himself* as the go-to expert on all manner of heart disease using bad science, covert deception, and fear.

In reality, the father of the "diet-heart hypothesis" was not a cardiologist or even an M.D. Keys had earned his Ph.D. in the 1930s studying salt-water eels. His nutritional credentialing rested on the fact that, during WWII, the military assigned him to design the ready-to-eat meal that could be stored for years and shipped to millions of soldiers. Dr. Keys named his pocket-sized meal the K-ration, after himself. When the war was over, the Minnesota public health department hired Keys to study the problem of rising rates of heart attacks. But ego got the better of him.

At his first scientific meeting he presented the idea that in countries where people ate more animal fat, people died of heart disease more often, suggesting a possible causal relationship. But his statistical work was so sloppy (see figure on the following page) that he was lambasted by his peers. Rather than cleaning up his act, Keys vowed vengeance: "I'll show those guys."[232] More than anything else, it seems, Keys wanted folks to think he had single-handedly discovered the cause of heart disease. And so did the country's margarine producers, who in Keys had found the perfect spokesperson. Though Keys's work failed to convince professional scientists (at least for the first decade or two), the margarine industry knew he still had a shot at convincing the man on the street. If the public thought butter and other animal fats would "clog their arteries," they could be persuaded to buy margarine instead.

It wasn't long before the American Heart Association, which depends on large donations of cash from the vegetable oil industry, jumped on the bandwagon with Keys. They took his sloppy statistics and ran with it, eventually con-

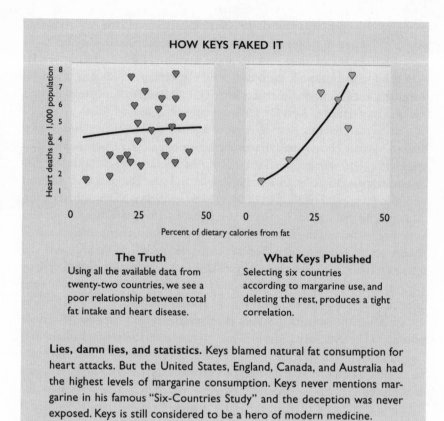

HOW KEYS FAKED IT

The Truth

Using all the available data from twenty-two countries, we see a poor relationship between total fat intake and heart disease.

What Keys Published

Selecting six countries according to margarine use, and deleting the rest, produces a tight correlation.

Lies, damn lies, and statistics. Keys blamed natural fat consumption for heart attacks. But the United States, England, Canada, and Australia had the highest levels of margarine consumption. Keys never mentions margarine in his famous "Six-Countries Study" and the deception was never exposed. Keys is still considered to be a hero of modern medicine.

vincing most doctors that steak is a "heart attack on a plate" and that margarine made from hydrogenated vegetable oils (full of trans fat) was healthy. Within a decade, grocery store shelves were loaded with ready-to-eat foods, and Americans were buying. No longer insisting on fresh food from small farmers right in our neighborhoods, we'd been convinced that products made in distant factories were safer, healthier, and better. And they were also cheaper. But even Keys had his doubts about eating them.

"Oops! Everything I Said About Saturated Fat Was Really About Margarine." —Paraphrasing Ancel Keys, Ph.D.

By 1961, under increasing scientific scrutiny, Keys began to waver in his support for his own (now publicly accepted) diet-heart hypothesis.[233] Scientists had pointed out Dr. Keys's misleading use of scientific terms. In public, he fingered animal fat as the culprit behind the rising rates of heart attacks. But in his laboratory and human experiments, he didn't use animal fat.[234] His subjects were fed margarine made from partially hydrogenated vegetable oil. And what was in the margarine? Trans fat—a full 48 percent!

Trans fats are the infamous artery-hardening molecules that have been banned from restaurants in New York City and elsewhere due to their now well-known associations with heart disease. These fats do not exist in foods that nature makes. (*Trans* describes a chemical bond between two molecules, not a molecule *per se*. More on this below.) While nature makes healthy versions of trans-containing fats, the trans fat that's been banned is the byproduct of an industrial process called *hydrogenation*. And so, for Keys to conclude from studies that used hydrogenated vegetable oil that animal fat causes heart disease is utterly nonsensical.

Unfortunately, the public never heard the straight story. Because margarine also contains saturated fat (made during the same hydrogenation process that generates trans fat), the food industry was handed the opening they needed to put an anti-saturated-fat spin on Keys's findings. Ignoring the presence of trans fat (and other distorted fats in margarine), spokesmen simply blamed saturated fat. And on TV, Keys equated saturated fat with animal fat, completing the deception.[235] This ingenious spin on the facts is akin to poisoning rats with strychnine-laced milk and then blaming the deaths on the milk.

The anti-saturated fat, anti-cholesterol ball was rolling along nicely, and there was so much money being made selling "healthy" low-cholesterol, low-fat processed foods, that the rolling ball wasn't going to be easy to stop. All the news reports you've heard on the hazards of saturated fat and cholesterol are supported in large part by studies that evaluated the effects of hydrogenated vegetable oil, which is full of unnatural molecules that aren't found in butter, steak, or any natural food.[236]

With so much junk science saturating the media, professionals who give nutritional advice need to go beyond the sound bites to discover the truth for themselves. While it's easy to go with the flow and tell patients to "cut out animal fat," doing so turns well-meaning healthcare practitioners into unwitting participants in an ongoing campaign to sell high profit-margin manmade substitutes for natural foods—substitutes which, in turn, make people sick.

Lipid Scientists to the Rescue

In an earlier chapter, I suggested that our health took a turn for the worse when we stopped talking about food the way farmers and chefs do and adapted the language of scientists. The scientists are not the problem. The problem arises when we use scientific terms without a true understanding of what we're saying. Case in point: the story I just told you about the media scaring us away from saturated fat coming from foods like butter and cream when the food in the studies actually was margarine and was, therefore, loaded with trans fats that only recently—fifty years down the road—we've learned are bad for our health.

These days we so frequently hear such terms as *trans* and *polyunsaturated* it's easy to forget that those are chemical descriptions of compounds with specific types of molecular bonds and conformations—details most non-chemists wouldn't be able to describe. So when the young man restocking salad dressing on grocery store shelves insists the dressing is healthy because it's high in polyunsaturates, or your server at the local restaurant extols the merits of omega-3 in canola, it's best to take this nutritional advice with a grain of salt. In 1961, when Ancel Keys brought national attention to lipids and their role in human health, he was hailed as *Time* magazine's Man of the Year. In the sixty-plus years since the lipid discussion took center stage of the nutrition conversation, the heart-health cover stories have reflected a consistent fascination with fats, but they have delivered a completely inconsistent message: "Cholesterol: And Now the Bad News" was a cover story in 1984, arguing that eating cholesterol is bad for you.[237] But by 2014, *Time* reported, in an article entitled "Ending the War on Fat," that doctors were now suggesting butter is okay.[238] What—or who—are we supposed to believe?

In my view we should only listen to the group of people who actually spend their careers studying fat: lipid scientists, who focus solely on learning more about various lipids (fats) and their respective roles in human health. In the decades we've been trying out different kinds of fats in different combinations—from Rip Essylstein's near-zero fat, Engine 2 Diet, to the South Beach Diet (only fish and plant-based dietary fats), to Atkins's emphasis on animal fats—the American public has never heard from a single lipid scientist. That's a real shame, because lipid scientists have plenty to say on the matter. And because they know more on this topic than anyone else, what they have to tell you could save your life.

A Cause of Heart Disease You Might Have Missed

If there's such a thing as a lipid science rock star, then I would consider Gerhard Spiteller to be something like Elvis Presley, Jim Morrison, and Mick Jagger rolled into one. This brilliant Austrian scientist has been quietly getting to the bottom of the role of fats in heart attacks for nearly half a century. A superstar among super-geeks whose resume includes teaching and research positions at MIT, Innsbruck, and other prestigious universities, he is lead author of over 130 published scientific articles. While other members of the lipid research community have studied and written extensively about lipid peroxidation and its potential role in arteriosclerosis, it was Dr. Spiteller, who, in his 2000 article, "Oxidation of Linoleic Acid in Low-Density Lipoprotein: An Important Event in Atherogenesis," definitively points us in the right direction.[239] In this meticulously researched article, Dr. Spiteller makes the case that it is processed polyunsaturated fats, not saturated fat or cholesterol, that deserve the blame for the stiffening of arteries throughout the body. (We'll learn more about what polyunsaturated fats are, and where they come from, later in this chapter.)

I'm going to guess that until now you'd never heard of Dr. Spiteller. Lipid scientists, as a rule, don't land their own TV shows. They are not asked to comment on the latest medical story on morning news programs. They do not wind up on the cover of *Time* or in any other mainstream magazine. Unlike living the life of a heart surgeon, or a brain surgeon, or a cardiologist, spending your career in a windowless lab studying fats isn't likely to impress people at a dinner party. Let's face it: for most us, "lipid scientist" is hardly synonymous with "sexy."

This explains why the general public—even those who study nutrition and health—don't usually get to hear what lipid scientists have to add to the nutrition dialogue, a conversation that, at least lately, largely concerns itself with the good-fat/bad-fat question. But what about other researchers and medical professionals? Surely, even the jocks of the medical world would take the time to acquaint themselves with the latest findings coming from those lipid researchers who know far more about how fats behave in the body than anyone else, right?

Wrong. By and large, the guy driving the Porsche Carrera to the surgical suite to thread another stent into another artery of another patient is almost guaranteed to be thirty years, or more, behind in his knowledge of nutrition and its role in the etiology of the arterial disease that, indirectly, paid for his house, his upcoming trip to Italy, and his children's Ivy League college educations. In fact, by the time you've finished reading this chapter, it's likely that you'll know far more about the causes of heart disease than your local heart surgeon or cardiologist. You'll understand what lipid scientists have been telling us—and what the research has supported for years—cholesterol and saturated fat are not your heart's enemy; industrial fat products, the vegetable oils, are.

Industrial fat products like vegetable oils are toxic to your arteries because they contain delicate polyunsaturated fatty acids (PUFAs) that are particularly prone to oxidative damage, especially when exposed to heat and when separated from the antioxidants that would otherwise help protect them from that oxidative damage. I know, that's nowhere near as catchy as "cholesterol clogs your arteries." But it is what the research evidence supports.

So, as lipid scientists have long argued, I submit that natural fats and cholesterol have been a part of the human diet for millennia and are not the problem. The historically recent rise in arteriosclerosis and heart disease is the result of an historically recent invention of the food industry—refined, bleached, and deodorized vegetable oils. By revealing how certain fatty acids are changed by heating and processing, Dr. Spiteller offers us a chemically indisputable definition of good fats versus bad.

Over the rest of this chapter, I'll discuss these concepts and show how eating heat-damaged fatty acids leads to plaque building up in your arteries. But first I want to show you the consequences of Keys's pet theory, and why anyone who villifies saturated fat is helping to support both the sickness and the junk-food industries.

HOW THE CHOLESTEROL THEORY CREATED A SICKNESS EPIDEMIC

In the 1950s, Ancel Keys and others popularized the idea that fat clogs our arteries the way grease clogs the pipe under a kitchen sink. And although the vast majority of all available research tells us that this concept is no longer tenable, the medical community, by and large, insists on sticking to that story. True, over the years we've modified this model a bit, but the central idea is that somehow the body is flawed and unable to deal with natural fats. All of this comes from failing to appreciate the chemical sleight of hand that Dr. Keys pulled off when he described his experiments using the term *saturated fat* while referring to margarine—but everyone thought he was talking about butter.

Let's take a moment to look at some of the ongoing consequences of this single misdirection.

Prior to Keys's campaign, people ate far more saturated fat and cholesterol-rich foods than we do today, but heart attacks were so rare they were almost unheard of.[240, 241] Over the past century, as butter consumption dropped to less than one quarter of what it was (from eighteen pounds per person per year to four), vegetable oil consumption went up five-fold (from eleven pounds per person per year to fifty-nine).[242, 243] In 1900, heart disease was rare.[244] By 1950, heart problems were killing more men than any other disease.[245] Now, at the dawn of the second millennium, heart disease is the number-one cause of death in both men and women.[246]

Natural fat consumption: down. Processed fat consumption: up. Heart disease: up—*way* up. Forget for a moment what the "experts" are saying, and ask yourself what these trends suggest to your inner statistician. The next time you go to the grocery store, see how many foods you can find that don't contain vegetable oil as an ingredient. What do you make of the fact that while watching TV at home, you catch a sixty-second health spot espousing the benefits of some low-cholesterol spread, followed by a commercial for a cholesterol drug, then another one for erectile dysfunction? What does this scenario say to the critical thinker in you?

What's been dropping us like flies is not any upsurge in saturated fat consumption, but an upsurge in consumption of *two major categories* of pro-inflammatory foods: vegetable oils (a.k.a. unnatural fats) and sugar. Cutting both from your diet will not only protect your heart, it will help protect you from *all* chronic diseases.

To help you understand why it's completely unscientific to blame natural fat for heart disease, I will appeal to your inner chemist, showing you why natural fats are beneficial. But first, I want to give you just a little bit of the history of these oils and tell you why vegetable oil has managed to work its way into nearly every product the majority of Americans eat every day. Food manufacturers use vegetable oils for the same reasons other manufacturers use plastic: it is easy to manipulate chemically, the public can be taught to ignore the consequences of its use, and best of all, it's cheap.

The First Bad Fat

In the late 1800s, Emperor Napoleon III offered a prize for a butter substitute to feed his army and "the lower classes."[247] The goal was a product that cost very little and wouldn't rot on extended sea voyages. After some experimentation, a chemist named Hippolyte Mege-Mourie found that squeezing slabs of tallow under pressure extracted oily elements that fused into a solid when churned together with skim milk. The dull gray material had a pearly sheen and so Mege-Mourie called it margarine, after the Greek *margarites*, meaning "pearl." It didn't taste good, but it was cheap.

Not cheap enough for America, however. Raising, housing, feeding, breeding, and milking cows is an expensive enterprise compared to growing plants. By the turn of the century, chemists had found a way to reinvent the reinvented butter by starting with material nearer the bottom of the food chain: cottonseeds. There were sacks and sacks of them lying around without much use. In fact, the tiny black seeds were hard to store because, if left alone, they would ferment and make a terrible stink. Chemists recognized that odoriferous volatiles meant the oil was reacting with oxygen, and they smelled opportunity. The reactive nature of the oil meant that it had the potential to be chemically modified for a variety of purposes and, soon enough, they found a way to spin this worthless byproduct of the textile industry into solid gold. Thus began a happy relationship between chemists, farmers, and petroleum companies that continues to this day.

To make the liquid cottonseed oil more like butter, they needed to thicken it into a solid paste. Chemistry offered two options: either tangling bunches of oil molecules together or making the individual molecules less flexible and more stackable. The first option creates a primordial form of plastic, too inedible to pass off as food. So they chose the second option. They engineered a transformation of the fatty acids in the oil, ironing them almost flat with heat, pressure, hydrogen gas, and a nickel catalyst. The key to making the product appear edible was the catalyst, which prevented the molecules from tangling up into plastic. When the oils get squashed flat in this process, their double bonds change from the natural

PARTIAL HYDROGENATION SQUASHES FATS FLAT

The chemical process of partially hydrogenating an unsaturated fatty acid may turn cis-shaped fatty acids into trans or convert the unsaturated bond into a saturated bond. Either outcome leads to a flatter shaped molecule with less fluid characteristics than the original cis-configuration, unsaturated fatty acid. Food maunfacturers exploit this to make butter substitutes.

bent and flexible configuration to something stiffer. And thus, *trans* fat was born.

We call partially hydrogenated fatty acids *trans* fat after the type of bond that holds the carbon atoms together. Naturally occurring fatty acids contain bonds in a cis configuration. In this configuration, fatty acids are highly flexible, which prevents crystallization (solidification), and so the molecules behave as liquids. Partial hydrogenation does two things: it irons some cis-configuration bonds completely flat (by saturating the bond with hydrogen) and switches others around to trans. Converting a cis fatty acid to saturated or trans makes it a stiffer and more stackable molecule. This is why partially hydrogenated vegetable oils solidify like butter (which contains naturally stiff and stackable saturated fats). Cottolene was the first major brand to be successfully marketed in the United States, over a century ago. It didn't taste quite like butter, but it was cheap. This process is still used to make "butter" for the "lower classes" today.

Now, most experts agree that consumption of inexpensive butter substitutes such as margarine and shortening is bad for our health. Nevertheless doctors are generally loathe to recommend butter to their patients. So what do people use instead? Some of the most dangerous food products in the store.

NATURE DOESN'T MAKE BAD FATS

One of the fundamental concepts of this book is that physical beauty isn't, as it turns out, in the eye of the beholder. Beautiful living things are the manifestations of the immutable laws of natural growth, rules grounded in mathematics. These rules apply everywhere, even at the molecular level.

Biomolecules, including fatty acids, cholesterol, and DNA, typically twist into either hexagonal or pentagonal configurations to facilitate their interaction with each other and with water. Processing distorts the fatty acids in vegetable oil so they can no longer assume the typical five- or six-sided geometry. Like Chinese finger traps, our enzymes pick up these distorted fatty acids and then can't let them go, which hampers cellular function so profoundly it can kill your cells. And if you eat enough trans fats, cellular dysfunction will impair so many cells in so many tissues that the cumulative effects will disrupt basic functions (like blood circulation or your body's ability to fight infection) and eventually kill you. Vegetable oils rarely kill children, but they can disrupt normal metabolism so profoundly that a child's *dynamic symmetry* is lost, and their skeletal proportions become imbalanced.

No food represents such a full spectrum of molecules—from healthy to distorted and extremely toxic—as fat. Good fats are some of the best foods you can eat. And some of the healthiest, most robust people on the planet live in cultures whose diets are highly dependent on natural fats, like animal fat. But take those good-fat foods away and replace them with foods high in refined carbohydrates and distorted fats, and the same problems we have in our country begin to crop up around the world: weight gain, heart troubles, mood disorders, other chronic diseases, newborn children exhibiting organ and facial deformation, and other hallmarks of physical degeneration. So far, establishment medicine blames milk and meat. But I blame toxic, distorted fats (and sugar). Fortunately, the principle behind avoiding toxic,

GOOD FATS AND BAD	
Good Fats These traditional fats can handle the heat involved in processing or cooking.	**Bad Fats** These industrial-era fats cannot handle the heat involved in processing or cooking.
■ Olive oil ■ Peanut oil ■ Butter (Yes, butter!) ■ Macadamia nut oil ■ Coconut oil ■ Animal fats (lard, tallow) ■ Palm oil ■ Any artisanally produced unrefined oil	■ Canola oil ■ Soy oil ■ Sunflower oil ■ Cottonseed oil ■ Corn oil ■ Grapeseed oil ■ Safflower oil ■ Non-butter spreads (including margarine) and the so-called trans-free spreads

distorted fats is easy to remember: *Eat natural fats and avoid processed ones.* This formula works because nature doesn't make bad fats; factories do.

The seductive flavors of fat-rich foods tempt us for good reason. Unlike sugar—which offers no nutrition—a meal complete with animal fat actually helps us absorb and taste other nutrients. This is why butter makes other foods taste so delicious.[248, 249, 250, 251] And because animal fats contain cholesterol—a natural appetite suppressant—they satisfy in a way that little else can.[252, 253, 254] In contrast, vegetable oils impair vitamin absorption and do little to suppress appetite, so you eat more and get less nutrition.[255]

When you worry about chemicals hidden in modern food, you might first think of monosodium glutamate (MSG), pesticide residues, and contaminants, like mercury. But compared to bad fats, those are small potatoes. Of all the dietary changes attending modernization, nothing compares to what we've done with fats and oils. Over the past one hundred years in the United States, our fat intake has gone from largely animal-based and natural to plant-based and so unnatural that our bodies can't adapt. Thanks to Dr. Keys and his associates in industry, and also in the AMA, we have been tricked into questioning our own senses, convinced that our health depends on staying away from these once-prized sources of sustenance and allowing ourselves to be herded into buying

FOODS LOADED WITH PRO-INFLAMMATORY FAT (DON'T EAT THESE)	
Margarine	This is a classic "one molecule away from plastic" food that backyard animals won't eat. Very little in here other than trans fat and twisted fatty acids that are worse than trans. Don't let kids near it; it interferes with normal bone growth and sexual development.
Salad dressing	Aside from water and vinegar, most store-bought salad dressing is pure vegetable oil plus sugar and flavoring agents.
Rice milk	One serving contains one teaspoon of vegetable oil and just under an ounce of liquified rice. There's nothing else to this stuff—except the synthetic vitamins. We tell diabetics not to eat rice, so why would drinking it be a good idea?
Soy milk, soy cheese, soy-based meat products	Processing damages the soy bean's cell membrane, releasing PUFAs, which are rapidly oxidized to harmful MegaTrans fats. Whole soy based meat beans can be part of a healthy diet.
Breakfast cereals	Most breakfast cereals are extruded, pressed, flaked, and/or puffed. The slurry is then hardened with a coating of vegetable oil, which acts like a protective varnish that can maintain the product's shape and prevent dampness from making it soggy.
Nuts (Oily nuts only. Raw or dry roasted nuts are good for you, but read labels carefully.)	Nuts are often cooked in "peanut and/or vegetable oil." Peanut oil would be fine, but since it costs five to ten times more than vegetable oil, I doubt they use much peanut. Nuts are more vitamin good for you, and amino-acid–rich when eaten raw.
French fries	Restaurants can reuse frying oil for a week or longer. These oils can turn so toxic that they are often too degraded to be recycled as biodiesel fuel.
Crackers and chips	Many patients assume that since crackers are bland, they are healthy. (This always makes me sad. Blandness indicates an absence of nutrients.) Factory-made crackers and chips are fried in oils that can be used over and over, increasing the concentration of the worst kind of pro-inflammatory fats: MegaTrans.
Granola	Up to half the calories in granola may come from vegetable oil.
Soft breads, buns, and most store-bought muffins	I saved these for last because, though the total unnatural fat content tends to be low, most people eat a lot of these products in a typical week, and they constitute a major source of trans and especially harmful pro-inflammatory MegaTrans fats.

tasteless, processed, "neutral" vegetable oils instead. Without even realizing it, we've traded in healthy fats for toxic ones, and now it's making us sick.[256]

THE TROUBLE WITH VEGETABLE OIL

What do you suppose would have happened if, several decades ago, an unknown lipid scientist conclusively proved that an artificial fat molecule present in margarine, as well as all kinds of other products for sale in every grocery store in the country, was deadly, and was very likely causing disease, growth defects, and premature mortality? And what if that scientist had had the opportunity to present this public health information to Congress? Would Congress have responded? Would their corporate supporters—companies as powerful as Unilever, Monsanto, and ADM—have recalled the millions of products containing the toxin this scientist had discovered? Would they have halted their production lines, given up their subsidies and, if necessary, torn up millions of acres of corn which (no longer devoted to the production of margarine) would no longer be needed? Would they have abandoned margarine production and gone back to making real butter, trading in the cash cow of margarine products for actual, milk-producing cows? Or rather, would the corn product freight train roar straight through the scientist's warnings, and even pick up speed as agribusiness marketing engineers frantically shoveled disinformation into the firebox?

We don't have to guess at the answer, because there was such a scientist, and her findings were brought to Congress—way back in 1988—to warn of the dangers of trans fat, present in hydrogenated oils.[257] We can only presume that the politicians who learned of Dr. Mary Enig's research had little personal experience with cheap butter substitutes or the convenience foods that contain them. But the rest of us were eating plenty of the stuff and we continued to do so decades after Enig's warnings because we had never heard them. Only after European countries outlawed trans fat did we finally hear that it might be bad for our health.

Why did it take the United States so long to take trans fat seriously? Earlier, I mentioned that scientific discoveries that are incompatible with commercial interests have a tough time making it to the papers. Trans is just one example. Cigarette smoking, another. Asbestos, another still. And I'm guessing that if there's something you and your family might be eating every day that scientists already know is deadly, you'd like to know about it now, not thirty years from now. That's why I'd like to tell you the truth about vegetable oil.

Vegetable Oil Should Not Be Heated

Vegetable oils contain mostly heat-sensitive *polyunsaturated* fats. When heated, these fragile fats turn into toxic compounds including trans fat.[258] The heat sensitivity issue means that all processed vegetable oils, and all products that contain vegetable oil, necessarily contain trans fat. Canola oil degrades so rapidly that a testing company, needing to find the purest canola oil to use as a standard against which other oils could be compared, couldn't locate any canola oil even from pharmaceutical-grade manufacturers with a trans fat content lower than 1.2 percent.[259]

This means that vegetable oil, and products made from vegetable oil, contain trans fat—even when the label seems to guarantee them trans free. But because heat so readily distorts their fatty acids, vegetable oil and products made from vegetable oil also contain something that is worse for us than trans. Before we get to that, I'd like to take a moment to compare and contrast the various fatty acids and their ability to handle heat.

FAT VERSUS OIL: WHAT'S THE DIFFERENCE?

Lipid is a generic term for both fats and oils. If the lipid is solid at room temperature, it's called fat. If it's liquid, it's oil. Butter is solid, so it's called a fat. In general, lipids made of stiff, inflexible saturated fats are solid and those made of fluid, flexible unsaturated fats are liquid. However, to describe butter (and other animal fat) as "saturated fat" is not strictly correct, because many fatty acids in butter are not saturated.

All storage fats (as opposed to fats in cell membranes and other actively functioning fats) exist in a chemical assemblage called a triglyceride. A triglyceride is made with three fatty acids that dangle like keys from a chain made out of glycerol, a short molecule to which each of the fatty acids is bound. The fatty acids can be any combination of saturated, monounsaturated, and polyunsaturated. Butter carries more saturated fatty acids in its triglyceride chains than vegetable oil, but not all are saturated fat. If they were, butter would be as stiff and solid as wax. Vegetable oil actually contains saturated fatty acids, but nowhere near as many as butter. The different blends of saturated and unsaturated combine to generate the final melting point of the fat.

WHY VEGETABLE OILS ARE PRONE TO OXIDATION

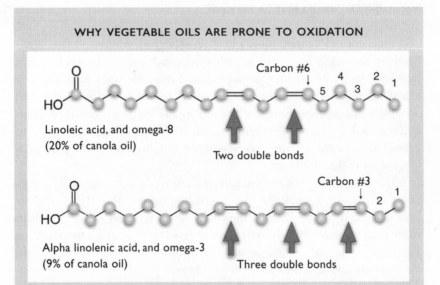

Polyunsaturated fats (PUFAs) have two or more double bonds, hence the "poly." The two molecules shown here are the two most common PUFAs found in canola and other vegetable oils, linoleic and linolenic acid. If a fatty acid has two double bonds near one another, the molecule becomes highly susceptible to attack by oxygen, particularly when heated as in processing and cooking. If it has three double bonds near one another, as does linolenic acid, it's even more vulnerable to an attack by oxygen. The products of these oxidation reactions are the damaged, distorted molecules that make vegetable oils so toxic.

Who Can Take the Heat? Cooking-Fat Basics

For the purposes of cooking, we want to pick the kinds of fats that can take heat. On that count, saturated fats (present in butter, coconut oil, lard, and traditional fats) win hands down. Why? Because they can resist a kind of heat-related damage called *oxidation*. Thanks to their shape, saturated fats have no room for oxygen to squeeze in, and even high heat can't force these tough molecules to be more accommodating. Monounsaturated fats have room for just one oxygen molecule to sneak in. But it's not easy, so monounsaturated fat-rich olive oil resists the harmful oxygen-induced molecular rearrangements and is still okay to cook with. Polyunsaturated fat—now that's another story. Polyunsaturated fat has *two* places where oxygen can chemically react, which makes oxygen not twice as likely to bind with the fat molecule, but *billions* of times more likely. This exponential increase in reactivity with oxygen is true of molecules generally, not just fats. TNT (trinitrotoluene) has six places where oxygen can react, making it so reactive it's literally explosive! But we're not cooking with explosives in our frying pans, are we? Actually, in a sense, we are, though on a slightly less dramatic scale. And it is those explosive oxidative reactions that we need to avoid.

The oils extracted from seeds that get processed into vegetable oils are composed primarily of polyunsaturated fatty acids, or PUFAs. If you want to remember which type of fatty acid most readily reacts with oxygen, just remember this: "*PUFAs go Poof!*"

Biology makes use of this reactivity. Enzymes in plants and animals fuse oxygen to polyunsaturated fats on purpose to change them from one shape to another. For example, fish oil isn't anti-inflammatory per se. Enzymes in the human body oxidize the PUFAs in fish oil to convert them into specific compounds that turn off pro-inflammatory enzymes. But this mutability also means polyunsaturated fats are more capable of being accidentally altered, and thus heat is a threat to their utility.

Where Does Vegetable Oil Come From?

Vegetable oil is the lipid extracted from *corn, canola, soy, sunflower, cottonseed, safflower, rice bran,* and *grapeseed*. Vegetable oil doesn't come from broccoli, and it doesn't equate to a serving of greens. It is found in almost all ready-made foods, from granola and squishy-soft baked goods, to rice milk and soy milk, to vegetarian cheese and meat substitutes, to frozen meals and side dishes, even salad dressings that say olive oil on the front label. I once purchased a package of dried cranberries only to discover, after I brought it home and read the label, that they were coated with vegetable oil.

There's a reason these oils are particularly temperature sensitive. Seeds stay dormant over the cold winter. But come spring thaw, the heat-sensitive PUFAs wake up in response to warming, facilitating germination.[260] To protect the PUFAs from damage as the ground warms and the sun's rays beat down on them, the plant has loaded its seeds with antioxidants. Unfortunately, refining these oils ultimately destroys both healthy PUFAs and their complementary antioxidants, converting them into distorted, unhealthy molecules. So what was once healthy in the seed isn't healthy in the bottle.

Canola Oil: Just Another Vegetable Oil

When I advise my patients to avoid vegetable oils, they often tell me that they only use canola oil, as if it were somehow exempt. I can't blame them for thinking this; the canola industry goes to great lengths to present their product as heart healthy, and the American Heart Association plays right along. They claim that canola oil is rich in anti-inflammatory omega-3 essential fats. And there's a grain—I should say *seed*—of truth to that claim. There's just one problem: omega-3 is a PUFA, which means it is easily distorted when exposed to heat. And since the omega-3 in canola seeds has *three* places for oxygen to react, it's really, really reactive. Canola oil still in the seed may indeed be full of omega-3, but factory-processed canola oil, *even organic-expeller-pressed*, contains mutated, oxidized, heat-damaged versions of once-healthy fats.[261] Canola consumption has been shown to cause the same health problems as the rest of the vegetable oils.[262, 263] If we could somehow get canola oil out of the seed without exposing it to heat, it would be good for us. But nobody can.

Well, that's not entirely true. In the old days, flax and rapeseed (a relative of canola) were gently extracted in the home using a small wedge press. Over the course of a day, the wedge would be tapped into the press a little further until, ever so slowly, the golden oil would start to drip, fresh and full of natural antioxidants and vitamins. These oils were *not* used to fry food, and therefore never exposed to damaging heat. If you aren't up for installing a wedge press in your kitchen, a few small enterprises can provide flax, hemp, and other healthy omega-3 rich oils—none of which should ever be used for cooking.

"Stop the Presses!" Oil Seeds Plead,
"You're Squeezing Me Too Hard!"

If we took a stethoscope and placed it to the side of a giant factory press as it applied more and more intense heat and pressure to a batch of tiny oil seeds, we might very well hear muffled cries indicating that, rather than being treated like little ambassadors of a heart-healthy diet, the seeds were being processed and refined like so much machine oil. In fact, one of the initial steps in making vegetable oil involves the use of hexane, a component of gasoline. If you were to get up close and catch the stench of the initial extract, you might never imagine it could be cleaned up. Making these stinky oils palatable requires a degree in chemical engineering; it takes twenty or so additional stages to bleach and deodorize the dark, gunky muck. And don't be fooled by so-called health products containing "expeller-pressed" oil; that only means the manufacturer didn't use solvents to maximize extraction.

Organic, expeller-pressed oil has gone through all the usual hazardous steps in the process of being "refined."

Olive oil, palm oil, and other oils that are good for us (see page 132) have mostly saturated and monounsaturated fatty acids, which are not so fragile. They are also easily extracted at low temperatures. Vegetable oils come out less readily, and are more prone to side reactions that polymerize and mutate the fat molecules. So getting them out creates a witch's brew of toxic lipids, only some of which will be removed. The rest, you eat.

Chemical analysis shows that even bottles of organic, expeller-pressed canola oil contain as much as 5 percent trans fats, plus cyclic hydrocarbons (carcinogens) and oxyphytosterols (highly damaging to arteries).[264] Of course, natural fats are all okay before they're processed and refined, so there's no harm in eating corn, soybeans, sunflower, and other tasty seeds.

Inflammation and Free Radicals

Maybe 5 percent trans (and other mutant fats) doesn't sound that scary. The real trouble is not so much that there's bad fat in the bottles (and other products). The real trouble has to do with the fact that after you eat these distorted, mutated fatty acids, they can reproduce inside you.

Imagine a zombie movie, filmed at the molecular level, except the mutant fatties don't stumble through your bloodstream in slow motion. Using *free radicals* (defined in the next section), mutated PUFAs convert normal fatty acids into fellow ghouls at the rate of billions per second.[265] I call this conversion-on-contact *the zombie effect* because, as every horror-movie connoisseur knows, when a zombie bites you, you become one of *them*. When a throng of molecular miscreants starts hacking away at your cells, things can really get scary. Their ability to damage normal PUFAs makes this class of oxidized PUFAs more dangerous than the trans fat we've all heard about on the news. Since they're a lot like trans, only worse, I call them *MegaTrans*.

There are many technical names for MegaTrans, including peroxidized fats, lipoxygenases, oxidized fat, lipid peroxides, lipid hydroperoxides, and a few others. Think of them all as different gangs of bad fats. While some of these toxic fats are in the trans configuration and others aren't, that's not the point. The point is these toxic fats are all gangsters with one thing in common: they're really bad for you. They contaminate all foods with trans fat and, in fact, all foods made from vegetable oils. They're bad because they lead to the formation of free radicals, which not only turn normal polyunsaturated fatty acids into mutants, but can also damage almost any part of your body: cell membranes, chromosomes, other fats—you name it.

The Reason Vegetable Oil Inflames Your Arteries

Free radicals are high-energy electrons that are involved in every known disease. They cause disease by restructuring nearly every molecule they come into contact with, converting biologically functional molecules into dysfunctional or even toxic molecules. Why would they do this? After all, the human body sometimes employs free radicals in order to perform basic physiologic functions like killing bacteria. It all boils down to a kind of loneliness—at the atomic level.

Imagine a set of neighboring molecules in your cell membranes as a village of polyamorous communes in the middle of a forest in Upstate New York. The electrons who are the members of these communes agree on one rule: we must always maintain an even number of members so that no one electron will ever feel left out; everyone should have a partner. Now imagine a circumstance where one elec-

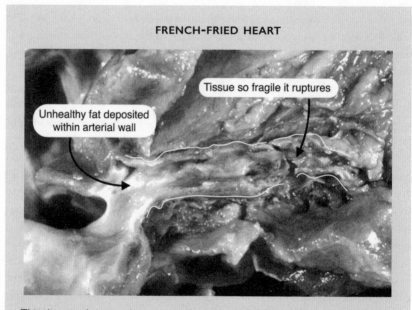

FRENCH-FRIED HEART

Tissue so fragile it ruptures

Unhealthy fat deposited within arterial wall

This dissected artery shows some fatty deposits, but of far greater concern is the effect MegaTrans has had on the arterial wall as free radical cascades have literally fried the arterial tissue. The artery and surrounding heart muscle are greasy and fragile, much like crispy fried food. When that fragile tissue tears and bleeds into the artery, it creates a clot. That's a heart attack.

HOW FREE RADICALS DAMAGE MEMBRANES

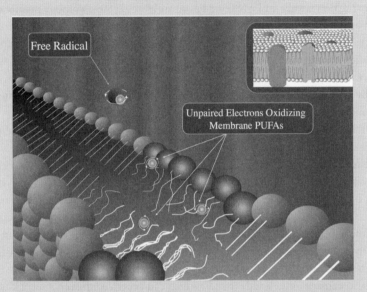

This is a closeup view of a cell membrane under attack. This particular section of membrane is composed of PUFAs. (The insert in the upper right is a cross-section of the same membrane.) Once the radical strips an electron from one of the PUFAs, it initiates a cascade reaction across the membrane, releasing more damaging unpaired electrons. In addition to mangling and distortion membrane PUFAs, the cascade reaction can damage hormone receptors, nutrient channels, and other proteins in the membrane, disrupting membrane function and putting the entire cell at risk.

tron decides to pursue an acting career and clears out one night without notice. Immediately, the unpaired electron it left behind goes berserk, racing through the halls of the commune, busting down doors, breaking walls, and completely disturbing the commune's essential structure as it desperately seeks out a new lover. The unpaired electron has been (free) radicalized—turned into a free radical. This commune now has two serious problems. One, it's no longer the commune that it once was; it's been beaten up and rendered entirely unrecognizable. And two, because it's breaking the cardinal even-number rule it has to do something about it. It chooses to solve the problem by passing the abandoned lover electron to another commune, and letting them deal with the consequences.

Those consequences are predictable. Whether the newly introduced electron ousts another lover from his bed or fails to find anyone willing to partner with him, in no time commune number two will have to deal with a lonely electron knocking down walls and wreaking havoc and forcing the commune members to hold an emergency meeting. Until such time that a patchouli-wearing therapist antioxident, such as the totally groovy vitamin E, shows up to say, "Whoa, dudes. I'll take your extra lover . . . it's all good . . . I've got another therapist friend I work with called vitamin C and, like, the whole even-number lovers thing will be, like, totally restored," this chaotic process will continue, leaving each and every affected commune permanently changed—and not for the better.

Chemists call this series of reactions a *free radical cascade*. Free radical cascades damage normal PUFAs, turning them into ugly molecular ghouls (the zombie effect). Just a little MegaTrans in the bottle of canola oil can become a lot of MegaTrans after you—or the cereal/donut/frozen dinner manufacturers—cook with it. On the plus side, free radical cascades make your food extremely crispy. (Free radical cascades also happen to play a role in the polymerization reactions that make plastic solid. This is probably the origin of the well-intentioned, but not strictly scientific, assertion that "margarine is one molecule away from plastic.") On the minus side, free radical cascades make your arteries extremely crispy. They will also damage other bodily tissues, which can generate *inflammation*, a kind of chemical chaos that interferes with normal metabolic function.

In the frying pan, MegaTrans reacts with oxygen to generate one free radical after another. Frying in vegetable oils doesn't so much cook your foods as blast them with free radicals—fusing molecules together to make the material stiff and inflexible.

WHY MEN GET HEART ATTACKS BEFORE WOMEN

Men get heart attacks ten to fifteen years on average before women. Why would that be? The only explanation cardiologists offer is that "women are just more perfect organisms."[266] While I tend to agree, I also believe there's more to the story. The real reason is that men have more testosterone, which makes them produce more red blood cells, so that men also have more iron in their blood.[267]

Iron acts as an accelerant, activating oxygen in ways that make it more likely to damage the linoleic acid and other fragile PUFAs traveling in lipoproteins right alongside iron-rich red blood cells.[268] Does this mean men are doomed to get heart attacks? Of course not! Aside from cutting vegetable oil, eating plenty of antioxidant-rich fresh vegetables will slow the reaction between iron and PUFA fats, rendering them less explosive and preventing the process of lipid deposition inside a person's arteries.[269, 270]

HOW CAN SOMETHING SO BAD TASTE SO GOOD?

If fast food fries and other crispy treats are so awful, why would nature allow them to tempt our tongues so tantalizingly?

Fast-food flavors are not real. Were they not doped with MSG, sugar, and other chemicals, you'd realize how flat those curly fries and meat nuggets taste. They're crispy, yes, but they lack flavor complexity. What happened? Processing and cooking with vegetable oil destroys complex nutrients and deadens flavors. (Flavor ligands become fused, rendering them either unrecognizable or too large to fit into your taste bud receptors.) You can get all the tangy, zesty, savoryness that you love in fast food from traditional cooking methods that enhance food flavors naturally by making nutrients more bioavailable.

Traditional cooking methods often make nutrients more bioavailable and are, for that reason, anti-inflammatory. Cooking with vegetable oil, on the other hand, destroys complex nutrients. So aside from the fact that foods cooked in vegetable oil will deposit loads of "zombie" fats into your tissues where they can, with little provocation, blast your tissues with free radicals, foods cooked with vegetable oils will also carry fewer vitamins and antioxidants than foods cooked using traditional methods and better oils.[271]

Free radicals can fry your cell membranes, damaging your arteries and, as I suggested earlier, eating foods fried in vegetable oil may very well precipitate a heart attack. But something happens before you have a full-blown heart attack: your arteries stop responding to normal body stresses. It's called abnormal *endothelial function*. And there's a test for it.

HOW YOUR DOCTOR CAN TELL
IF YOU HAVE FRENCH-FRIED ARTERIES: ERECTILE
DYSFUNCTION AND ENDOTHELIAL FUNCTION

In 1999, a team of lipid scientists in New Zealand wanted to see what eating deep-fried food does to our arteries in the short term. They planned to feed subjects french fries and then test them to see if their blood vessels were still able to regulate blood flow normally (this ability is called *endothelial function*). The test is performed by slipping the patient's arm into a blood pressure cuff, then squeezing it to cut off the blood flow for a few minutes. Normally, on releasing the cuff again, the oxygen-starved arteries open wider so blood can come rushing back in, just like you would suck in more air after holding your breath for a while. This dilation response depends on the endothelial cells lining the blood vessels which have to be healthy enough to generate the nitric oxide that makes arteries dilate. If endothelial cells can't make nitric oxide, or if the nitric oxide they make gets destroyed too soon, a person's circulatory system can't work correctly.

Male sexual function depends on healthy endothelial function, for reasons that pertain to arterial dilation and the obvious tissue expansion facilitated by such dilation. What may be less obvious is, if a person has erectile dysfunction (ED), they (most likely) have endothelial dysfunction, meaning their health problems extend beyond the bedroom. Specialized centers can perform an endothelial function test on anyone. This easy test tells your doctor how healthy your arteries are and how readily they can deliver blood in response to exercise or other activities.

The scientists in New Zealand acquired week-old frying oil (rich in MegaTrans) from a typical restaurant and made a batch of fries. Four hours after study subjects ate the fries, they slipped their arms into blood pressure cuffs to test their endothelial function. The effect of the oil was unmistakable. Before the fries, the subjects' arteries had dilated normally, opening 7 percent wider. Afterward, there was almost no dilation—barely one percent.[272]

(You might be wondering if the results were affected because the scientists used week-old frying oil. Well, the truth is, although law requires that fryer oil be replaced weekly, lots of restaurants use the same oil for more than a week. One restaurant owner told me of a new oil that extends this time to two weeks or even longer.[273] So we have to believe that the week-old oil used in the study was, like it or not, a good example of what our fries are cooked in when we order them at a restaurant.)

What this test tells us is that after eating food fried in vegetable oil, your blood vessels won't work right. You may feel lethargic. Men may suffer from temporary ED. As the authors point out, exercising after a fast food meal will also stress your heart.[274] Why? MegaTrans free radicals attack the nitric oxide signal that arteries send when they sense oxygen levels are low. Without that signal, your muscles don't get the oxygen they need. The most active muscles will be the most affected—and your heart is always active.

Men with ED have sick endothelial cells that can't generate normal amounts of nitric oxide. Viagra works by helping sick endothelial cells in the penile arteries generate nitric oxide as if they were healthy. Nasty frying oil temporarily inhibits that ability. You could call it anti-Viagra. But listen up, boys: if you keep eating foods made with vegetable oil (especially if you also eat too much sugar), you'll damage those endothelial cells so much that even Viagra won't work anymore.

The New Zealand study was performed on young people with healthy arteries, but what might happen to a person whose arteries are older, or already damaged? After reading the study, I started asking patients admitted to the hospital for heart attacks what they'd eaten last. So far, *everyone* has told me they ate something fried in vegetable oil. One Japanese man had eaten fried fish, which goes to show you: the use of vegetable oil can turn an otherwise healthy meal into a 911 emergency. That winded feeling you get when you try to exercise may be a sign that you are just out of shape. But it may mean that MegaTrans has already damaged your arteries.

The Best Test for Arterial Damage

An endothelial function test will tell you something about the health of your arteries. But there's an easier way to determine whether or not they've been damaged. If you've been eating vegetable oil and sugar-rich foods, you can be certain they have. Some people want proof, of course. It's like spending money: some of us know when we've been spending more cash than we're bringing in, and others of us have to look at that bank statement to confirm the bad news. So if you can't get an endothelial function test, but you still want to test the condition of your blood vessels, there are several other things you can do.

One is to have your doctor check your fasting blood sugar level. If it's 89 or higher, you may have *prediabetes*, a condition in which your cell membranes have become too rigid to take in glucose as fast as they normally could. (This often leads to insulin resistance and full-blown diabetes.) And what makes cell membranes stiff? MegaTrans-instigated free radical damage, nutrient deficiency, and sugar. It's also not a bad idea to check your blood pressure. Normal levels range from 80 to 120 over 50 to 75. Higher than 130/80 (while relaxed) can indicate abnormal endothelial function. You can also get a test of your liver enzymes. Elevated liver enzymes occur when MegaTrans explosions damage liver cells. Finally, you can get a cholesterol test. But ordering the right test and then interpreting the test correctly requires some knowledge of the way fats circulate through your body, a physiologic function I call *the lipid cycle*.

Introducing the Lipid Cycle

The lipid cycle describes the process by which fats are packaged into particles that travel through your bloodstream in order to be delivered to various body tissues that either make immediate use of them or store them for later.

Your body needs to control and regulate every nutrient in your diet. For example, regulating calcium involves vitamins D, K2, and A and hormones estrogen, testosterone, and calcitriol, among others. To keep your blood sugar in range, the body requires insulin, glucagon, growth hormone, and leptin, among others. And to keep your sodium balanced, the body requires hormones aldosterone, renin, and angiotensin, among others. Meanwhile, your body also needs to regulate things like oxygen and carbon dioxide levels, temperature, pH, and hydration. And this is just the tip of the iceberg. Your body is the ultimate multitasking expert, and, to keep everything coordinated, your cells are designed to be absolute control freaks.

Doctors go to school to learn about these and other precision control systems that enable our body's cells to work together and put nutrients to best use. But for some reason, it doesn't dawn on most of us that the body would have systems in place for controlling fat and cholesterol utilization as well. Instead, we allow ourselves to be led to believe that keeping fat and cholesterol out of our bloodstream almost entirely, using extremely restrictive diets or drugs, is the best way to prevent heart attacks.

I prefer to understand the methods by which the body controls where fats and cholesterol go. To that end, I'd like to show you the model I've created from the best currently available evidence that shows how the body safely ferries dietary fat (from natural sources) through the bloodstream, just as it does with every other nutrient. And I'd like to help you avoid those elements of a modern diet that disrupt your body's ability to control these nutrients, thus increasing your risk for arterial disease.

How the Lipid Cycle Is Supposed to Work

If you eat like the average American, somewhere around 30 percent of your dietary calories probably come from fats.[275] After your food is broken down by enzymes in the intestine, the fat and most other nutrients get absorbed into intestinal cells (called *enterocytes*). Here, fat and fat-soluble nutrients are prepared for circulation through the bloodstream. You can eat all the fat and cholesterol you want, and none of it will get into your arteries without first being wrapped inside a special layer of protein. When they're working as designed, the special proteins suspend all the fats inside them in the solution of our bloodstream, and this is what prevents dietary fat from clogging our arteries. The resulting little blobs of fat wrapped in protein are called *lipoproteins*.

Lipoproteins are designed rather like microscopic M&Ms. Just as the can-

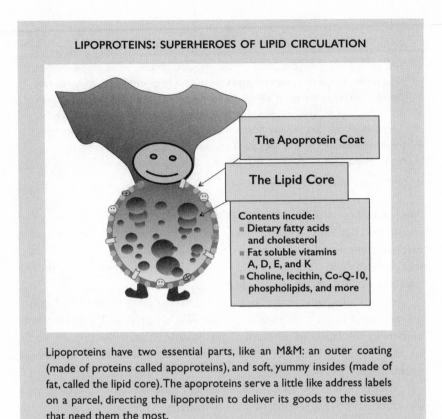

LIPOPROTEINS: SUPERHEROES OF LIPID CIRCULATION

The Apoprotein Coat

The Lipid Core

Contents incude:
- Dietary fatty acids and cholesterol
- Fat soluble vitamins A, D, E, and K
- Choline, lecithin, Co-Q-10, phospholipids, and more

Lipoproteins have two essential parts, like an M&M: an outer coating (made of proteins called apoproteins), and soft, yummy insides (made of fat, called the lipid core). The apoproteins serve a little like address labels on a parcel, directing the lipoprotein to deliver its goods to the tissues that need them the most.

dy's coating prevents the chocolate inside it from getting all over your hands, the protein coat enables lipoproteins to circulate throughout your body without getting their messy insides smeared on your arterial walls. Of course, lipoproteins don't carry chocolate. If your diet is healthy, your lipoproteins are full of essential nutrients—all kinds of good stuff.

When intestinal cells are preparing the lipids from your last meal for entry into the bloodstream, they don't throw just any old kind of protein over the fats, kick the little particle out into circulation, and say, "Good luck!" The cells of our bodies must be able to recognize lipoproteins as sources of fatty nutrients. So the protein coating (called an *apoprotein*) also serves as a kind of barcode describing the particle's origin and contents.

Lipoproteins made in the intestine are called chylomicrons. They con-

LIPOPROTEINS: THE GOOD AND BAD

The LDL and HDL your doctor talks to you about refers to two types of lipoproteins: **low-density lipoprotein** and **high-density lipoprotein**. During such discussions, you'll typically hear that LDL is "bad" and too much will damage your arteries, and that HDL is "good" and cleans your arteries. These characterizations are inaccurate. LDL, HDL and other lipoproteins (chylomicrons, VLDL and IDL) each play important roles in making sure the fat-soluble nutrition from your food gets distributed correctly.

tain some cholesterol, but mostly they contain triglycerides, other fatty nutrients (like lecithin, choline, omega-3 and omega-6, and phospholipids), varying amounts of fat-soluble vitamins, and antioxidants. Other tissues that participate in the lipid cycle make other types of lipoproteins, all with the same general design: a blob of fat wrapped in protein.[276]

As with any package delivery service, the accuracy of this labeling system is critical to the success of the whole delivery process. If anything were to damage the label (we'll return to this idea soon), the lipoprotein would fail to carry out its function, and the whole system would be thrown out of whack.

After the packaged lipoprotein leaves an intestinal cell, it travels through the bloodstream for several hours, completing many circuits. As it floats along, it deposits its fatty nutrients into the tissues that need them most.

Hungry tissues get fed by signaling endothelial cells lining their smallest blood vessels to place special proteins on their surface, which act like tiny fishing rods set to snag lipoproteins as they float by. Once snagged, the particle may unload some of its payload into the endothelial cell or, alternatively, the endothelial cell may open up a tunnel-like structure right through its center to allow the lipoprotein to pass from the bloodstream, through the endothelial cell, and directly into the hungry tissues.

Hours after a meal, the amount of fat in circulation drops as lipoproteins either exit circulation or give up their fat and shrink (gradually decreasing in size and increasing in density as they travel). Eventually, the liver picks up the shrunken, high-density remnants and sorts through the contents to recycle anything useful while discarding any waste. Unwanted or damaged fats exit by way of the liver's bile system back into the intestinal tract for disposal.

The lipid cycle can take any of several different routes. Fats can enter the circulation by way of the intestine (as lipoproteins called chylomicrons) or by way of the liver, or even by way of the fat under your skin. There are actually multiple points of entry, and even the brain may participate. The fats can exit the cycle by being transported into a hungry cell anywhere in the body, or by being exported out of the body through the liver's bile system. The liver is like a transfer station. It sorts through the incoming lipoproteins to separate the good fats from the bad. When it has collected enough good fats, the liver fashions its own lipoproteins (called VLDL, for "very low density lipoprotein"), complete with new identifying labels, and sends them back into the bloodstream again. These particles go through another arm of the cycle, following the same series of steps, delivering cargo piecemeal or transporting it to a final destination intact. Those particles that deliver cargo piecemeal eventually get small enough to be picked up by the liver again, where they will be disassembled and their fats either discarded or recycled once more.

One loop of the lipid cycle starts in the intestine and distributes lipids you just ate. Another starts in the liver and distributes lipoproteins your liver made. And a third loop starts in the *periphery*—that is, the rest of the body—and distributes lipoproteins made by the skin, brain, and other organs. Each of the three sources (intestine, liver, and periphery) manufactures its own brand of lipoproteins complete with its own proprietary labels.

How the Lipid Cycle Feeds Your Brain

The lipid cycle is an amazingly efficient system that allows cells to order up the delivery of fatty nutrients. It functions a little like Uber, the on-demand transportation service.

Here's how. Say, for example, a brain cell (named Fred) needs more omega-3 fatty acid. No problem! Like a passenger using the Uber app to request a nearby driver, Fred the brain cell makes a request that one of the circulating lipoproteins stop by and deliver omega-3. Fred does this by releasing a stream of a specific type of apoprotein called APO E into the bloodstream. Soon enough, one or more of the APO Es Fred released will encounter one or more of the body's fat-rich lipoproteins. When they meet, APO E inserts itself into a lipoprotein particle (one APO E per particle) and can now serve to direct the particle back to Fred, waiting patiently in the brain.

The APO E need not give the nutrient-carrying lipoprotein specific directions on how to find Fred in order to serve its purpose. Instead, because the APO E acts as a little handle sticking out of the lipoprotein it's riding in, it simply waits to circulate through the brain, where Fred, waiting with open arms (a receptor for APO E on his surface) will be able to grab the lipoprotein particle by its inserted APO E as it floats by.

Once Fred the brain cell has retrieved the APO E, he can help himself to all the omega-3 and whatever other fats might be on offer in the particle, and then release the lipoprotein back into circulation.

Of course, other cells in the brain (or elsewhere) may be requesting omega-3 (or other fatty nutrients) at the same time using the system. Unlike Uber, where a driver is assigned to you specifically, this is a first-come first-serve system, and other cells can poach Fred's APO E before it ever gets back to him. But the body works as a cooperative unit and eventually another APO E containing particle (with APO E perhaps made by another cell) will float by Fred to deliver the omega-3 he ordered.

As efficient as this system is, it has one important vulnerability. The APO E lacks the ability to distinguish good fats from bad. So if a person's diet is loaded with MegaTrans fat, their lipoproteins will be too—and that's what Fred will get delivered to him, whether he likes it or not.

Obviously, this intricate and ancient internal fat-distribution system is amazing and complex. And I don't mean to imply, by describing it to you, that I know everything about the way it works. I don't. But let me tell you a secret: neither do the drug manufacturers who tell us we need to get our LDL numbers down, and they have just the pill to do it.

When everything works properly, when all the connections are made without a hitch, your arteries stay wide open, pretty, pink, and clean. But when the system breaks down and the connections can't be made, the lipoproteins can't exit the bloodstream, your cholesterol numbers may climb, and the particles eventually break apart, dumping their contents into the bloodstream, where they damage epithelial cells. Repeat this process over and over, and the accumulating lipids give your arteries a yellowish, irregular, lumpy appearance that is conspicuously unhealthy (see the illustration on page 152). This is the disease we call atherosclerosis.

Lipid Cycle Breakdown Leads to Atherosclerosis

Atherosclerosis refers to hardening of the arteries. It is the diagnosis doctors give you when you've got plaque building up in your circulatory system. When your diet disrupts your lipid cycle and fats don't get where they need to go, your cholesterol numbers will often start to go out of whack. Your LDL can go up, and your HDL can go down. Neither is good, as they are both warning signs that damaged lipoproteins may be damaging your blood vessels.

The key concept here is that the underlying problem—the reason your numbers go out of whack—is not eating too much cholesterol or saturated fat. It's eating foods that disrupt the lipid cycle. So the real secret to preventing (and reversing) heart disease is avoiding foods that disrupt the lipid cycle.

What are those cycle-disrupting foods? You guessed it: foods rich in vegetable oils (and sugary foods as well). These foods disrupt the lipid cycle by damaging the very fragile proteins on their surfaces, the apolipoproteins, which

---

HOW I INTERPRET A STANDARD LIPID PANEL

The best test available to gauge the health of your lipid cycle is a properly interpreted particle size test (see page 157). If you can't afford this test, you can still get a lot of information from a standard test. Here's how I interpret the results:

Your cholesterol profile contains four different numbers: total cholesterol, LDL, HDL, and a triglyceride value. The two numbers I'm most interested in are the triglyceride and HDL levels. HDL should be over 45 in men and over 50 in women (I've seen it as high as 108). I like to see LDL less than three times the HDL value. This ratio, together with triglyceride levels less than 150, tell me a person's fat-distribution system, lipoproteins, and diet are healthy. I don't worry about a high total cholesterol number if the ratio of LDL to HDL is within an acceptable range. On the other hand, if triglycerides are above 150 and/or the HDL level is below 40, it's very likely that your lipoprotein cycle is disrupted.

---

serve to help direct the particles during their journey through the lipid cycle.

Let's take a closer look.

Bad Diet Disrupts the Lipid Cycle
by Damaging Apoproteins

As we saw in the figure on page 147 entitled "Lipoproteins: Superheroes of Lipid Circulation," the apoprotein, the protein layer encasing the round lipoprotein shown in the picture, serves as a kind of address label that helps to ensure that the particle's contents end up someplace useful in the body. I believe

HOW DYSFUNCTIONAL LIPOPROTEINS CAUSE ATHEROSCLEROSIS

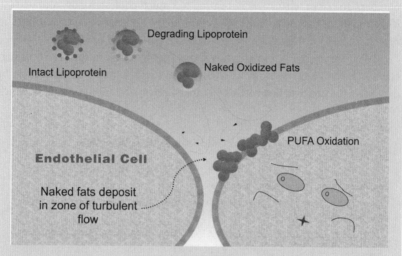

The endothelial cell on the right is worried because naked oxidized fats from degraded lipoproteins are landing on him and oxidizing his membrane PUFAs. PUFA oxidation can disrupt cell metabolism or even kill the cell (see "How Free Radicals Damage Cell Membranes" on page 141). When this kind of damage affects many endothelial cells, it can lead to the first state of athero-sclerosis, called "The Fatty Streak."

the key to preventing and reversing heart diseases lies in this idea: damage to those lipoproteins' labels disrupts the lipid cycle, which, ultimately, leads to atherosclerosis.

To better understand how damaged lipoprotein labels can cause such disruption, imagine a six-year-old girl traveling back and forth across the country by plane between the homes of her divorced mom and dad. Suppose that this young child is traveling unchaperoned and carries an identification tag on a string around her neck displaying her name, the addresses of both parents, and contact information. If the receiving parent wasn't at the airport, this tag would enable airport officials to know who she was, where she was coming from, and where she needed to go. But if the tag were to get damaged so that the words became unintelligible, she'd be lost.

If your lipoprotein particles have their labels damaged, they can get lost, too. Like vagrant children hopelessly tugging the shirtsleeves of every stranger they see, lipoproteins missing proper identification are given the cold shoulder from cells unable to recognize them. These orphaned lipoproteins float aimlessly through the bloodstream, begin to disintegrate, and ultimately collect onto the lining of your arteries (see illustration on the opposite page), where they cause problems.

What damages lipoprotein labels? One of the most important factors appears to be vegetable oil. Since 1977, lipid scientists have been writing about linoleic acid oxidation in lipoproteins. Citing articles published that year and in the 1980s by himself and by others, Dr. Spiteller, the Austrian lipid scientist, writes, "Oxidatively modified LDL is no longer recognized by the LDL receptor."[277] And how does LDL get oxidatively modified? MegaTrans fat generates free radicals that char the lipoprotein's surface, rendering it unrecognizable by the LDL receptor. The more MegaTrans-rich vegetable oil you eat, and the worse your diet in general—low in antioxidants and particularly low in naturally occurring vitamin E—the faster the LDL label (the apoprotein coat by which each LDL particle is identified) gets oxidized.[278, 279]

HOW BAD DIET CAN MAKE HDL GO DOWN

Another factor that damages lipoprotein labels is sugar. As I'll discuss in Chapter 9, sugar adheres to things by a process called *glycation*. Over time, this stiffens cell membranes, leading to prediabetes and consistently elevated blood sugar levels. Whenever blood sugar levels are high, it creates an opportunity for sugar to gum up the protein labels on your lipoprotein particles. And that's a problem.

In 1988, researchers working in Lyon, France, discovered that when the labels on HDL particles got jammed up with sugar, they simply fell off.[280] The study was done in a test tube, where the denuded HDL particles adhered to the glass. In your body, the naked fat would be exposed to blood. That's no good, and I'll explain why below. First let me point out that one of the common findings in diabetic patients is a low HDL level. One possible explanation is that the excessive sugar in their blood has knocked the coats off their HDL, and the naked particles have fallen out of circulation.

EATING MORE FAT CAN MAKE LDL CHOLESTEROL GO UP, AND WHAT TO DO IF IT DOES

You might be thinking, "You had me at butter." However, the reality is, eating more fat can sometimes make LDL cholesterol go up, whether it's healthy fat or not. How your body responds to adding fats into your diet depends on many factors, including activity, age, sex, hormones like insulin, leptin, thyroid, cortisol, and whether or not you're simply eating too much. So it's difficult to predict what will happen to your LDL until you run the experiment.

I don't see LDL as a bad thing. What I worry about is whether or not your body is able to control where fats and cholesterol in LDL will end up, and thus successfully prevent the particle and its contents from depositing inside your arteries. However, when most doctors see LDL cholesterol going up they consider this a red flag indicating that their patient either needs to change his diet or needs to take a cholesterol pill, or both. If your doctor thinks your diet is a problem and you disagree, then the conversation around your LDL can cause you unnecessary stress. I'd like to help prepare you for that conversation beforehand by teaching you about the test I use to determine if your body has lost control of its lipoproteins (see page 157).

HOW BAD DIET CAN MAKE LDL AND TRIGLYCERIDES GO UP

And what does sugar do to LDL? In 1990, another experiment investigated just that. This time, the labels didn't fall off, but rather became so deranged as to be illegible and unrecognizable to hungry cells.[281] As a result, these sugar-encrusted (glycated) LDL particles stayed in circulation too long, which would explain why some diabetics have high LDL levels: with so many undeliverable LDL packages floating around, they just start adding up.[282, 283] (When LDL levels are high because of glycation, then high LDL is a problem, as we'll see.)

Most prediabetics and diabetics have high triglyceride levels. High triglycerides suggest a serious problem with all the lipoproteins in your body. Triglyceride is not a lipoprotein, it is a component of all lipoproteins. Triglycerides are carried in both LDL and HDL particles. But the vast majority of triglyceride is carried by chylomicrons (the lipoprotein particles your gut makes right after a meal) and *very low-density lipoproteins* (VLDL), which your liver makes from recycled fats. These plump nutrient carriers want to deliver their cargo into your hungry cells. But, like all lipoproteins, they can't do the job all alone. They need a special enzyme—think of it as a dock worker—to pick the fatty acids up and carry them into the cell. A study done in 1990 showed that sugar interferes with the function of this enzyme.[284]

WHY LOWERING LDL DOESN'T DO MUCH TO PREVENT HEART DISEASE: IT'S NOT THE TRUCK—IT'S THE CARGO

Getting your LDL down well below average—to, say, 70—still leaves you with very nearly the same risk of heart attack you'd have at an LDL of 150.[285] Your risk goes down, but very little. For example, if your risk of heart attack is 20 percent when your LDL is 150, cutting that number to under 70 will drop your risk down to roughly 15 percent. Meanwhile, your risk of cancer,[286] infections,[287] depression,[288] anxiety,[289] hemorrhagic stroke (bleeding in the brain)[290] and dying (if you have severe kidney disease)[291] all go up significantly. In the decades before pharmaceutical companies created the blockbuster class of cholesterol lowering drugs called statins, doctors didn't pay much attention to LDL.

What they looked at was HDL, the so-called "good" cholesterol, because statistical evidence showed high HDL correlated with a very low risk of heart attack.[292] Get your HDL up to 60, and even if your risk of heart disease was previously a whopping 20 percent, you've just slashed your risk to less than 2 percent. Meanwhile, your risk of those above named diseases also goes down. Pretty good deal, huh? (By the way, if your HDL is low and you follow the Human Diet outlined in Chapter 13, you will almost certainly see your HDL climb within three months.)

The online risk calculators cardiologists use (and you can use, too) to determine your chances of heart attack don't even ask for your LDL level.[293] So why do we talk about LDL at all? You probably already know the answer. There's no drug to raise HDL but there are drugs to lower LDL: the statins (Lipitor, Zocor, Crestor, Vytorin, and their generic equivalents). If you sell one of these drugs, and you can use statistics and sleight of hand to convince people that getting LDL down is the strategy for living a longer life, you're spinning straw into gold.

While researchers funded by pharmaceutical corporations have been busy trying to produce evidence condemning LDL, a particle that's been with us for as long as we've been human, lipid scientists like our "rock star" scientist Dr. Spiteller have been performing a chemical inspection of the cargo carried *inside* LDL and other nutrient-carrying lipoproteins. This investigation has enabled us to gain insights into what's really causing heart attacks.

As an analogy, you could say that the researchers for pharmaceutical corporations are like investigators who, following a terrorist attack in which a government building was blown up, focused all their attention on the truck that blew everything up: *Are yellow trucks somehow uniquely explosive? Is it the size of the truck that made it detonate?* Dr. Spiteller chose a different avenue of inquiry: *What if we consider what the vehicle is carrying? Maybe it's not the vehicle itself but, rather, its cargo.* Maybe it's not the truck that's so dangerous but the hundreds of pounds of explosive petrochemical fertilizer and diesel fuel inside it!

Dr. Spiteller focused his investigation on the most prevalent PUFA in all vegetable oils—linoleic acid, a kind of omega-6.[294] His interest in linoleic acid was piqued because, as a lipid scientist, he understood how easily linoleic acid oxidizes and how damaging it can be. His research suggests that the total amount of LDL in a person's bloodstream is practically irrelevant. What matters to our health, and particularly to our risk of heart attack, is how much oxidized linoleic acid is present in LDL.

And I would agree. Over the years, I've found that people who eat foods fried in vegetable oil can have very low LDL, particularly when they're taking one of the statin drugs, but still often suffer one or more heart attacks. I've also learned that the best indicator of oxidized linoleic acid is low HDL and high particle counts. (For more on particle counts see "The Best Cholesterol Test" on page 157.)

So if you have high blood sugar, that sugar may shred the lipoprotein coats beyond recognition, or simply rip them off the particles' backs. If the particles ever do make it to a cellular dock, sugar keeps them from completing the delivery. With so many barriers to getting nutrition into hungry cells, it's no wonder people with diabetes feel hungry all the time.

As you can see, there is plenty of evidence that sugar can gum up, jam, or simply confuse the otherwise perfectly orchestrated choreography of fat and nutrient delivery that is the lipid cycle. Inevitably, this leads to a lot of misdirected—and, as far as the body is concerned, missing—cargo. How much of a problem is this? That depends on what kind of material has gone missing. If a shipping company misplaced a truckload of paper towels, the authorities could tell the HazMat units to stay home. If, on the other hand, they lost a couple pounds of high-grade uranium, there would be cause for concern. In your body, one of the most dangerous things a lipoprotein can carry is oxidized, pro-inflammatory fat—MegaTrans. When that gets spilled inside your arteries, your body calls on its own HazMat unit.[295] But in pre-diabetics and diabetics, so much bad fat is released (either all at once or over time) that the cleanup crews can't keep up, and arteries wind up getting injured by free radical cascades and, literally, fried (see illustration on page 141).

THE BEST CHOLESTEROL TEST: WHEN IT COMES TO LDL CHOLESTEROL, SIZE MATTERS

If your LDL number is high, say 160, that may or may not be a problem. Likewise, if your LDL is low, say 70, that may or may not indicate you're in good metabolic shape. What matters more than these numbers is the size of your LDL particles, because that's the best proxy we have to assess how well the LDL particles function. Bigger LDL particles are healthier LDL particles. Why? For the simple reason that healthy LDL particles can deliver the fat they're carrying efficiently. They enter the bloodstream, do a delivery job or two (which reduces their size), and are then easily recognized by the liver, which plucks the little particles out of circulation and refills them with more cholesterol and lipid supplies, making them big again.

But what happens when the liver can't recognize the smaller, partially empty lipoprotein (what lipidologists call a "remnant" particle) because the particle's protein coat (which displays vital information identifying the particle and it's cargo) has been damaged by oxidation? These smaller, orphan particles are now forced to wander through the bloodstream looking for a home until the same oxidative process that damaged their coats forces them to precipitate out of circulation and onto the delicate surfaces of your arterial walls. A regular cholesterol test can't tell you how many of these little, wayward particles are floating around destined to cause damage, but a particle-size test can! (See Chapter 14 to learn how to talk to your doctor about ordering one of these tests.)

The diet/heart disease story is a fairly simple one. Sugar and vegetable oil combine forces to destroy lipoproteins. First, the one-two punch of oxidation and glycation reactions rusts and sugar encrusts the delicate equipment on the surface of the lipoprotein (the apoproteins), which function as a kind of navigation system, preventing lipoprotein particles of all kinds from getting to their destination. Eventually, like damaged sputniks falling out of orbit, they crash land on the insides of your arteries.

FLUSH THE CLOG CONCEPT:
THE PROBLEM IS PLAQUE INSTABILITY

When a single lipoprotein lands in your arteries, it does not automatically cause a heart attack or stroke. However, if your diet is high in vegetable oil, then the fallen lipoprotein particles pile up like so much useless debris, polluting every avenue, side street, and back alley of your circulatory system.

The damage wrought by MegaTrans is nothing as peaceful as litter quietly blowing through the streets. At a molecular level, it's more like Darth Vader's evil forces strafing the surface of Yoda's home planet with white-hot streams of free radicals. Large swaths of the cell membrane are scorched as "zombie" fats spawn and free radicals propagate across the surface, incinerating everything they touch—ion channels, sugar transporters, hormone receptors (see illustration on page 140). This disables, and ultimately destroys, functional cells. This is how free radicals fry arteries. Over the years, the damage can become so advanced that during open heart surgery it is visible to the naked eye. It looks a lot like fried chicken skin.

And it's about as crispy and weak as fried chicken skin, too, and tears more easily than the unfried version. Free radical chain reactions weaken the underlying collagen scaffolding and fuse molecules together, polymerizing the arterial walls into a kind of crunchy protein plastic. Now the artery can easily rupture and bleed.[296] If blood ever contacts collagen directly it will clot, plugging up the artery. And that's how you get a heart attack or a stroke. So it's a blood clot, *not fat*, that shuts off the flow of blood. That's why ER doctors treat heart attacks and strokes with clot busters, not fat busters.

What does plaque have to do with any of this? Think like your body. Your arteries are under continued attack from MegaTrans and sugar. Although your entire vascular tree is being damaged, some sections are getting fried so badly they are in danger of rupture. Your body tries to patch these badly damaged sections with matrices of protein, calcium, and cholesterol. Most of these patches do just fine, holding the arterial section together for the rest of your life. These sturdy, calcium-reinforced plaques are called *stable plaques*.

The image of a clogged artery cutting off blood to your heart is scary. In reality, however, that's almost never what causes a heart attack or stroke. In fact, if the arterial plaques that the body has built to repair damaged arterial surfaces were perfect—permanent fixes that would remain forever stable—they would pose little threat at all. Your body has a way of responding to arterial narrowing by growing more arteries elsewhere, what doctors call collaterals. As we age this process of rerouting arterial pathways goes on all the time. Your heart muscle and other tissues are perfectly fine with this solution, as long as they continue to get a sufficient, uninterrupted supply of blood.

Stable plaques only cause problems when continued inflammation weakens the plaque material so that within the stable plaque, small patches develop that are more prone to spontaneous rupture. These weakened areas are called *unstable plaque*. Unstable plaques can also form over broad areas of an artery but are not as thick or as hard; cardiologists call them *buttery plaque*. Whether the unstable areas are large or small, they are dangerous because they can burst open, bleed, and clot.

Plaque can grow so thick that it will narrow a section of an artery enough to be visible on an angiogram. A cardiologist will typically point a finger at a picture of the narrowed section, tell you how you are a ticking time bomb, and schedule you for bypass surgery or stenting. But that one thick plaque is not the real problem. If you have such a thick, stable plaque that it's visible on an angiogram, it's a sure thing that your entire vascular tree has been damaged, and there's really no way to tell where you might develop a clot. If I had my way, instead of hearing, "You need surgery to save your life," people would hear, "You need to get off vegetable oil and sugar immediately. But if you're unwilling to do that, then I'll need to crack your chest open and replace as many of these damaged arteries as I can with cleaner blood vessels from somewhere else in your body."

HOW FAST FOOD CAUSES BIRTH DEFECTS

Eating vegetable oil doesn't just mess up your arteries. Those disruptive free radicals can interfere with nearly everything a cell might need to do, leading to almost any disease you can name.[297, 298]

At no point in our life cycle is this disruption more devastating than while we're developing in the womb. In 2006, when researchers tested the blood of mothers whose babies were born with congenital spinal and heart defects, they found evidence of oxidative stress,[299, 300] exactly what you would expect to find in someone eating lots of vegetable oil. In 2007, an article in *Genes to Cells* showed how oxidative stress can disrupt hormone production and interfere with hormonal responses, suggesting that women who consume vegetable oil while pregnant are increasing their child's risk of all kinds of growth deformities and disease.[301] So if you are pregnant or plan on getting pregnant, banish vegetable oil and foods containing vegetable oil from your kitchen, and get the stuff out of your life.

A PLAY-BY-PLAY PICTORIAL OF A HEART ATTACK (OR STROKE)

The story of a heart attack, illustrated here, begins with degraded lipoproteins dropping out of circulation, landing on the lining of your blood vessels, where they attract a cleanup crew of white blood cells. But sometimes, during the cleanup procedure, oxygen ignites a free radical reaction so large that the underlying collagen is exposed to flowing blood. Whenever collagen contacts blood, clots form. If the clot is large enough to disrupt arterial flow, it may cause a heart attack, stroke, or venous thrombosis (a blood clot in your leg).

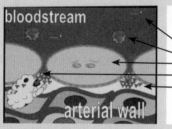

1. Degraded Lipoprotein Contents Attract a White Blood Cell

■ Oxygen
■ Lipoprotein
■ Endothelial cell
■ Degraded lipoprotein contents (MegaTrans fat)
■ Collagen layer of the arterial wall

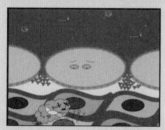

2. MegaTrans Kills the White Blood Cells

The white blood cell does its job by ingesting lipoprotein detritus, including MegaTrans. This overwhelms the white blood cell. Pro-inflammatory enzymes leak from its body into the tissue that supports the arterial wall, weakening it.

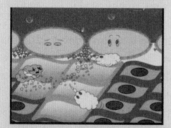

3. Inflammation Attracts More White Blood Cells

The dying white blood cell sends out pro-inflammatory chemokines, chemical signals that summon white blood cells from the surrounding tissue. Meanwhile, the leaking pro-inflammatory enzymes continue chewing through collagen, creating a soft area in the arterial wall. This is *unstable plaque* (see text).

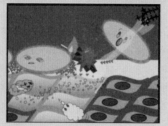

4. Oxygen Reacts Explosively with Mega-Trans.

Oxygen molecules and MegaTrans molecules with identical spin states meet, react, and explode. This dislodges and endothelial cell, exposing the underlying collagen layer. Thin wisps of collagen dangle into the bloodstream where they attract platelets. The dislodged endothelial cell knows there is more trouble ahead.

5. The Free Radical Reaction Continues

After detonating, the free radical cascade spawns more and more MegaTrans, many of which match the spin state of ordinary oxygen present in abundance in the bloodstream. As the reaction grows in strength and the explosion becomes more powerful, the collagen layer is further damaged and weakened.

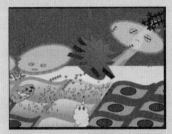

6. A Race Against Time

The inflammatory reaction has triggered the gathering white blood cells to release collagen-destroying enzymes. Now, platelets must coat the collagen layer before the enzymes so weaken the supporting arterial wall collagen that the pressure in the artery creates a tear.

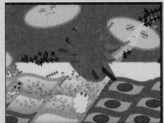

7. Worst-Case Scenario

If a tear forms, the mixture of pro-inflammatory chemicals generated by the gathering white blood cells would be exposed to flowing blood in the artery, creating an enormous clot. If this is an artery in the brain, the result would be a stroke. If in the heart, a heart attack. Let's hope the platelets can clot the area off in time.

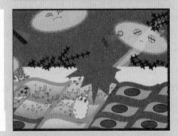

8. The Tipping Point

Today is not a good day for this person's blood vessel. The unstable plaque has ruptured into the bloodstream, and the pro-inflammatory mixture will now generate a sizable clot, shown in the next frame.

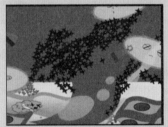

9. Deadly or Not?

There is no test to see if your arteries contain unstable plaque that can lead to this kind of clot. The commonly performed angiogram only shows narrowing that results from a buildup of thick, older plaque. Stable plaque has been hardened with a matrix of calcium, proteins, and cholesterol and is therefore unlikely to rupture.

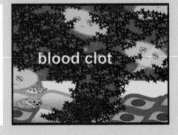

blood clot

GENETIC EXPERIMENTATION—ON YOU

You may have noticed the various cut-off levels over the years to identify people at "high risk" of a heart attack. Years ago, if your total cholesterol was 300 or less, your doctor would have said you were fine. Soon, that number was lowered to 200. Now people also watch their LDL, "safe" levels of which have been lowered from 200 to 160, to 130, to 100, and now 80. Currently, the average person's LDL level is still about what it's always been, around 120 to 130.[302] The controversial 2013 revision of the cholesterol guidelines means nearly half of the United States population between the ages of forty and seventy-five can now be labeled "high risk."[303] And drug companies are raking it in. According to Harvard's Dr. John Abramson and former *New England Journal of Medicine* editor Dr. Jerome Kassirer, the reason our medical leadership plays along, unflinchingly insisting that there's no potential harm from pushing these numbers so low, may stem from financial conflicts of interest.[304, 305]

So what's a good number? As I've said, I like to see LDL less than three times the HDL value. If it's higher, you may have prediabetes and fat-encrusted arteries. Keep in mind the really important number is your fasting blood sugar level—and we'll learn more about that in the next chapter.

The war against cholesterol is not without casualties. Women with the lowest cholesterol levels have five times more premature births than women with higher levels.[306] Even when carried to term, babies of mothers with low cholesterol are often born smaller, with abnormally small brains. Remember, epigenetic alterations can accumulate over generations. So when these small-brained babies have babies of their own while on low-cholesterol diets themselves, it's anybody's guess what the outcome of this ongoing experiment will be.

And it's not just baby's developing brain we need to worry about. In the next chapter you'll learn of the mounting evidence that, due in large part to the fact that it is such a fatty organ, our own brains are uniquely susceptible to the damaging effects of vegetable oil.

CHAPTER 8

Brain Killer

Why Vegetable Oil Is Your Brain's Worst Enemy

- Vegetable oils attack the brain at seven distinct vulnerability points using seven distinct strategies.

- All seven strategies are at work in causing autism and other childhood neurologic disorders.

- Vegetable oils make your brain more susceptible to damage by sugar.

- Eliminating these oils will enable symptoms of all sorts of brain disorders to improve, from autism to Alzheimer's.

- There are five specific kinds of foods you should eat to optimize brain health.

These days, when we look at someone who is overweight, we tend to reflexively make the connection between their body's condition and their diet. But it's now abundantly clear that body size is just one of many consequences of an imbalanced diet, as many metabolic disorders clear up when people eat better and restore normal weight. By the time you finish this chapter, my hope is that when you see a person suffering from depression, Alzheimer's, or even when you encounter a child with a learning disorder, you will likewise think about diet—both as a cause and as a cure. I sincerely hope that you will come to understand why, if you care about your mental health, the single most important product to avoid is a staple so ubiquitous it goes largely unnoticed. I'm talking, of course, about vegetable oil.

In the last chapter we learned that dietary vegetable oil can transform ordinary fatty acids into a kind of atomic tornado, tearing through cellular structures and leaving molecular wreckage in its wake. We also saw that lipid scientists have been publishing papers on this topic for decades, trying to warn us that vegetable-oil-rich diets can cause dangerous oxidative stress and are an under recognized cause of heart disease and accelerated aging. But the most terrifying thing about vegetable oil is that it's also destroying the organ most susceptible to oxidative stress, our brains. It's no exaggeration to say that vegetable oil attacks your family legacy at both ends of the generational spectrum, robbing your children of their physiologic birthright and erasing memories from our parents' and grandparents' minds.

Vegetable oil is undoubtedly the most unnatural product we eat in any significant amount. Keep in mind, GMOs (genetically modified organisms) are generally the starting point in the production of vegetable oil, and things just go downhill from there. Thanks to vegetable oil's inherent ability to inhibit life, vegetable oils are the chemicals that preserve a Twinkie for years on end. More than any other ingredient, vegetable oil is what puts the "junk" in junk food. A patient of mine on Kauai told me that the *paniolos* (Hawaiian cowboys) used to cure hide leather to make their saddles using cottonseed oil, but did they eat the stuff? *Ho, brah, dat's lolo* ("crazy"). They didn't eat it, and neither should you.

NO BRAINER: VEGETABLE OIL IS THE PERFECT BRAIN-EATING TOXIN

Vegetable oil, the perfect brain-eating toxin, promotes brain disorders both directly and indirectly by impacting these systems:

1. **Gut.** Inflammatory reactions in the gut influence brain health by way of the microbiota, the immune system, and leaky gut.

2. **Lipoproteins.** These serve as Trojan horses distributing the toxins to the brain and other target organs.

3. **Arteries.** Vegetable oil disrupts the regulation of blood flow through the brain.

4. **White blood cells.** Vegetable oil turns our immune system against us, causing food and infectious diseases to trigger nerve degenerating reactions.

5. **Nerve cellular architecture.** Vegetable oils cause an overload of oxidative reactions inside the cell, leading to the accumulation of intra-cellular trash. When this affects our white matter, we lose our mobility. When it affects our gray matter, we lose our personalities, and our connections to the world.

6. **Gene replication.** Vegetable oils impair brain development through direct mutagenic effects on DNA and altered epigenetic expression.

If you've read *Grain Brain, Cereal Killer, Sugar Crush, Sweet Poison, The Sugar Blues, Fat Chance, Sugar Nation, The Starch Solution,* or any of the other excellent books delineating the relationship between excess dietary sugar and poor health, particularly mental health, then you're well aware of the fact that sugar in any form can have toxic effects. But fructose, glucose, sucrose, starch, and other members of the sugar-sweet gang only have one weapon at their disposal, glycation, which we'll discuss in the next chapter. Vegetable oil has multiple strategies by which it wreaks havoc in your body. Like a seasoned general, it knows your weaknesses and probes every vulnerability point for the opportunity to get into your brain and dismantle your cognitive functioning. These are: (1) attack the gut; (2) deactivate the defense systems; (3) counterintelligence; (4) cut off supplies; (5) fire bombing; (6) blow up the roads; and (7) identify theft.

STRATEGY ONE: ATTACK THE GUT

Vegetable oil often initiates its attack on the brain by first attacking the gut. More and more researchers are appreciating the connection between gut and brain function. Inflammation in the gut causes heartburn, which is just the tip of the inflammation iceberg and should serve as a kind of red flag telling us that whatever we're eating is harmful. Unfortunately, many people wrongly attribute heartburn in spicy foods to the spices, and simply ignore the warning signs. Others quiet the gastric flames with heartburn medications and antacids, but these do nothing to block the damaging effects of MegaTrans fats on the gut. As you'll see, when these bad fats exit the stomach to make their way further down the digestive system, the impact on your microbial flora can have mind-altering effects.

How Vegetable Oil Causes Heartburn

Vegetable oil gets into the body via the gut. Every bite of food you swallow lands first in the stomach. The stomach releases acid and gently massages it through the food with peristaltic action, the name given to the squeezing of the intestines that serves to both help break food down and propel it forward through the digestive tract. The acid aids digestion by activating digestive enzymes and killing off pathogenic bacteria, ultimately enabling us to extract as much nutrition as possible from our diets. But in the presence of vegetable oils, stomach acid interacts with otherwise beneficial compounds in our food in such a way as to incite oxidative reactions that lead to the formation of MegaTrans fats that cause damage to the stomach lining.

In 2001, a pair of Israeli lipid scientists aware of the tendency for PUFAs to react with iron—present in high concentrations in all types of meat—wanted to evaluate whether stomach acid would accelerate or delay oxidative reactions. In a study entitled "The Stomach as Bioreactor"[307] they combined turkey meat with soy oil, the most commonly used vegetable oil worldwide, and varying amounts of acid. What they discovered was disturbing. They found that acid levels similar to those in the human stomach accelerated the reaction between soy oil and the iron in turkey meat, rapidly transforming the linoleic acid in soy oil into harmful MegaTrans fat (lipid peroxidation products). Another group of scientists whose work appeared in the *Saudi Journal of Gastroenterology* wanted to compare the effects of different fats on a stressed-out gut. Using mice as subjects, they reduced the bloodflow to the stomach to simulate the effect of emotional stress on the gut. Half the mice were fed oleic acid, the predominant component of olive oil, and the other half got the same component of vegetable oil studied by Dr. Spiteller—linoleic acid. The mice who got the vegetable oil ingredient, linoleic acid, developed lesions, whereas the mice who got the olive oil did not.[308] And a third group of lipid scientists[309]—aware that antioxidants can sometimes have the opposite of the desired effect and will, depending on the chemicals they're surrounded by, potentially act as pro-oxidants—evaluated the antioxidant vitamin C. Using a model stomach, they tested how various levels of vitamin C would affect the chemical reactions between iron (in meat) and linoleic acid. Surprisingly they found that adding just a little vitamin C to the mixture accelerated iron's ability to react with linoleic acid and led to more MegaTrans fat being formed than when they added no vitamin C at all. On the other hand, adding a lot of vitamin C slowed these reactions down again, leading to less MegaTrans fat being produced than when vitamin C was absent, which is more like what you'd expect. Taken together, these three articles suggest that cooking iron-containing foods in vegetable oil could be an important cause of inflammation-related gastrointestinal disorders including heartburn, gastritis (stomach lining inflammation), and ulcers. Throw the other variables into the mix, like vitamin C in certain concentrations, or stress, and you might be throwing gasoline on a fire.

Vegetable oil's irritating pro-inflammatory effect on the stomach lining is just the beginning; there's another twenty-eight feet of digestive tract to go and no shortage of evidence that vegetable oil can irritate and inflame every inch. For example, a 2009 article published in the journal *Gut* showed a powerful connection between linoleic acid consumption and a serious colon disorder called ulcerative colitis, which affects nearly a million Americans and which can cause bouts of bloody diarrhea. It is often confused with appendicitis, and for some unlucky patients, the only effective treatment is removal of the colon. The authors of the study concluded that simply cutting down the intake of linoleic acid could immediately reduce the number of people suffering from this painful, disfiguring disorder by 30 percent.[310]

What you can take away from this is that if you have heartburn, gastritis or other digestive symptoms, one of the simplest things you can do as a first proactive step is to eliminate the vegetable oil in your diet. I'm not saying that vegetable oil is the only possible cause of these symptoms, but eliminating vegetable oil is certainly the most important first step to take toward reducing digestive discomfort, no matter what other factors may be involved. In my decades of clinical experience I've found that vegetable oil consumption, and the attendant MegaTrans-induced inflammation, makes people more susceptible to developing food sensitivities and autoimmune reactions. If you are thinking about cutting out gluten, dairy, or other common foods but haven't yet eliminated vegetable oils, I'd recommend you consider cutting out vegetable oils first. Cutting out vegetable oil is far easier to accomplish than limiting your exposure to nearly ubiquitous toxic food contaminants, or avoiding any side effects of medications that you're not able to discontinue, and is an essential first step toward eliminating intestinal parasites and other infections.

The downstream effects of vegetable-oil–induced stomach inflammation can potentially be quite serious. Persistent stomach inflammation might lead to gastritis, or an ulcer, or cancer. Inflammation can also reduce your ability to produce adequate stomach acid, which can in turn limit the ability of beneficial bacterial colonies to stake their claim of intestinal territory. A scarcity of do-gooder bacteria in the gut can leave you open to all manner of pathogenic invasion, which can result in bacterial diarrhea (like Salmonella, Shigella, and C-diff), blood born infections, and (particularly in the very young or very old) even septic shock. Inadequate acid production also interferes with the absorp-

MOST FISH OIL SUPPLEMENTS CONTAIN MEGATRANS

You may have heard that marine oils are a good source of the essential, heart-healthy, brain-building omega-3 fatty acids, and it's true. Unfortunately, trying to extract long-chain omega-3 fats out of living organisms while keeping their molecular structure intact is a little like trying to put lightning in a bottle. Omega-3 fats are even more prone to oxidation reactions than omega-6 because (given equal fatty acid lengths) omega-3s typically have an additional double bond.[311] This extreme oxidizability mandates gentle treatment of the oil, i.e., cold-pressing and no refining or processing. Even so, after thirty days, you'd be better off saving your money for real seafood, because, as a group of lipid scientists in New Zealand investigating the safety of marine oil products explain, "Even oil stored in the dark at 4 degrees Centigrade may oxidize unacceptably within a month of storage." The New Zealand group's conclusion: "Consuming purchased supplements entails risk of exposure to unacceptably oxidized oil."[312]

My conclusion: get your omega-3 fix from real foods, like sushi, oysters, grass-fed butter, raw nuts (especially walnuts) and seeds, and lots of green leafy vegetables. By the way, another group of researchers found that fish oils react with stomach acid to form three potent genotoxic and cytotoxic compounds: 4HNE, 4HHE, and malonaldehyde.[313] Little wonder that at least half my patients tell me that fish oil supplements give them indigestion!

tion of vitamins (including antioxidants that ameliorate the dangerous effects of vegetable oils in your bloodstream) and prevents digestive enzymes from doing their job—because many enzymes must be activated by acid. This in turn can lead not just to malnutrition but also to bacterial overgrowth and inflammation in the lower digestive tract, producing bloating, constipation, diarrhea, and intolerances to certain foods—all of which indicate inflammation somewhere in the small or large intestine, or both. Because the intestine contributes greatly to the overall function of your immune system, and houses the microbiota, which also contributes greatly to your overall health, this means that frequent heartburn is a red-flag symptom potentially indicating widespread damage to several body systems.

Severe heartburn is enough to make you miserable all by itself. It hurts. It disrupts sleep. It can make every meal feel like a game of Russian roulette. But more concerning still is the recent evidence of a link between heartburn and poor mental functioning. A 2016 study published in *JAMA Neurology* reported that older men using antacids to control their digestive symptoms had a 78 percent greater risk of dementia. The authors open the door to the possibility that these cognitive effects may be due to the medication. I find this explanation less compelling than the possibility that heartburn is the tip of the iceberg, indicating widespread inflammation resulting from the long-standing conflict between the human body and the pro-oxidative effects of vegetable oil.[314]

There are several deservedly influential books that argue that a healthy microbiota is a necessary prerequisite to normal brain health.[315] Conversely, they argue, an unhealthy microbiota compromises the gut lining leading to leaky gut, which, in turn, interferes with nutrient absorption and immune function in ways that directly impair mood, cognition, and memory. These popular books have brought the general public a great deal of valuable information about the role of diet in cultivating a healthy microbiota.

One of the most talked about dietary factors is grains. Lately, many physicians and researchers have shown a link between gluten and mental illnesses. In so doing they cast light on an important connection between diet and health. While I believe there is a lot to be gained by limiting refined grains and thus reducing your intake of blood-sugar-elevating empty calories, I am not yet convinced that the gluten itself is inherently toxic to the beneficial organisms living in our gut. (For more on this topic, see Chapter 14). I have, however, long suspected that vegetable oil might be directly damaging to our tiny microbial friends because of its now well-established pro-inflammatory effects that begin the moment you ingest any food containing vegetable oil. Over the past decade I've encountered plenty of circumstantial evidence to this effect, but I never had direct evidence showing that oxidized fats—which is principally what makes vegetable oils so unhealthy, the fact that they are oxidized—can completely reorder the power structure among microbial populations in the gut until I happened upon an article entitled "Obese-Type Gut Microbiota Induce Neurobehavioral Changes in the Absence of Obesity" and did some digging into the diet the researchers studied.[316]

What I found was that by feeding mice oxidized, damaged fats, researchers so profoundly altered the gut flora of the mice that it significantly altered their emotional state of mind.

How Vegetable Oil in the Gut Disrupts the Microbiota: An Inside Job

It's no fun to be fat. Of the many problems associated with obesity, the one my patients tell me bothers them most is that they feel bad about how they look, and that makes them feel hopeless and discouraged and unmotivated to sustain difficult habit change. Since 2003, researchers have found increasing evidence that the brain function of obese and normal weight people is fundamentally distinct: "Functional studies report deficits in learning, memory, and executive function in obese compared with nonobese patients."[317] Executive functioning requires being able to break down complex tasks into their individual components and gives you the ability to plan ahead. A lack of such skill is associated with anxiety and depression, which should not come as much of a surprise. After all, if you're not great at strategizing but are being forced to do so for work or a wedding—or even to go grocery shopping for the week—it can be pretty stressful, and failing at it can get depressing. If that sounds like you or someone you know, you may be relieved to hear that scientists have discovered evidence that those elements of your personality may not be nearly as personal as you might think. They may be a complication of an unhealthy balance of microbes growing in your gut. Research shows that the health of your microbiome has a direct effect on your own ability to view your circumstances and your body in a positive light. In other words, what you see in the mirror is at least in part mediated by tiny creatures living inside you.[318, 319, 320, 321, 322]

This is a compelling idea, and it's not just theoretical. One of many studies that substantiates this idea was performed with two groups of mice whose gut flora had been obliterated by large doses of antibiotics. Each group received an inoculation of microbiota isolated from either obese or normal-weight donor mice. Two weeks after the transplant, both groups underwent a battery of tests to evaluate memory and anxiety states. The mice given the obese mouse microbiota showed "significant and selective disruptions in exploratory, cognitive, and stereotypical behavior," engaged in excessive marble burying (a measure of anxiety), spent less time exploring an open field, and failed to freeze—stop what they're doing to listen—when a novel sound was played. They also failed other tests of memory and learning ability. The mice given normal-weight mouse microbiota, on the other hand, passed all of these tests with no problem. While the differences were subtle, they were significant and not mediated by excessive weight.[323]

So does this suggest that people with excess weight could benefit from what's called fecal transplant therapy, sterilizing their guts with antibiotics and infusing a bacterial slurry extracted from a skinny friend via a nasogastric tube into their stomach? It will be years, if not decades, before scientists can recommend such a radical and potentially dangerous procedure. But there may be an easier and safer way to accomplish the same beneficial shift in your microbiota: cut vegetable oil out of your diet.

In the anxious mouse study, the authors tell us they used obese mice as donors of the microbiota which ultimately transformed the study mice into little nervous wrecks. This made me wonder what it was that made the mice obese in the first place—was it their diets or a genetic tendency? It turns out that the obese donor mice were not genetically obese, but rather they were made obese through diet.[324] And what kind of diet? A very important question, since we know it was the very same diet that bred the microbes that made the experimental mice anxious and impaired their ability to learn. Well, the diets that the obese and the normal mice were fed were nearly identical except for one important factor: the amount of oxidized fats (MegaTrans) formed from the reactions between sunflower oil and lard stored for months on end in pelleted chow containing iron, copper, and ascorbate—all known to incite oxidation reactions during extended storage with PUFA and monounsaturated fats.[325] This study applies to you because although you are not living off stale, rancid rat chow that has been oxidized through months of storage, in a way you kind of are, because the oxidized vegetable-oil-rich foods typical of an American diet contain the very same blends of oxidized fats. Keep in mind, these compounds not only turned calm happy rats into skittery anxious little rodents, they also made them fat. Other toxins may impact the microbiome in a similarly negative way, like chemotherapy or infection or radioactivity.

By the way, getting at the root of what was actually in the study's food was not easy. But this is the kind of mining operation a good scientist has to do with these kinds of studies. You have to seek out with a divining rod the actual useful conclusions buried in a poorly constructed study. If you look hard enough you find out what they really did conclude; in this case, that the mice were fed not just any high-fat diet, but a high toxic–fat diet.

Thanks to research studies like this, people who never would have thought about mental health as something their diet could impact are now waking up to the potential links. And there are many surprising connections.

STRATEGY TWO: DEACTIVATE THE DEFENSE SYSTEM

The second way vegetable oil attacks your brain is by disarming its antioxidant defense system. Of all the organs in your body, the brain is most dependent on a steady stream of fresh antioxidants to defend against oxidative stress. But because vegetable oils can deplete your brain of its antioxidants, they can also compromise this most important brain-defense mechanism, leaving your delicate nerve cells subject to destructive free radical reactions and potentially devastating inflammation.

How Vegetable Oil Uses the Brain's
Physiology Against Itself

You already know that antioxidants are vital to your health, but to understand the vital role they play in the maintenance of your brain's health, you first need to understand a little about how the structure and function of your brain make it uniquely vulnerable to oxidative damage and, therefore, particularly dependent on antioxidant protection.

The brain runs on electricity. Keeping the grid online requires a constant supply of fuel. Although your brain represents just about 2 percent of your total weight, it uses a full 20 percent of the calories you're burning each minute while you sit quietly at rest. Brain cells, like all cells, produce energy by oxidizing (burning) a variety of fuels in little chambers called mitochondria.

Cell physiologists have recently found that our mitochondrial reaction chambers have a nasty habit of leaking explosive material into the surrounding cellular cytoplasm.[326] Called *superoxide anion,* this explosive material is a kind of activated oxygen molecule that escapes the boundary of the mitochondrial membrane during the transfer of electrons inside the mitochondrial electron transport chain. A little like sparks flying out of a furiously hot fireplace, superoxide anions are an unavoidable byproduct of the process of mitochondrial energy production. It seems that, just as in the outside world, the production of energy in the body comes with an inherent cost of some kind of hazardous waste.

Because of the nature of its construction, superoxide anion leakage in a brain cell creates a particularly troubling scenario. Thirty percent of the dry weight of your brain is composed of very long-chain PUFAs, some of the most highly combustible materials in the living world. DHA and AA (docosahexanoic acid and arachidonic acid, both PUFAs) are so reactive that the body uses them to respond quickly to emergencies like blood vessel breach and bacterial invasion. The brain needs them for entirely different reasons, however. These long and jointed fats are also extremely fluid and flexible, making them the perfect material for use in the connection points between nerves, called synapses.

Your thoughts are made of electric impulses. As an idea is about to manifest, electricity in the brain travels down the length of a nerve until it reaches a synapse. At the synapse, it must jump from one nerve to the next, or the thought you were about to have will evaporate before it can ever form.

All communication between nerves happens through the action of com-

pounds called *neurotransmitters* that a nerve ending releases into the space between it and the neighboring nerve it's talking to, called the *synaptic* cleft. Here's
how they make the connection between two nerves: at the terminal end of nerve
number one, neurotransmitters, including dopamine and serotonin, sit waiting
inside a bunch of tiny globules, called vesicles. Upon stimulation by an electrical
impulse coming from the head of the nerve, the vesicles in the tail end of nerve
number one immediately fuse with the cell's outer membrane, dumping their
neurotransmitter contents into the synaptic cleft. There, the neurotransmitters
can reach nerve number two and bind to a receptor that regenerates the electric
impulse on the receiving end of the synaptic cleft. For this process to work, the
vesicles must be flexible, like microscopic water balloons. And the only kinds of
fatty acids that are capable of fusing fast enough to make this all happen—literally at the speed of thought—are those extremely fluid, flexible, and unfortunately unstable long-chain PUFAs.[327]

The nature of the brain's uniquely fragile construction combined with its
intense mitochondrial energy production puts your brain in a perpetually pre-
carious state.[328] This is why, more than any other type of cell, brain cells must
do a near-perfect job of defending against the inevitable high-energy atomic
releases from the mitochondria. And the only defense mechanism cells have
at their disposal are the antioxidants. Think of antioxidants as a kind of force
field that absorbs and neutralizes free radicals that would otherwise threaten the
integrity of your brain. Without a constant supply of fresh antioxidants, sparks
flying out of the mitochondrial chamber may ignite free radical reactions in the
nerve cell membrane, damaging large sections of the cell and interfering with
basic metabolic functions. When enough cells are damaged and malfunctioning
all at once, we develop clinical symptoms. In the immediate term that would be
something along the lines of a migraine or a seizure. But as the brain ages, much
more serious problems begin to take shape.

Psychiatrists and neurologists have begun to pay more attention to the
important role these oxidative reactions play in major diseases affecting their
patients. A 2009 review article—an analysis and conclusion of recent relevant
research written by a group of neurologic researchers in Milan, Italy—advises
doctors to be aware of the harms of oxidative stresses in the nervous system.
"Oxidative stress (OS) leading to free radical attack on neural cells contributes
calamitous role [sic] to neuro-degeneration" leading to "loss of cognitive function in AD [Alzheimer's], PD [Parkinson's], MS [multiple sclerosis] and ALS
[amyotropic lateral sclerosis, a.k.a Lou Gherig's disease]."[329] And in 2014, from
the field of psychiatry, an article entitled "Oxidative Stress and Psychological
Disorders" echoed the same idea, concluding that "accumulating evidence implicates free radical-mediated pathology, altered antioxidant capacity, neurotox-

icity, and inflammation in neuropsychiatric disorders."[330] I feel we've reached a point in medical science where it's clear that when depleted of antioxidants, the brain suffers a slow death by oxidative stress. This bolsters what other doctors and authors have suggested, which is: if you want to know what's damaging the brain, look no further than oxidative stress.

On the one hand it is encouraging that so much important research is being done to show doctors and patients that something as simple as controlling oxidation reactions can help with such a vast array of otherwise not very treatable disorders. On the other hand, I find it discouraging that the authors of otherwise excellent articles such as these continue to look to antioxidant supplements or pharmaceuticals as their primary source of therapeutic solutions. We just saw in the previous section that antioxidant supplementation can produce the opposite of the desired effect, serving as a pro-oxidant, depending on the chemical milieu. So it seems to me that a safer and more productive intervention would come from, once again, looking to the scientists who specialize in lipid oxidation—the lipid scientists.

As I'll discuss in a moment, their research has shown that when your diet is high in vegetable oils, no matter how many antioxidants you get from your food or supplements, they may not even reach the brain to aid in the constant battle of protecting its tissues from the ravages of oxidative stress.

How Vegetable Oils Intercept the Delivery of Antioxidants to Your Brain

Thus far, we have seen that most researchers now agree oxidative stress plays a major role in just about every brain disease you can name, and that the brain's unique physiology makes it uniquely susceptible to oxidative stress. Now let's take a look at how pro-oxidative vegetable oils knock out the brain's antioxidant defense system at every stage of the process.

Polyunsaturated fats—the type of fats most common in all the vegetable oils—are uniquely prone to oxidative reactions. As I just described, this is the very same kind of molecule that makes up 30 percent of your brain by dry weight. And as we saw in Chapter 7, oxidative reactions readily transform PUFAs into dangerous free radicals that smash into molecules randomly, transforming them, zombie style, into high-energy molecules that are themselves capable of generating more free radicals in a cascading fashion. Your survival and reproduction depends on a working, functional brain, so it's little wonder that your body has built-in defenses that try to protect it from oxidative damage. To that end, your body depends on two lines of antioxidant defense: (1) enzymatic antioxidants, produced in almost every cell in your body; and (2) diet-derived antioxidants that you must get from the foods you eat.

Antioxidant enzymes that directly catch and neutralize reactive oxygen molecules are your body's first line of defense against oxidative stress. They use metals like zinc, copper, iron, or a sulfur-containing amino acid to trap high-energy, so-called *excited* oxygen molecules, handing off some of those oxygen molecules' energy to other molecules, effectively calming them down. The enzymes act a little like bouncers whose job it is to deal with drunken belligerent patrons—but with one key limitation: they can only deal with a specific class of free radical, characterized by a specific size, and a specific electron spin state. Think of them as bouncers who are only allowed to deal with customers between the ages of twenty-eight and thirty. These antioxidant enzymes must be in close proximity to the troublemaking "excited" oxygen molecule to catch it before it smashes into something else and thereby generates a secondary free radical. The enzyme "bouncers" are trying to deal with free radicals preemptively by going after the excited oxygen before it can cause more free radical trouble.

While the oxygen-derived free radicals are limited in possible shapes and sizes, technically called spin states and energy levels, the secondary free radicals generated by the excited oxygen can assume any one of a great number of possible shapes and sizes. To defend against these secondary free radicals, the body is armed with a second line of defense—the non-enzymatic radical scavenging antioxidants. This defense team is composed of a much more varied set of molecules than the first line of defense, to deal with the fact that the enemy whose spin states and energy levels it must match takes so many myriad forms. Like the dangerous molecules they must be prepared to stop, they come in water-soluble and fat-soluble forms. Since the 1922 discovery of vitamin E, a fat-soluble antioxidant, we've codified thousands of other compounds with antioxidant properties, including familiar vitamins A, C, and E, and less familiar plant phytochemicals like allicin (from garlic), cinnamic acid (from cinnamon), and cocoa and chocolate flavonoids. There are quite possibly millions of molecules with potentially useful antioxidant capabilities. And that's good news, because collectively, they can step in and calm down just about any kind of free radical that might form. On a whole-foods diet rich in flavor-intense vegetables, herbs, and spices, you can be assured your body is flush with all manner of antioxidants—those we know and those we have yet to discover.

So now you understand not only why antioxidants are so vitally important to the health and function of your brain, but also why a whole class of antioxidants that are not produced by the brain must be ingested through diet. Once absorbed they have to be delivered to your brain so they can join in the fight against oxidative stress. And here we have yet another point of vulnerability, because the same lipoproteins your body uses to deliver fat-soluble antioxidants and other lipid nutrients to the brain (and other body tissues) will also, on a bad diet, deliver more ammunition to the enemy, feeding the oxidative cascades that put your brain at risk.

You might be wondering, If vegetable oils and other harmful distorted fats are so bad for us, particularly for our brains, why doesn't the body just reject them or deal with them somehow? Can't the body recognize how harmful these substances are and somehow detoxify them before they reach the brain to do their damage?

This is a great question. And the answer is that, much like asbestos or mercury, the human body has not adequately adapted to deal with high levels of what is in evolutionary terms a very novel toxin. For millions of years, when lipoproteins delivered their goods, they would be delivering only the naturally occurring, healthy versions of fats. Only in the past century or so have we had the industrial technology now used to extract fragile PUFA fats from the seeds that created them. This industrial processing strips out many of the antioxidants nature intended to accompany them. As I discussed in Chapter 7, it also mutates a small but significant portion of the fragile PUFAs into MegaTrans fat,[331] molecules that are known to initiate free radical cascades (i.e., known to cause oxidative stress).

When these distorted MegaTrans fats hitch a ride inside your lipoproteins they don't just sit quietly, like stowaways. They necessarily interact with whatever antioxidants are also present in the lipoprotein[332, 333] (which would have had to come from your diet). Through this interaction the antioxidants are able to mitigate some of the damaging effects of the distorted MegaTrans fat. But the price they pay for this interaction is their lives. Like bees guarding the nest, the non-enzyme antioxidants can only sting an intruder once. After that, they're permanently out of commission. So by the time the lipoprotein vehicle arrives in the brain to deliver its cargo, many of the antioxidants that should be part of the delivery are conspicuously absent.[334] What the brain gets instead is a truck full of what it takes to be natural fat—remember that these distorted fats are so novel the brain has no mechanism for rejecting them—so it must accept the delivery.

While the method by which lipoproteins cross the blood-brain barrier is still being studied, we already know that when the arriving lipoproteins are devoid of antioxidants they can cause oxidative stress and inflammation in the central nervous system. In 2015, researchers at the Linus Pauling Institute in

CAN VEGETABLE OILS LEAD TO "EMOTIONAL EATING"?

You've probably heard that sugar is addicting, which is one of the reasons people have such a hard time weaning themselves off junk food. But what if junk food contained a major ingredient that could lower your self-esteem, make you feel hopeless, and make you far more critical of your body every time you looked in the mirror—a perfect recipe for emotional eating?

According to a recent study appearing in the *Public Library of Science*, oxidative stress (an inevitable consequence of a high-vegetable-oil diet) correlates with lower "emotional IQ."[335] The study, conducted on a sample of fifty female psychology students, investigated the possible correlation between each participant's antioxidant enzyme activity and parameters of emotional intelligence.

What the researchers found was that the women showing the highest antioxidant enzyme activity scored significantly higher in six variables: optimism, self-regard, reality-testing, stress tolerance, happiness, and impulse control.

In the next chapter, I'll discuss in detail how vegetable oil and sugar work together to predispose you to weight gain and metabolic syndrome. This study shows how the combination of sugar and vegetable oil form a perfect, biochemical weapon of addiction—reminiscent of "impact boosting" used by cigarette manufacturers—to turn junk foods, and other processed foods, into effective delivery systems of metabolic disease.

Corvallis, Oregon, investigated this problem using a zebrafish model.[336] (Zebrafish have a similar antioxidant requirement to humans, and unusually large nervous systems for their size.) They discovered that inadequate brain antioxidant supply (the focus of this study was vitamin E) translates to damage of the essential DHA, an omega-3 fatty acid that composes roughly 15 percent of the dry weight of a human brain. When the deficiency occurs during brain development, growth of the nervous system is disrupted and, in this fish model, leads to abnormal motor responses to light. And since we now know that the human brain demonstrates what neurologists call neuroplasticity (the brain's ability to grow and change) well into old age,[337] it makes sense that oxidative insult that impairs development in youth would likewise impair basic nervous system function and other aspects of neuroregeneration as we age.

So far, I've been talking about processed vegetable oils that were not used for griddle frying or subjected to extended heat. When you turn the heat on these fragile fats, the percentage of distorted fats contained in the vegetable oil you consume grows dramatically. This translates to a higher percentage of distorted fats in your lipoproteins, and an ever greater reduction in the antioxidants available for your brain.[338]

If your head is spinning from all this chemistry, the take-home is quite simple: since for every instance of vegetable oil use there's a far better and tastier alternative, why not just go with a healthier, tastier fat? Switch out the canola oil dressing for an olive oil alternative. If you can't find one, make one yourself (see recipes in Chapter 13). Instead of the usual brand-name mayo, have a taste of Primal Kitchen's new mayo product, which I can tell you is pretty good. At your local restaurant, where they no doubt fry the fish in a vegetable oil or "blended oil," ask if they can cook yours using butter. If you want to make yourself a batch of home-fries, make sure it's either peanut oil or (if you can afford it) duck fat, and that you change the oil after every couple uses.

The other takeaway from all this is that since flavor-intense vegetables tend to be great sources of antioxidants and cooking diminishes antioxidant content, just about everyone could benefit by having more fresh, raw veggies in their diet. Studies show that most flavor-imparting phytonutrient compounds also have antioxidant capacity that protects fragile PUFA fats against oxidative damage.[339] Of course, leaders of the vegan community like David Wolfe, Dr. Caldwell Esselstyn and his son Rip, Dr. Michael Greger, and Gene Stone have been telling us this for years. Given the almost unavoidable presence of vegetable oil in restaurants and supermarkets, making sure that your diet is consistently plant strong is a great way to defend yourself against the brain killers that may sneak their way onto your plate.

STRATEGY THREE: COUNTERINTELLIGENCE (GET THE BODY TO TURN ON ITSELF)

It's impossible not to notice the popularity of gluten-free diets these days—now that some supermarkets have entire aisles stocked only with gluten-free products. The argument behind these diets is that, in its most basic form, modern-day wheat bears little resemblance to its distant ancestor, the wheat cultivated ten thousand years ago. Proponents argue that modern wheat triggers inflammation, an overactive immune response, and plays a role in nearly every disease you can name, including brain diseases like Alzheimer's, Parkinson's, schizophrenia, depression, and more. As the gluten-is-bad-for-you idea has caught on—between 20[340] and 30 percent[341] of Americans are making a conscious effort to avoid products containing gluten—so too has the idea that gluten may not be good for your brain.

I agree with the idea that gluten is a real problem for a substantial number of American consumers: the statistics that claim 1 to 2 percent of us suffer from celiac disease[342] and that another 4 to 6 percent[343] have some level of gluten sensitivity seem reasonable. Where I disagree with the leaders of the anti-gluten phenomenon is with the cause-and-effect relationship.

The anti-gluten folks tell a simple story: gluten is the underlying cause of a substantial portion of modern disease. You know my argument: pro-inflammatory fat found in vegetable oil is public health enemy number one. I don't see the body's reaction to gluten as the underlying problem; I see it as a symptom. Gluten intolerance is a serious condition. But as a doctor, I think of it very much the same way as I think of other allergies.

That's why, when I see a child allergic to cats, I don't say, "Well, cats are just dangerous and we should probably all be avoiding them." The same applies when I see a child allergic to bees or peanuts or shellfish or eggs or soy or grasses or dust mites or newspaper ink or shoe leather glue or any of the hundreds of allergens doctors like me encounter on a regular basis. When I see anyone with an allergy of any kind, my first thought is that something has gone awry with my patient's immune system. Their immune system has developed a hyper-reactivity to a common protein. I don't use their allergic reaction as evidence that there is something inherently dangerous about bees or peanuts or shellfish or eggs or soy or grasses or dust mites or newspaper ink or shoe leather glue—or anything else. A recent CDC report[344] shows that all these allergies, not just gluten, are on the rise. Have these proteins all changed or has something changed about our reaction to them?

I think it's the latter. The immune system in the gut sees more foreign substances in a day—from food, bacteria, and viruses—than the systemic immune system sees in its lifetime. (Substances that the immune system treats as dangerous are called *antigens*.) The most important thing the gut immune system needs to do is be able to ignore most of them. The ability of the immune system to ignore non-threatening agents is called *immune tolerance*. And lately, our immune systems—especially those of our children—have become increasingly intolerant. Why would that be?

As we learned earlier in this chapter, vegetable oil causes inflammation in the gut, the very place where white blood cells of the immune system are doing their darndest to discriminate between the proteins you want to digest and absorb and proteins indicating the presence of potentially pathogenic bacteria (and other toxins). White blood cells play key roles in the military defense system of your body, patrolling your tissues twenty-four-seven in search of invading pathogens. When they find one, they launch an attack, literally engulfing bacteria and digesting them nearly completely. White blood cells that have ingested bacteria then travel back to central command (in your lymph nodes), where they present the bits and pieces of the bacterial outer protein coat to the white blood cell generals. These bits and pieces are analyzed and used as templates to generate antibodies that will be able to recognize the invader and destroy it more easily the next time. Surely the fact that these white blood cells are floating in a toxic vegetable oil broth won't in any way impair their ability to profile suspect bacteria and weed them out before they can pass the gates of the intestinal wall, will it?

Of course it will. The white blood cells can't see what's in your stomach; they can't see anything. All they can do is look for familiar patterns in amino acid and sugar molecules. They don't know bacterial protein from pea protein from peanuts. They only know what they've learned from the progenitor white blood cells that handed them a description of a suspect that was seen in the area of inflammation in the past. The more often your intestine has been subject to episodes of inflammation, the more frequently your white blood cells will need to haul off different suspects into the interrogation room for questioning. Many interrogations are followed by the addition of a photo to the "most-wanted protein" scrapbook. Unlike the criminal justice system in the outside world, which only has to catch the bad guy once and his photo comes down off the wall, your immune system needs to remember his description for life, because bacteria have twins. Lots of twins. The very same pathogen can reappear time and time again. As you might imagine, the more protein profiles are compiled into the scrapbook, the more likely it is that white blood cells might misidentify a food-derived protein as matching the description of a previously booked criminal. Not an easy job for a white blood cell walking the beat of the intestine. And the job is made more complicated by the continued presence of vegetable-oil-induced inflammation.

One critical piece of evidence supporting the case that vegetable oil induces significant immune system disruption comes from a 1997 study in Taiwan entitled "Effects of Dietary Oxidized Frying Oil on Immune Responses of Spleen Cells in Rats." Scientists fed one group of rats a diet containing 15 percent fresh soy oil, and fed another group of mice the same quantity of soy oil that had been used to make several batches of french fries—replicating the conditions in a typical restaurant. The feeding experiment lasted six weeks. Then, they evaluated the animals' immune system function by examining the reaction of white blood cells in the spleen to a compound from bacterial cell membranes. They chose the spleen because it's one of the locations where white blood cells congregate to exchange the latest immunological information—sort of like a briefing room for white blood cells. Their work showed that white blood cells of the rats exposed to oxidized oil overreacted significantly, and the authors concluded that "dietary oxidized frying oil may increase spontaneous spleen cell proliferation and B cell activation, which may have significance in the development of altered immunological functions." They go on to suggest a potential link between such environmentally induced immune dysfunction and the recent "rapid increase in prevalence of certain immunological diseases such as allergic diseases and auto-immune disease."[345]

Wherever white blood cells patrol for pathogens, flooding their environment with pro-inflammatory oils is like asking these patrollers to search for bad guys in the midst of a thick fog while intoxicated. They get edgy, are quick to pull the trigger, feel confused—and the next thing you know, you have a corrupt force who has a tough time defending their choices about the innocent citizens they've unintentionally attacked. And when these otherwise well-meaning patrollers are forced to work in an impossible environment, they can go so far as to attack your body's own proteins. This is the essence of all auto-immune disease. By inciting chaos, vegetable oil confuses the immune system and ultimately gets the body to turn on itself in ways that can lead to auto-immune brain disorders like multiple sclerosis, Lou Gehrig's disease, Parkinson's, and all the other neurodegenerative processes we now understand result at least in part from auto-immune attacks.

STRATEGY FOUR: CUT OFF SUPPLIES

Once vegetable oils burn through your brain's supply of antioxidants, antioxidant depletion can impair the ability of your brain to increase blood flow on demand, a process dependent upon normal endothelial function (the mechanism by which your body regulates blood flow, first introduced in chapter 7). By disrupting endothelial function and limiting blood flow, vegetable oil cuts off supplies to the most active regions of your brain. This necessarily means that, whatever mental task you may be trying to accomplish, you can feel as if you're not keeping up. What is more, as you're about to see, vegetable oils can even put chronically overworked sections of your brain at risk for tiny strokes.

Vegetable Oil Causes Brain Cramp

To understand how critical it is to maintain sufficient blood flow, it helps to realize that thinking hard—when learning a new task or concentrating on a complex problem, for instance—is effectively an athletic endeavor. By simply opening your eyes, you increase the blood flow to the area of your brain that processes visual input by 20 percent.[346] If you sequentially tap your fingers against your thumb as fast as you can, you increase the blood flow to the motor cortex by 60 percent.[347] So you might suspect that, just as you need better blood flow to support an athletic muscle, if you want to get better performance out of your brain to brighten your mood, enhance concentration, and improve cognitive abilities, blood flow is where it's at. If you are healthy, your body can readily increase blood flow to the brain without increasing heart rate or blood pressure. How does your brain do this? Exactly the same way your muscles get more blood in times of increased need: by selectively dilating arteries in the tissues working the hardest. Arterial dilation instantaneously allows more blood to flow independent of any increased work on the part of the heart.

Just as endothelial function is essential to normal heart health and male sexual function, we now have two different lines of evidence supporting the idea that better endothelial function in your brain enables you to think more nimbly and sustain concentration for longer.

The first line of evidence comes from studies evaluating nitric oxide, the molecule (first introduced in Chapter 7) that sends a message to the muscles surrounding arteries to slacken, thus permitting dilation.[348] When fuel supplies in a cluster of cells are running low, they produce nitric oxide. The nitric oxide in turn signals to nearby blood vessels that they need to dilate now in order to deliver more of the oxygen, glucose, glutamate, and other raw materials your brain cells need to maintain focus on the subject at hand.[349]

Studies show that nitric oxide signaling, and the blood flow increases it stimulates, play a central role in nerve cell maintenance, growth, and repair.[350, 351, 352] Most pertinent to anyone looking to enhance their aptitude for learning, nitric-oxide-induced blood flow also makes forming new memories physically possible as it plays a key role in what neurologists call long-term potentiation, a process required for assembling and reinforcing new synaptic connections throughout the entire cerebral cortex, striatum, and hippocampus.[353, 354]

Another line of evidence supporting the direct link between blood flow and better brain power comes from studies on the antioxidant enzymes that support endothelial function by reducing oxidative stress and, in so doing, protect nitric oxide.[355] Neuroscientists at University College, London, recently discovered a fascinating connection between an antioxidant enzyme system called CAT (for catalase) and several major markers of high cognitive functioning. They found "CAT activity correlated with . . . adaptability, stress management, [and] general mood."[356]

On the heels of these discoveries linking bloodflow to cognitive function, in 2014, a collaboration of scientists led by researchers at the California Institute of Technology hypothesized that the feeling of brain fatigue you can get from trying to learn something new or thinking too hard about the same subject for too long may simply be a failure of your brain to deliver those raw materials on demand—literally, the food for thought. "We present a model of cognitive cost based on the novel idea that the brain senses and plans for longer-term allocation of metabolic resources by purposively conserving brain activity." In other words, if there's no fuel, there's no thought. They continue: "We suggest that an individual's decision of whether or not to incur cognitive costs in a given situation can be fruitfully understood as one of decision-making strategy: an agent will only commit limited resources in cases where the payoff is worth it." In other words, reduced bloodflow to the brain reduces motivation for learning.[357]

This research has powerful implications for your ability to complete mentally demanding tasks. When you've been working on a project for a while—be it reading or doing your taxes—and get to a point where you feel you just can't concentrate any longer, it may be a direct result of blood flow failure. Very much in the same way that an overtaxed muscle will twitch briefly before giving way, nerve cells of the cerebral cortex involved in running the task appear to be forced, by lack of fuel, to simply tap out for the moment, leaving you no choice but to take a break.

So what's all this new research into blood flow and brain function got to do with vegetable oil? Earlier in this chapter we discussed how vegetable oil's ability to generate oxidative stresses can often overwhelm all our antioxidant defense systems. And since antioxidants protect nitric oxide, that means they are likely to interfere with endothelial function. What's more, you may recall that in Chapter 7 I explained how New Zealand researchers demonstrated that a single meal of fries cooked in week-old vegetable oil can cause endothelial dysfunction lasting up to twenty-four hours, disrupting the ability of muscles to get the oxygen they need on demand.[358] Multiple studies report that vegetable oil consumption is followed by a kind of diet-induced arterial aging.[359] While brain endothelial function after the ingestion of used frying oil has yet to be tested, there's every reason to believe the effect would be the same. So when you feel fatigued or like you're having a brain cramp, perhaps you literally are. Just as with a muscle cramp, when your ability to deliver nutrients and flush out waste products can't stay apace with the biochemical demands of a muscle under exertion, the same physical limits are being imposed on your brain. On a related note, I've encountered athletes who make incredible performance gains in strength simply from cutting out vegetable oil. Why would that be? All athletes know that explosive bursts of muscular activity require intense concentration to sustain them. And I suspect that these anecdotal reports of massive, rapid strength gains may be made possible thanks to an improved ability to focus on physically demanding tasks.

So if you choose to load up on foods fried in vegetable oil right before you're scheduled to take your IQ test, guess what: you got one question wrong before you even picked up the pencil. The sharpness of your mind—your thoughts, your focus, your ability to form and recall memories—all depend on adequate moment-to-moment blood flow, and, thus, vegetable oil blocks your mental flow.

In other words, when you lose the vegetable oil, you free your mind.

Migraines and Mini Strokes

In the previous chapter, I explicitly warned men with erectile dysfunction (ED) to wake up to the fact that the condition is telling them something very important about their cardiovascular health. I don't need to tell these men why Viagra can be a really good thing. But it can be a bad thing when it allows men with ED to brush aside a symptom indicative of a serious problem with their cardiovascular systems. In my perfect world, women would tell their pharmacologically ready-to-go partners, "I have a headache. And I'll keep having a headache until you take your cardiovascular health more seriously."

Well, ladies, I'm sorry to say it's your turn for some bad news. If that headache you're laying claim to is legitimate and the result of a migraine, we need to talk. Just as erectile dysfunction is a symptom to be taken seriously, if you're a woman with a history of migraines, then you need to know about the latest research warning us that female migraine sufferers may be at significantly increased risk of stroke—*no matter your age!*[360, 361, 362]

I'm not talking about the kind of stroke your grandmother is likely to have. Those are typically associated with arteriosclerosis and very often occur in areas of the brain on the lowest rung of the blood supply pecking order, the so-called watershed areas that largely depend on diffusion for their nutrient supply. For the purposes of this discussion let's define stroke as an event in which an area of brain is denied its requisite blood supply and is damaged to the extent that you can see it on an MRI. By that definition, young women with a history of migraines should be every bit as concerned about strokes—and what role their diet plays in their brain health—as their grandmothers.

In the previous section I described a link between impaired endothelial function in the cerebral cortex as a potential explanation for the feeling of mental burnout that makes you need to take a break. But what if you're driving? Or taking an exam? Or your boss is breathing down your neck? Or for whatever reason, you simply can't respond to your brain's polite request for relief?

If you've developed a migraine enduring a prolonged stressful situation, it may have been a result of vegetable oil intake forcing endothelial dysfunction to graduate to the next level, represented by a bioelectric phenomenon called *cortical spreading depression*.[363] This isn't depression as in feeling the blues; it refers to a marked reduction in normal brain electrical activity. When this disturbance occurs in the gray matter—the thinking, feeling, and dreaming part of your brain—it interferes with information processing in the affected area, often producing what's called an *aura*—a sensory aberration that manifests in different ways depending on location. For many migraine sufferers the location is the part of the brain at the back of the skull that processes vision, called the *occipital cortex*.[364] This is where you get flashing lights (called *scotoma*) or tunnel vision. If the brain area malfunctioning is the somatosensory cortex, a tactile aura will occur, often beginning as a tingling in the arm or the face and tongue. Auras in other areas of the brain will commonly impair a person's speech or cause weakness in half of the body.

Wherever it occurs, the electric disturbance results from severe, prolonged endothelial dysfunction reducing blood flow to the point that it forces nerve cell metabolism to slow so much that energy production drops.[365] If those energy levels drop below a critical threshold, the neurons can essentially go into spasm, like a docked fish flopping around as it fights for air, biochemically overexciting themselves almost to death.

In the 1990s neuroscientists used PET scanners on migraine patients during the aura just preceding a migraine to better understand the pathophysiology of an attack. They discovered that the aura phase of a migraine is associated with a dramatic reduction of blood flow in the affected area of the cerebral cortex.[366, 367] While the triggers for migraines are variable and often unpredictable—MSG, red wine, dehydration, hormone fluctuations, stress—the duration of the aura is remarkably consistent: ten to thirty minutes.

The aura begins with a reduction of cerebral blood flow in a small segment of gray matter, and the phenomenon quickly spreads. The initially impacted section soon grows electrochemically unstable, and suffers abnormally prolonged electric pulses. In response, the blood vessels in this localized area constrict, reducing blood flow even further—perhaps in a kind of last-ditch attempt to shut down abnormal nerve activity in this defined area before it either triggers a seizure or kills the affected neurons. This constriction, however, means that nearby areas will now lack adequate blood as well, causing these surrounding sections to be similarly affected. This, in turn, expands the area of disturbance to the next adjacent brain region, and the next, and the next, and so on. (Hence the "spreading" in cortical spreading depression.) The disturbance expands across the brain at a rate of one to two millimeters per minute over the course of ten to thirty minutes until an entire lobe has been affected. At this point, for unknown reasons (perhaps because the muscles contracting the arteries have run out of the calcium or other fuel required to sustain the constriction), the blood vessels suddenly dilate. This dilation opens the floodgates, allowing blood to come rushing back in, arresting the spreading depression. It also coincides precisely with the point in time that many patients in the studies report developing pain and other common migraine symptoms such as nausea, light and sound sensitivity, and fatigue.

The dilation and restoration of blood flow successfully halts the spreading depression phenomenon, but this desperate attempt by the nervous system to quash the electrical storm takes its toll. The nerves deprived of oxygen were barely getting blood for ten to thirty minutes, and now are badly damaged. While cut off from their energy supply, numerous cellular activities had to grind to a screeching halt, causing buildup of intracellular toxins and the increased membrane permeability that permits leakage of valuable supplies. The affected nerves then release inflammation-promoting chemicals called *cytokines* to signal emergency repair crews. While cytokines are necessary for the damaged nerves to get the attention they require, the inflammation diffuses to delicate nerve endings in the lining of the brain (called the *meninges*), sensitizing them. This, neuroscientists believe, is why migraine pain is usually accompanied by hyper-responsiveness to light, sound, and other sensory input—even including the pulsations of the brain's own blood vessels.[368]

It makes sense that the symptoms attendant to this spreading depression event sound a lot like the symptoms of a stroke. Both result from diminished blood flow. Given this, neurologists in multiple academic centers began to wonder about a link between migraine and abnormal brain MRI findings they'd been attributing to atherosclerotic stroke, called *deep white matter hyper-intensities*. These are bright areas that appear on MRI images of the brain to look like shining craters on the surface of the moon. The question of a possible link between migraine and stroke occurred to these scientists because many white matter hyper-intensities showed up in women without any of the typical risk factors for stroke: smoking, diabetes, hypertension, and atherosclerosis. What they did share was a history of migraine.

To investigate the possibility that these abnormalities could develop as a direct result of migraines in the absence of other risk factors, they designed a nine-year study following two groups of people, both men and women, 203 with migraines and 83 without (to serve as a control group). The study, published in *JAMA* in 2012, showed no obvious link in the men. The women, however, told quite a different story.[369]

Thirty percent of the women who had a history of migraines developed ten or more lesions within the nine-year span of the study. Of those without a history of migraine, only 9 percent developed as many lesions. Among the women with migraine, white matter hyper-intensities were also more diffusely distributed than among controls, which were generally localized to the watershed areas of the brain, just as you'd expect with atherosclerotic strokes. The younger the subject with globally dispersed lesions, the more likely it was that she had the diffuse lesions. The authors theorized it might be a matter of different strokes for different folks. While members of the younger group were developing mini strokes as a complication of their migraines, those in the older group were more likely developing silent embolic strokes due to atherosclerosis.[370]

So what are we to take from all this?

Although failure to achieve an erection may mean that you're simply not in the mood, and although a migraine might be nothing more than the natural consequence of stress or hormone fluctuation, in the context of a modern diet where vegetable oil is so ubiquitous it's difficult to avoid, migraines, just like ED, should serve as a reminder that it's always the right time to get vegetable oils out of your diet. At least as much as you can.

STRATEGY FIVE: FIRE BOMBING

A brain whose supply of antioxidants has been cut off is like a forest during a drought, cut off from its supply of rejuvenating rain, a tinderbox vulnerable to the smallest spark of lighting. One thing that can spark off a firestorm of neurologic damage is a concussive injury; even a mild concussion can instigate damaging inflammation and oxidation. But continuing research now indicates that a diet rich in vegetable oils may, in a very literal way, also add fuel to the *slow-burning* fire of oxidative stress associated with chronic progressive diseases, including Alzheimer's.

Vegetable Oil Accelerates Oxidation

Hollywood loves blowing things up. How many times have you watched the scenes where the movie's hero is walking toward the camera, triumphantly, while the background expands in a brilliant orange ball of fire as a building or a car or a bridge or what-have-you explodes, usually in super slo-mo. On the other hand, how many times have you watched the scene where the hero walks toward the camera while in the background a large metal object quietly grows covered in rust, or a heap of bananas develop brown spots indicating ripeness, or a fallen tree gradually rots. My guess is you've never seen such a scene. But though a rotting pile of bananas doesn't make for a thrilling action movie trailer, chemically, these imperceptibly slow reactions represent the same process that drives an explosion: oxidation. The major difference between an explosion and the other oxidative processes is time. Explosions happen in the blink of an eye. Ripening, rotting, and rusting occur over days or months or years.

Oxidation reactions are ongoing in our bodies all the time. We breathe oxygen because, thanks to mitochondrial enzymes, we can harness the power of oxygen to turn fat and sugar into chemical energy with a high degree of efficiency. But nothing in this universe is 100 percent efficient. So sometimes oxygen goes about its business in our bodies without enzymatic supervision, generating random reactions that our bodies do not want. It's these random oxidation reactions that rust and rot us slowly from the inside out, playing a primary role in the natural aging of the body. Wrinkles, stiffness, presbyopia (the loss of near vision resulting from a stiffening of the lens of the eye)—all the drawbacks of getting older—come at least in part from the accumulated damage of decades of oxidation reactions. (The two most important age-promoting reactions are called *lipid peroxidation* and *protein-lipid glycation*.)

I'd like to tell you that the Human Diet can completely halt oxidation and its effects on your body, allowing you to live for hundreds of years, if not indefinitely. But that wouldn't be true. What is true is that a vegetable-oil-free/high-antioxidant diet, along with plenty of restorative sleep and exercise, is the best strategy to slow the oxidation in your brain so you can remain sharp and independent, ideally, until the day you die.

The two factors most powerfully impacting whether you spend your final decades living your life as you'd have it or lose yourself in the devastation of moderate or severe Alzheimer's are: (1) the rate at which your brain is exposed to oxidative damage; and (2) your brain's ability to control oxidative damage.[371] Every day of your life, your brain is engaged in a battle for control over oxidation, and the rate at which your brain ages depends largely on the daily balance of that battle. If oxidation wins the day, your brain is moved a little further toward premature aging. If oxidation is kept in check—and you keep oxidation in check day by day and year by year—then you get to keep your wits and your memory and your sense of self, ideally, for the rest of your life.

The Flammable Mind

A blow to the head, even a small one, can trigger nerve cell injury. The injury exposes extremely oxidizable membrane PUFA fats to pro-oxidative compounds, rapidly oxidizing vast quantities of PUFAs and potentially overloading the antioxidant capacity of the brain. Because of the uniquely volatile nature of the brain's biochemistry, a relatively mild force can quickly cause massive cellular destruction. This interaction between oxidation-vulnerable PUFA structures of the brain and novel pro-oxidative distorted PUFAs from our diet is, I believe, what's behind many of the life-changing personality and mood alterations some people develop after a concussion.

Back in the 1990s, I noticed that my patients who'd gone to the emergency room after mild head trauma, and then been cleared to safely go home based on normal CT or MRI brain scans, would sometimes come to my office still impaired and not sure why. One patient, a nurse who had hit her head on an open kitchen cabinet at home a few days earlier, found herself staring blankly at a bottle of lidocaine she was supposed to prepare for the doctor she was assisting, her memory of the details of a procedure she'd performed thousands of times completely blanked out. Another, a secretary in the local university English department, had been struck while crossing the street by a slow-moving car that, in his words, "barely knocked my head" but came to me weeks later wondering if there was a connection between that minor accident and the sudden onset of headaches, dizziness, and attention deficits that had made it impossible to keep up with the usual routines of his job and were worrisome enough that he began to question his sanity.

At that time, the only explanation I could offer was based on what an attending neurosurgeon told me while on call with the hospital's trauma team back in medical school. It was after midnight in a dimly lit hospital radiology reading room as we were waiting for a victim of a New Jersey Turnpike motorcycle accident to finish his forty-minute run through the CAT scanner. The neurosurgeon explained that even with a normal scan—done primarily to catch life-threatening bleeding—the patient's brain might be seriously impaired. Such radiographically invisible forms of damage result not so much from the initial physical impact, which causes compression, but from the secondary rebound and expansion as the soft, fragile brain sloshes back and forth inside the skull, stretching the long, slender axons that conduct electricity from one nerve cell body to one another.

Later that same night, because it turned out the patient's brain was bleeding and the mounting pressure could kill him, the surgeon instructed me on how to drill a hole in the skull to help release the buildup of fluid. It's a straightforward procedure: just drill through a certain spot like you'd drill through drywall, while being extremely careful to avoid poking too far through the other side. What I remember most was when he encouraged me to "appreciate the texture" of the man's living brain by reaching my pinky finger through the little burr hole. It was terrifyingly soft, exactly like the bowl of oatmeal I had eaten for breakfast that morning in the hospital cafeteria. After experiencing the delicate structure of the brain, literally firsthand, it was easy for me to appreciate how even a mild knock like bumping your head on a cabinet could stretch, or even tear, axons.

As with any insult to body tissue, a brain injury precipitates an inflammatory reaction that can persist for days, weeks, or even months. This post-trauma inflammation can give rise to any number of post-concussive symptoms, even following a seemingly minor bump to the head. Happily, as the inflammation subdues, the cognitive deficits diminish and finally disappear.

Except, that is, when they don't. Sometimes problems continue to wax and wane for years, never allowing the head-injured person to return to full capacity at home or work. Sometimes symptoms will even worsen over time. This begs the question: Why do some people with seemingly minor impacts develop significant and worsening problems while others with more serious trauma fully recover? I think the difference lies in part in the post-concussive conditions that either facilitate or disrupt the dynamic processes of healing in the hours, days, weeks, and months following the initial injury.

Many concussive injuries compromise cell integrity. When this happens, enzymes whose function it is to oxidize PUFA fats within the cell in a highly controlled beneficial manner escape from their confined location within the cell. Once released, these enzymes can now interact with PUFA fats in the nerve cell membranes where their pro-oxidative properties are not at all beneficial and are, in fact, quite harmful. Because 30 percent of the brain's weight is comprised of these PUFAs, this enzymatic activation accelerates the normal low-grade pitter-patter of oxidative stress and rouses it into a full-blown storm of oxidative reactions.[372]

In those cases where a person walks away from major head trauma without suffering cognitive problems, it's likely because their membranes were preloaded with antioxidants that helped to contain the free radical reactions, inhibiting oxidative reactions and "cooling" the inflammation thought to be responsible for the "injury after the injury" catalyzed by the initial concussive event. The brain armed with a rich supply of antioxidants and free of pro-oxidative MegaTrans is poised to defend itself against the ravages of oxidative stress and can more quickly get to the business of repairing damaged tissues. Mechanical engineers design helmets to protect the skull from an initial concussive event; an anti-oxidative/anti-inflammatory diet is designed—as just one of its many benefits—to protect the concussed brain itself, and help it heal.

A Formula for Predicting Accelerated Aging

Emergency room staff know the phrase well: *time is brain*. They're talking

about time between the onset of stroke symptoms and the threading of a catheter into the internal carotid artery to release clot-busting drugs. But the phrase
applies aptly to a head-injured person's need to control oxidation reactions. Seconds count, as every second that goes by, every single free radical initiates a
chain reaction capable of oxidizing billions of fragile membrane PUFAs.[373] You
can express the problem as a formula. The quantity of oxidative damage a damaged brain experiences would be called oxidative stress (OS). The amount of
time before OS is controlled would be called time (T). Multiply the two together
and the product becomes the total amount of oxidative type damage (OTD) an
injured brain will suffer.

The formula would look like this: OS x T = OTD. Let's call this the healthy
brain formula. After a concussion, a brain with a lower OTD score will heal
more quickly and more completely than a brain with a higher OTD score, no
matter how old the patient, how severe the impact, or how long they're knocked
out.

In 2002 a brilliant humble Nigerian-born pathologist named Bennet Omalu showed the world what OTD looked like. In examining a thin section of a
deceased NFL player's brain, he found something very surprising: brown com-
ma-like splotches reminiscent of bats hanging from cave ceilings—*tau proteins*.
Tau proteins had long been recognized as a hallmark of Alzheimer's.[374] And
though the football player had died at forty-five, Omalu had found tau protein
concentrations consistent with "a ninety-year-old brain with advanced Alzheimer's."[375]

When he published his paper describing his findings, the now infamous
initial reaction from the NFL was one of denial. Dr. Omalu's conclusion couldn't
possibly be true. So years went by, and nothing changed. Only after more NFL
players and their families stepped forward to share their tragic stories—of memory loss, depression, anxiety, aggression, and even suicide—did the league finally take any action.

A critical part of that action was to change the guidelines that athletic trainers follow when dealing with players who have had their "bells rung." Since that
change, concussed football players are now examined carefully before they're
allowed to re-enter the game, as a secondary head trauma of an already concussed player can have multiplier effect on the player's already wounded brain,
diminishing his chances of a positive recovery outcome. My hope is that as more
team doctors and other medical professionals understand the important role
oxidative stress plays in traumatic brain injury (TBI) recovery, more steps will
be taken to coddle the post-concussive brain with a combination of stress reduction, plenty of restorative sleep, *and* dietary intervention to give the player every
possible chance of complete recovery.

Where Not to Fight Fire with Fire:
The Forest of PUFA-Rich Membranes

It's important that you fully understand how the healthy brain formula can help you to make the best real-world choices. And to do that, it's crucial to understand the relationship between your brain (particularly the PUFA fatty acids in your brain), the highly pro-inflammatory MegaTrans delivered to your brain through the consumption of vegetable oils, and the arsenal of protective, diet-derived antioxidants whose beneficent function is to protect plant and animal tissues, including the tissues of your brain, from oxidative damage.

Think of a healthy brain as a forest that gets plenty of rainfall. Everywhere you look, there are lush, verdant leaves, babbling creeks, ponds or marshes—the kind of forest that relaxes and restores the senses. The forest's health is a direct result of receiving all the moisture that its ecology has, over millennia, come to depend on and expect. The water—from rain, the water table, the moisture sustaining the soil where fungus recycles organic matter—is like antioxidants in the brain, an especially fitting metaphorical element, as moisture does in fact act as an antioxidant in the prevention of the wildly oxidative event of a forest fire. Now imagine lightning striking this healthy forest: this is a concussion. In our healthy, moist forest, a single lightning strike is unlikely to start a fire. And if it does, it probably won't be a major fire; it'll likely burn for a little while in a contained area and then burn itself out.

If a lush, moist forest is like a healthy brain, a brain without a rich complement of antioxidants is like a forest in a drought. The creeks that used to flow have been reduced to a trickle or, worse, a ribbon of cracked, dry mud. Brittle leaves and pine needles crunch underfoot. And the earthy scent of mushroom and loam is absent—just the smell of dust is in the air. It's as if the trees themselves sense what you sense, that this once verdant wonderland has been reduced to a tinder-box ready to go up in flames with the first spark. And that's exactly what happens when a single finger of heat lightning flickers down to touch the ground.

As long as we're in this forest, let's add one more metaphoric element: an abandoned meth lab in the middle of the drought-dry woods. Much like the MegaTrans fat in vegetable oil, a meth lab is something even drought-stressed forests have not had to deal with until very recently. You see, this drug lab is a real hazard, littered as it is with cans of accelerant—paint thinners, gasoline, and other dangerous flammables that, when the heat rises from the fire, are ready to explode.

Keep this metaphor in mind, because it's shorthand for understanding how, in the discussion of creating the best possible healing environment for a concussed brain, we must take into consideration not just vegetable oil *or* antioxidants alone but rather the two together. So now it should be easy to see that the best-case healing environment is a diet rich in antioxidants (fresh vegetables, herbs, and spices) and free of vegetable oils. A suboptimal environment is one in which the diet is either rich in vegetable oils and rich in antioxidants *or* absent of vegetable oils and low in antioxidants. And the worst possible dietary scenario is a diet absent in antioxidants but rich in vegetable oil—this creates the metaphorical dessicated forest with a meth lab right in the middle of it.

I'll be taking on sugar and its effects in the next chapter, but for now I should at least mention that MegaTrans fat and sugar, taken together, create a particularly volatile combination—let's say that two cans of two different chemicals in the meth lab are wildly explosive *when combined*. You'll learn more about why this combination is so deadly a little later on, and why reducing sugar while reducing vegetable oil consumption and increasing dietary intake of antioxidant-rich veggies during concussion recovery is a simple, low-cost, no-risk strategy to rebuilding the healthy rainforest of the brain.

Certainly, more research and more funding need to be focused on the very important question of how much we can improve TBI outcomes with diet. Until that happens, and until those findings are applied in a clinical setting, this physician will continue to cringe whenever I consider typical hospital food: the trays of canola-grilled overcooked meats, the canola or soy or cottonseed salad dressing, the whipped margarine on toast, the uninspiring tasteless vegetables, and the fruit punch and tapioca pudding topped with a dollop of hydrogenated vegetable oil. My antidote for this thought is the hopeful image of a future mixed martial arts superstar one day publicly attributing his or her speedy and full recovery to the caring and talented hospital chef who was allowed to cook for his patients *as if food really were medicine.*

STRATEGY SIX: BLOW UP THE ROADS

As you now understand, PUFAs are particularly prone to chemical degradation, which is why factory refining of PUFA-rich vegetable oils generates highly toxic compounds. The most toxic of these many compounds are present only in trace amounts in bottles off the shelf, but because of the zombie effect (discussed in Chapter 7), they multiply when reheated, and continue to multiply in your body even after you've consumed them. What makes these compounds so toxic to your brain? In addition to the mechanisms already discussed, they also cause the breakdown of the subcellular highways essential for normal nerve function, giving rise to delays in learning in early life, or, as we age, even dementia.

Vegetable Oil Deranges Traffic Flow
Inside the Nerve Cells

The idea that vegetable oil is a brain killer rests on the reality that it's swirling with toxic compounds. One of the worst is called 4-hydroxy-2-nonenal, or 4-HNE. Like many of the toxic fats produced by refining vegetable oils, 4HNE is derived from an omega-6 essential fatty acid our bodies require for optimal function, called linoleic acid. The processing steps (discussed in Chapter 7) squeeze the seeds too hard, distort their fragile fats, and lead to production of 4-HNE, along with other mutated versions of once-healthy PUFA fats. Present in trace amounts in bottles straight off the shelf, when the oils are used to cook your dinner, continued oxidation of the parent linoleic acid increases the concentration of 4-HNE by a factor of ten or more.[376] 4-HNE disrupts cellular function in so many ways and is implicated in so many diseases that entire journals have been devoted to describing its toxic effects.[377]

One of the most dramatic ways 4-HNE terrorizes our cells relates to the demolition of nerve cell highways, called *microtubules*. Without microtubules, it's difficult to form new memories. In a 2002 study conducted by researchers in Osaka, Japan, rats were given an anti-gout drug called colchicine to prevent the formation of new microtubules. These rats were unable to learn their way through a maze.[378]

The microtubules, in turn, depend on a protein called *tau*. As I mentioned in the previous section, a hallmark pathologic finding in brains of people who have died with either Alzheimer's or the accelerated form of Alzheimer's induced by concussions (called chronic traumatic encephalopathy, or CTE) are comma-shaped brown blotches pathologists call *tau protein tangles*. The job of tau protein is to stabilize the cellular microtubule highways similar to the way steel girders support the concrete and asphalt of an elevated roadway. Take away the girder, and the elevated roadway goes crashing to the ground. Take away tau protein, and the microtubule structure dismantles itself. As researchers in Rome described it in 2012, "Upon HNE modification, α- tubulin [a component of the microtubule] is structurally altered, and microtubules depolymerize. Therefore, cargo cannot reach its destination and the cytoskeleton is altered."[379]

But 4HNE doesn't just take away the tau girders stabilizing the neural highways, it also does something worse. It causes oxidative stresses that lead to modification of tau by phosphate groups. That modification changes tau protein's shape, making it less capable of stabilizing the microtubules, and prone to tangling and sticking to itself.[380] This leads to the development of *neurofibrillary tangles,* glommed up microtubules that not only fail to function as effective cellular roadways, but physically stick to other microtubules and block the flow of traffic.[381] When enough have become entangled with one another, the protein mass grows large enough to be seen under a microscope, in the form of those hanging bat-like structures.

This particular form of cellular disruption appears to play a role in causing the earliest objectively measured stage of Alzheimer's, called mild cognitive impairment (MCI).[382] While Alzheimer's is usually very obvious on an MRI because it causes gray matter losses and brain shrinkage, people with MCI often have normal brain volume.[383] What they don't have is the ability to make new synaptic connections. It turns out intact microtubules allow for the steady delivery of supplies essential for the development of new synapses, which are, in turn, essential for the development of new memories. This is why the common findings of MCI include things like repeatedly asking questions, making the same comments, or forgetting an important event— say, a big meeting or a friend's birthday, when that's something you wouldn't have done before.

If you're getting the feeling that I've declared war on vegetable oil, you're exactly right. But it's not for nothing. Now that you've seen up close the specific mechanisms by which vegetable oil robs your brain of the ability to form new memories, I hope that you feel like picking up a weapon and joining the fight. Nothing takes away your identity the way Alzheimer's does, with one possible exception: when the effects of vegetable oil reach past the individual and rearrange the genes that will help define the identity of your children, as in the case of Autism.

WHY THE AUTISTIC BRAIN IS UNIQUELY UNIQUE

The brains of autistic children can exhibit every manner of growth anomaly. They can be overly large due to a failure of non-contributing nerve cells to undergo the natural process of cell death that allows for normal structural development of the brain.[384] Children with autism can have unusually high numbers of local cellular connections and fewer long-distance connections.[385] They can have completely novel connections between two areas of the brain, or between an area of the brain and some other part of the body,[386] disrupting movement. Differences can be seen even at the cellular level, such as smaller cell bodies, or atypically low connectivity between nerves (called synapses).[387] The layers of the brain may not develop completely, so that the six distinct layers of gray matter are dimpled with interruptions where no differentiation is present.[388]

What does all this mean for the autistic child's day-to-day experiences? This is one of the most troubling mysteries for the parent of an autistic child, and one for which there is no easy answer. To help guide us, we can listen to, and learn from, children affected by autism who have the language to express themselves, who describe profoundly uncomfortable sensory reactions to input that most of us take for granted. When asked why autistic children perform repetitive behaviors, Carly, a young woman affected by autism who cannot speak but is eloquent on a computer keyboard, explains, "You don't know what it feels like to be me. When you can't sit still because your legs feel like they're on fire. It's a way for us to drown out all sensory input that overloads us all at once. We create output to block input."[389]

Autistic children tend not to make eye contact. Some have attributed this avoidance, perhaps wrongly, to a lack of interest in other people. Carly's story, and her continuing contribution to the autism discussion, tells us that sometimes this behavior may stem not from a lack of ability, but from a capability so acute that it leads to distraction. "Our brains are wired differently. . . . I see over a thousand pictures of a person's face when I look at them. That's why I have a hard time looking at people."[390]

Could Carly's sensory processing disturbances arise from one or more of the structural brain anomalies associated with autism? My sense is absolutely yes. And because, as with all autistic children, Carly's brain is unique—more so, by far, than those of non-autistic kids—each child's sensory experiences, capabilities, and impairments are their own.

STRATEGY SEVEN: IDENTITY THEFT

There was a patient I got to know during the years I was in Hawaii who I'll never forget because she almost always spent the entire office visit in tears. For good reason: her life was a mess. Once a successful realtor and part-time model, after having a son followed by a set of twin boys one year later, it seemed like nothing could go right for her. The first son was diagnosed with a learning disorder and Attention Deficit Disorder (ADD), and her twins were both on the autism spectrum. She lost her job, got divorced, gained 150 pounds, and though she tried to put a bright face on things, she did not seem like a happy woman.

I met her as the twins were entering puberty, their bodies flush with testosterone and not dealing with it well at all. In spite of the fact that the state provided her with four full-time in-home staff to cover twenty-four-seven care, bursts of unexpected violence were part of daily household routines. Lamps shattered. Tables upturned. On several occasions she came in with bite wounds to her hands requiring antibiotics. Once, she pulled out of her purse a clump of hair attached to a tiny section of her own scalp—torn off in the prior day's scuffle. She loved her children. She didn't blame the twins for their behavior. But she was devastated to a breaking point by the lack of normal human connection.

Many times she'd look me in the eyes and say "I know they're in there," and then she'd break down. I couldn't begin to grasp the depth of her loneliness, until one day she managed to follow the thought with "because they only act out at me. They never hurt the staff." That their anger had a consistent trajectory was her singular indication that she had any particular significance to her twins at all. She hung on to it like a lifeline.

I'd like to tell you that she implemented the Human Diet in her household and suddenly everyone got along, but she couldn't change the family's diet—even though she desperately wanted to; her life was too chaotic. This story has no happy ending. I don't retell it here because I believe that children on the spectrum cannot be as wonderful and loving as typical children. Most children on the spectrum are doing leaps and bounds better than my patient's twins in Hawaii. I tell the story of this woman's unending trial to make a very important point: there are some disorders that take your children away from you and you can never get them back. I want to stop that from happening.

And I believe we can.

What Is Autism?

The very first diagnostic manual for psychiatric disorders published in 1954 described autism simply as: "schizophrenic reaction, childhood type."[391] The next manual, released in 1980, listed more specific criteria, including "pervasive lack of responsiveness to other people" and "if speech is present, peculiar speech patterns such as immediate and delayed echolalia, metaphorical language, pronominal reversal (using *you* when meaning *me*, for instance)."[392] Of course, the terse language of a diagnostic manual can never convey the real experience of living with a child on the spectrum, or living on the spectrum yourself.

When I graduated from medical school, autism was so rarely diagnosed that none of my psychiatry exams even covered it and I and my classmates were made aware of autism more from watching the movie *Rain Man* than from studying course material. The question of whether autism (now commonly referred to as ASD) is more common now than it was then or whether we are simply recognizing it more often is still controversial. Some literature suggests that it is a diagnostic issue, and that language disorders are being diagnosed less often as autism is being diagnosed more. However, according to new CDC statistics, it appears that autism rates have risen 30 percent between 2008 and 2012. Considering that diagnostic criteria had been stable by that point in time for over a decade, increased diagnosis is unlikely to be a major factor in this 30 percent figure.[393]

Given these chilling statistics, it's little wonder that so many research dollars have been dedicated to exploring possible connections between exposure to various environmental factors and development of the disorder. Investigators have received grants to look into a possible link between autism and vaccines,[394] smoking,[395] maternal drug use (prescription and illicit),[396, 397, 398] organophosphates,[399] and other pesticides,[400] BPA,[401] lead,[402] mercury,[403] cell phones, [404] IVF and infertility treatments,[405] induced labor,[406] high-powered electric wires,[407] flame retardants,[408] ultrasound,[409] —and just about any other environmental factor you can name. You might be wondering if they've also looked into diet. But of course: alcohol,[410] cow's milk,[411] milk protein,[412] soy formula,[413] gluten,[414] and food colorings[415] have all been investigated. Guess what they've never dedicated a single study to investigating? Here's a hint: it's known to be pro-oxidative and pro-inflammatory and contains 4-HNE, 4-HHE, and MDA, along with a number of other equally potent mutagens.[416] Still haven't guessed? Okay, one last hint: it's so ubiquitous in our food supply that for many Americans it makes up as much as 60 percent of their daily caloric intake,[417] a consumption rate that has increased in parallel with rising rates of autism.

Of course, I'm talking about vegetable oil. In Chapter 2, I discussed in some detail how and why gene transcription, maintenance, and expression are necessarily imperiled in the context of a pro-inflammatory, pro-oxidative environment, so I won't go further into that here. But I do want to better acquaint you with the three PUFA-derived mutagens I just named because when they make it to the part of your cell that houses DNA, they can bind to DNA and create new, "de novo," mutations. DNA mutations affecting a woman's ovaries, a man's sperm, or a fertilized embryo can have a devastating impact on subsequent generations.

First, let's revisit 4-HNE (4-hydroxynonanol), which you may recall meeting in the above section on firebombing the highways. This is perhaps the most notorious of all the toxic fats derived from oxidation of omega-6 fatty acids, whose diversity of toxic effects requires that entire chemistry journals be devoted to 4-HNE alone. When the mutagenicity (ability to mutate DNA) of 4-HNE was first described in 1985, the cytotoxicity (ability to kill cells) had already been established for decades. The authors of a 2009

THE ECONOMICS OF GENETIC WEALTH

"I am autistic. But that's not who I am." This is how Carly, the autistic girl I mentioned earlier, describes the struggle between her autism and what she considers to be her true identity. I suspect many autistic kids would relate to that experience. While some people with autism are extremely capable, live independently, and contribute to the betterment of our world, most never really break out of their isolation.

And given that the lifetime cost of care for each child has recenly been estimated at $1.2 to $2.4 million, I think it's safe to say that if we, as a society, have the option of giving each child a better chance at typical health by reducing the rate of autism, we would benefit economically.[418]

And it does boil down to economics. Autism is, in my estimation, just another complication of the industrial diet, together with obesity, diabetes, sleep apnea, hypertension, Alzheimer's, and cancer. All these stem from the decision to ignore nutritional practices that fortified our ancestors with genetic wealth. This decision was economically driven. If what we want is cheap food, and the marketplace has spoken loud and clear in saying yes, we want cheap food, then that means we get industrial seed oils instead of grass-fed butter or extra virgin unrefined olive oil, or any of the other traditional fats that cost more to make.

How much more does healthy fat cost, compared to toxic fats? When I asked my friend, Chef Debbie Lee, a restaurant consultant, she estimated the cost of using olive oil in place of one of the vegetable oils would come out to roughly fifty cents a plate. We understand financial economics because you can hold a dollar in your hand. My hope is that we will some day see more value in the economics of genetic wealth and come to appreciate the immeasurable value of the gifts of a healthy body and mind.

review article explain that the reason it had taken so long to recognize that HNE was such an effective carcinogen was largely due to the fact that "the cytotoxicity [cell-killing ability] of 4-HNE masked its genotoxicity [DNA-mutating effect]."[419] In other words, it kills cells so readily that they don't have a chance to divide and mutate. How potently does 4-HNE damage human DNA? After interacting with DNA, 4-HNE forms a compound called an HNE-adduct, and that adduct prevents DNA from copying itself accurately. Every time 4-HNE binds to a *guanosine* (the G of the four-letter ACGT DNA alphabet), there is somewhere between a 0.5 and 5 percent chance that G will not be copied correctly, and that the enzyme trying to make a perfect copy of DNA will accidentally turn G into T.[420] Without 4-HNE, the chance of error is about a millionth of a percent.[421] In other words, 4-HNE increases the chances of a DNA mutation rate roughly a million times!

Second, 4-HHE (4-hydroxy-hexanal), which is very much like 4-HNE, his more notorious bigger brother derived from omega-6, but 4-HHE is derived instead from omega-3. If bad guys had sidekicks, 4-NHE's would be 4-HHE. Because 4-HHE does many of the same things to DNA as 4-HNE, but has only been discovered recently.[422] You see, when omega-6 reacts with oxygen, it breaks apart into two major end products, whereas omega-3, being more explosive, flies apart into four different molecules. This means each one is present in smaller amounts, and that makes them a little more difficult to study. But it doesn't make 4-HHE any less dangerous. 4-HHE specializes in burning through your glutathione peroxidase antioxidant defense system.[423] This selenium-based antioxidant enzyme is one of the three major enzymatic antioxidant defense systems, and it may be the most important player defending your DNA against oxidative stress.[424, 425]

Finally, there is malonaldehyde (MDA), proven to be a mutagen in 1984, but presumed to only come from consumption of cooked and cured meats.[426] Only in the past few decades have we had the technology to determine that MDA can be generated in our bodies as well.[427] And unlike the previous two chemicals, MDA is generated by oxidation of both omega-3 and omega-6. It may be the most common endogenously derived oxidation product. Dr. J. L. Marnett, who directs a cancer research lab at Vanderbuit University School of Medicine, Nashville, Tennessee, and who has published over 400 articles on the subject of DNA mutation, summarized his final article on MDA with the definitive statement that MDA "appears to be a major source of endogenous DNA damage [endogenous, here, meaning due to internal, metabolic factors rather than, say, radiation] in humans that may contribute significantly to cancer and other genetic diseases."[428]

There's one more thing I need to add about vegetable-oil-derived toxic breakdown products, particularly given the long list of toxins now being investigated as potential causes of autism spectrum disorders. Not only do they directly mutate DNA, they also make DNA more susceptible to mutations induced by other environmental pollutants.[429, 430] This means that if you start reading labels and taking vegetable oil out of your diet, your body will more readily deal with the thousands of contaminating toxins not listed on the labels which are nearly impossible to avoid.

Why all this focus on genes when we're talking about autism? Nearly every day a new study comes out that further consolidates the consensus among scientists that autism is commonly a genetic disorder. The latest research is focusing on *de novo* mutations, meaning mutations neither parent had themselves but that arose spontaneously in their egg, sperm, or during fertilization. These mutations may affect single genes, or they may manifest as *copy number variations*, in which entire stretches of DNA containing multiple genes are deleted or duplicated. Geneticists have already identified a staggering number of genes that appear to be associated with autism. In one report summarizing results of examining 900 children, scientists identified 1,000 potential genes: "exome sequencing of over 900 individuals provided an estimate of nearly 1,000 contributing genes."[431]

All of these 1,000 genes are involved with proper development of the part of the brain most identified with the human intellect: our cortical gray matter. This is the stuff that enables us to master human skills: the spoken language, reading, writing, dancing, playing music, and, most important, the social interaction that drives the desire to do all of the above. One need only have a few of these 1,000 genes involved in building a brain get miscopied, or in some cases just one, in order for altered brain development to lead to one's inclusion in the ASD spectrum.

So just a few troublemaker genes can obstruct the entire brain development program. But for things to go right, all the genes for brain development need to be fully functional.

Given that humans are thought to have only around 20,000 genes, and already 1,000 are known to be essential for building brain, that means geneticists have already labeled 5 percent of the totality of our genetic database as crucial to the development of a healthy brain—and we've just started looking. At what point does it become a foolish enterprise to continue to look for genes that, when mutated, are associated with autism? When we've identified 5,000? Or 10,000? The entire human genome? At what point do we stop focusing myopically only on those genes thought to play a role in autism?

I'll tell you when: when you learn that the average autistic child's genome carries de novo mutations not just in genes thought to be associated with autism, but across the board, throughout the entirety of the chromosomal landscape. Because once you've learned this, you can't help but consider that autism might be better characterized as a symptom of a larger disease—a disease that results in an overall increase in de novo mutations.

Almost buried by the avalanche of journal articles on genes associated with autism is the finding that autistic children exhibit roughly ten times the number of de novo mutations compared to their typically developing siblings.[432] An international working group on autism pronounced this startling finding in a 2013 article entitled: "Global Increases in Both Common and Rare Copy Number Load Associated With Autism."[433] (*Copy number load* refers to mutations wherein large segments of genes are duplicated too often.) What the article says is that yes, children with autism have a larger number of de novo mutations, but the majority of their new mutations are not statistically associated with autism because other kids have them, too. The typically developing kids just don't have nearly as many.

These new mutations are not only affecting genes associated with brain development. They are affecting all genes seemingly universally. What is more, there is a dose response relationship between the total number of de novo mutations and the severity of autism such that the more gene mutations a child has (the bigger the dose of mutation), the worse their autism (the larger the response). And it doesn't matter where the mutations are located—even in genes that have no obvious connection to the brain.[434] This finding suggests that autism does not originate in the brain, as has been assumed. The real problem—at least for many children—may actually be coming from the genes. If this is so, then when we look at a child with autism, what we're seeing is a child manifesting a global genetic breakdown. Among the many possible outcomes of this genetic breakdown, autism may simply be the most conspicuous, as the cognitive and social hallmarks of autism are easy to recognize.

As the authors of the 2013 article state, "Given the large genetic target of neurodevelopmental disorders, estimated in the hundreds or even thousands of genomic loci, it stands to reason that anything that increases genomic instability could contribute to the genesis of these disorders."[435] *Genomic instability*—now they're on to something. Because framing the problem this way helps us to ask the more fundamental question, *What is behind the "genomic instability" that's causing all these new gene mutations?*

In the section titled "What Makes DNA Forget" in Chapter 2, I touched upon the idea that an optimal nutritional environment is required to ensure the accurate transcription of genetic material and communication of epigenetic bookmarking, and how a pro-oxidative, pro-inflammatory diet can sabotage this delicate operation in ways that can lead to mutation and alter normal growth. There I focused on mistakes made in epigenetic programming, what you could call *de novo epigenetic abnormalities*. The same prerequisites that support proper epigenetic data communication, I submit, apply equally to the proper transcription of genetic data.

A FOUR-STEP PATH TO UNDERSTANDING
AND PREVENTING AUTISM

1. Acknowledge that autism is not an isolated disease, but rather one of a number of possible symptoms that arise with increasing frequency from an underlying problem, a ten-fold increase in de novo mutations (those muta-tions that neither parent had but the child does). Until someone comes up with a better name, let's call it De Novo Gene Mutation Syndrome.

2. Get to work learning how to prevent De Novo Gene Mutation Syndrome.

3. Understand that there will be no technological solution to De Novo Gene Mutation Syndrome.

4. Focus on identifying the healthy reproductive environment that has allowed DNA to produce healthy children with normally developed brains for thousands of generations.

What's the opposite of a supportive nutritional environment? A steady intake of pro-inflammatory, pro-oxidative vegetable oil that brings with it the known mutagenic compounds of the kind I've just described. Furthermore, if exposure to these vegetable oil-derived mutagens causes a breakdown in the systems for accurately duplicating genes, then you might expect to find other detrimental effects from this generalized defect of gene replication. Indeed we do. Researchers in Finland have found that children anywhere on the ASD spectrum have between 1.5 and 2.7 times the risk of being born with a serious birth defect, most commonly a life-threatening heart defect or neural tube (brain and spinal cord) defect that impairs the child's ability to walk.[436] Another group, in Nova Scotia, identified a similarly increased rate of minor malformations, such as abnormally rotated ears, small feet, or closely spaced eyes.[437]

What I've laid out here is the argument that the increasing prevalence of autism is best understood as a symptom of De Novo Gene Mutation Syndrome brought on by oxidative damage, and that vegetable oil is the number-one culprit in creating these new mutations. These claims emerge from a point-by-point deduction based on the best available chemical, genetic, and physiologic science. To test the validity of this hypothesis, we need more research.

DOES DE NOVO GENE MUTATION SYNDROME AFFECT
JUST THE BRAIN?

Nothing would redirect the trajectory of autism research in a more productive fashion than reframing autism as a symptom of the larger underlying
disease, which we are provisionally calling de novo gene-mutation syndrome,
or DiNGS. (Here's a mnemonic: vegetable oil toxins "ding" your DNA, like
hailstones pockmarking your car.)

If you accept my thesis that the expanding epidemic of autism is a
symptom of an epidemic of new gene mutations, then you may wonder why
the only identified syndrome of DiNGS is autism. Why don't we see all manner of new diseases associated with gene mutations affecting organs other
than the brain? We do. According to the most recent CDC report on birth
defect incidence in the United States, twenty-nine of the thirty-eight organ
malformations tracked have increased.[438]

However, these are rare events, occurring far less frequently than autism. The reason for the difference derives from the fact that the brain of
a developing baby can be damaged to a greater degree than other organs
can, while still allowing the pregnancy to carry to term. Though the complex
nature of the brain makes it the most vulnerable in terms of being affected
by mutation, this aberration of development does not make the child more
vulnerable in terms of survival in utero. The fact that autism affects the most
evolutionarily novel portion of the brain means that as far as viability of an
embryo is concerned, it's almost irrelevant. If the kinds of severely damaging
mutations leading to autism were to occur in organs such as the heart, lungs,
or kidneys, fetal survival would be imperiled, leading to spontaneous mis-
carriage. Since these organs begin developing as early as four to six weeks
of in-utero life, failure of a pregnancy this early might occur without any
symptoms other than bleeding, which might be mistaken for a heavy or late
period, and before a mother has even realized she's conceived.

If enough individuals can agree that the identity-robbing nature of
ASD is something we'd like not to invite into our lives; and if we can shake
loose this debilitating sense that the only action we can take against this epidemic is crossing our fingers with each pregnancy and praying that the little boy on the way will not be the one in forty-two who will be affected,[439]
then perhaps researchers will feel compelled to look into vegetable oil consumption as a contributing factor. And every bit as important—as research is driven
by consumer behaviors as much as anything else—if enough grocery shoppers
and restaurant goers indicate with their purchasing dollars that they know their

DE NOVO MUTATIONS IN MEN VERSUS WOMEN

A number of studies have shown that older fathers are more likely to have autistic children. According to a 2011 study, a fifty-year-old, when compared to a man younger than thirty, carries 2.2 times the risk of having a child with autism.[440] As I discuss in this chapter, some level of de novo mutations are inevitable, even in the context of a perfect diet. The reason children born to older fathers are more likely to develop autism is that de novo mutations accumulate in a man's sperm-producing cells (called *spermatogonia*) as he ages, so that the older he gets the more mutations a given sperm will carry. But, because vegetable oils are genotoxic, it's not that much of a leap to suggest that the more vegetable oil a man exposes himself to, the more mutations his spermatogonia produce. I would, therefore, expect that if a man is following a typical American diet, with up to 60 percent of his calories coming from vegetable oils, then his rate of de novo mutations will be much greater than a man following the Human Diet—vegetable-oil-free and packed with intense nutrition.

Remember the simple equation I put forth in my explanation of Alzheimer's, which described how vegetable oil's effects essentially speed up the aging process of the brain? The very same vegetable-oil-induced accelerated-aging processes occur in a man's testes every time he loads up on vegetable-oil-rich foods. To put it bluntly, this means that the testes a man carries with him into the fast food joint will be significantly older, physiologically speaking, than the mere half-hour it took for him to scarf down his burger and fries.

Monty Python does a skit where they sing about the preciousness of every single sperm, funny in part because a man's testes produce 1,500 sperm per second. But there is something miraculous about the accurate transcription of all the billions of lines of genetic code that will help define the physiologic identity of his children. And the more youth he can maintain in those miracle workers we call the spermatogonia, the better the odds for his child.

reproductive health depends on an antioxidant-rich, low-toxin diet, and specifically seek out vegetable-oil-free products, then the flow of research money will, in short order, begin to be redirected toward a better understanding of the role vegetable oil plays in robbing children of their genetic birthright.

Until the day researchers are directed to provide us with more evidence that would-be parents are well-advised to avoid vegetable oils, we can take this simple action on our own with the certainty that it will play a beneficial role in *all* aspects of your baby's development: steer clear of vegetable oils and continue to optimize your diet. By doing this, you're not so much rejecting the idea of a technological solution, but rather tapping into what is far and away the most sophisticated and effective baby-making technology that has ever existed: Mother Nature.

Now that you know what I think about Public Enemy Number One, let me tell you what I think about its conspirator, Public Enemy Number Two—sugar.

CHAPTER 9

Sickly Sweet

How a Carbohydrate-Rich Diet Blocks Metabolic Function

- Sugar is sticky, and that's why high blood and tissue levels can have toxic effects.
- The body knows sugar is toxic and releases hormones to regulate it.
- Eventually, too much sugar disrupts hormonal function.
- Too much sugar also disrupts basic cellular functions in ways that accelerate the aging process.
- Because grocery stores are full of foods that raise blood sugar, most people eat more sugar than they realize.

Now that I've made it abundantly clear that the vegetable oil present in so many foods is toxic to your health and your genetic legacy, brace yourself: you are about to be advised to throw out another ubiquitous product: sugar. Before you worry this will leave your kitchen cabinet bare, take heart. Processed foods made with vegetable oils are also the foods typically loaded with sugar, so cutting vegetable oil automatically helps you to cut sugar intake. And keep in mind that by cutting out these two deadly toxins, you'll be allowing your genes to operate as they should and immunizing yourself against chronic disease. Once you get rid of vegetable oil and sugar, and start eating the Human Diet, everything you ingest will help keep you young, slim, smart, and beautiful. I promise, even if you really love sweet stuff, cutting your sugar intake way down will not be a big deal. Getting rid of sugar allows you to taste the natural sweetness in foods that your palate couldn't previously detect. Not only do I get this feedback all the time from patients, I went through it myself. The only truly difficult part of getting sugar out of my life was the first step, accepting the fact that, because of my own chronic ailment, I had no choice.

A STICKY MESS

On August 5, 2002, I finished a cup of coffee sweetened with homemade caramel sauce and set off on a mission to retrieve a species of Hawaiian fern. The hike into the hills on the south side of Kauai took me up a steep grade through mud and three-foot grass that wound itself around the wheel of my wheelbarrow. When my knee started hurting, I figured it would get better later, as it always had. I was wrong. Way wrong. The pain would continue to get worse over the ensuing months and then worse still after a desperate surgery. Soon, I could barely make the journey from the parking lot into the grocery store, and it was a struggle just making it through my workday. Eventually, I discovered that a virus had taken residence in the fluid inside my knee. When I learned of the possible connection between sugar and immune system dysfunction, I had to make a choice: either tame my cravings for sweets or give up any hope of recovery.

How could sugar cause such a serious and unusual problem? What I had learned in medical school was that sugar was energy that could be "burned off" by exercise. Besides, the single nutrition course I took made it clear that my body's main enemy was cholesterol, not sugar and other carbs. Fortunately, my husband suspected otherwise. One day Luke handed me a newsletter he'd re-

EXERCISE AND SUGAR

If you are a competitive athlete or your job involves heavy labor, your hungry muscles act like sugar sponges, sopping the stuff from your bloodstream before the levels get dangerously high. But don't think, like I did, that exercise enables you to get away with eating junk. For one thing, that junk destroys your collagen (see Chapter 11). It also forces you to store fat. Even as a college-level cross-country runner burning thousands of calories during two-hour daily training sessions, my dorm-food diet was so low in nutrients that, in spite of all the exercise, I actually developed one of the earliest signs of diabetes, called trunkal obesity.

While far from fat at five-foot-four and 125 pounds, my waistline was surprisingly unflattering. Underneath rock-hard abs (I also did hundreds of sit-ups a day) my intestines were coated in omental fat, a very unhealthy form of fat that develops in everyone eating low-nutrient, high-carb, high-trans-fat, high-vegetable-oil diets. This gave me a classic "apple-shaped" figure even though I wasn't overweight. At age thirty-five, when I started eating better, I finally lost that omental fat and developed a more feminine waistline. (I also grew an inch taller!)

ceived from a friend and pointed to an article that said, "A half teaspoon of sugar puts white blood cells to sleep for four hours." The article was missing a few experimental details; there was no description of whether the study was done in a lab culture dish or in living subjects. Though I tend to be wary of articles missing those kinds of facts, it did prompt me to do a little research of my own. I started looking into the effects of sugar on living cells, and what I found was horrifying.

Of course, we need sugar in our bloodstream just to stay alive. Glucose is the only fuel that red blood cells— and a few other types— can use. But things go awry when you eat more than your body can deal with. Because sugar—in high concentration—is a rarity in nature, the human metabolism is simply not prepared for exposure to the 200-plus pounds the average American now consumes yearly.[441] In a different century, only the wealthy could indulge in sweets made with refined sugar. Now, sugar is a mainstay of the modern diet.

After my (long overdue) review of the literature on sugar's effects on body biochemistry, I found that the consequences of excess sugar consumption are disastrous, especially in childhood. As sugar seeps into your tissues, it coats the surface of cell membranes, with life-changing consequences. As a young girl, I would often sneak away to the corner candy store or munch on handfuls of the chocolate chips I would sometimes find hidden in the kitchen pantry, stressing my body's connective tissues already weakened by my low-fat, low-cholesterol, no-meat-on-the-bone diet. And the sugar encrusting my cells interfered with hormone receptor function, disrupting the complex series of physiologic developments scheduled to take place during puberty. As a result, I had no idea what all the fuss over boys was about until shortly after I went off to college.

SUGAR CHANGES HOW OUR HORMONES WORK

You may have heard that, on average, we gain ten pounds a decade after the age of thirty-five; women, in particular, start reporting that they can't eat like they used to. This phenomenon may be directly related to the biochemical effects of sugar binding to hormone receptors, jamming them, and rendering us insensitive to the hormone *insulin*. Once you are insulin resistant, blood sugar levels rise higher still, leading to diabetes and all its related disorders, including weight gain and circulatory and sexual dysfunction.

For the same reasons sugar jams hormone signals, it also clogs nutrient channels, weakening bone and muscle and slowing neural communication, which can impair mood and memory and lead to dementia. While all this is going on, sugar stiffens the collagen in your tendons, joints, and skin, causing arthritis and premature wrinkling, while interfering with the production of new collagen throughout your entire body. And because sugar changes the surface markers your white blood cells need to distinguish indigenous cells from invaders, it opens the door to cancer and infection.

How does sugar do all this?

Glycation: The Reason Sugar Is Bad for You

Ever notice how licked lollipops and half-chewed taffy have a tacky feeling? Sugar feels sticky because, once dissolved in water, it reacts with proteins on the surface of your skin to form easily breakable chemical bonds. When you pull your fingers apart and feel that sticky resistance, you're feeling the tug of those bonds being broken. The process by which sugar sticks to stuff is called *glycation*. Glycation reactions are reversible, but with enough heat or time, the temporary bonds become permanent due to oxidation reactions. The products of these later oxidation reactions are called *advanced glycation end products*, or AGEs. And that's a useful acronym, because AGEs make you *age* unnaturally fast.

When you toast bread, oxidation reactions generate AGEs in the proteins and sugars present in wheat. These AGEs change the bread from soft, pliable, and pale, to hard, stiff, and brown because the proteins and sugars form cross-links that stiffen the bread. The same thing happens inside your body as AGEs cross-link normally mobile proteins. This hardens your cells and tissues, making them brittle and stiff. Fortunately, at normal blood sugar levels, the reactions occur so slowly that cleanup crews of white blood cells keep them under control by breaking them down. The kidney cleans these AGEs from the blood and excretes them from the body. It is principally these waste chemicals that give urine its characteristic yellow color.

The clinical implications of having your tissues hardened by sugar-protein cross-links are vast and far-reaching. Cross-links turn the semi-permeable surfaces of arteries into impervious walls, preventing nutrients from exiting the bloodstream. When trapped nutrients can't escape your bloodstream, where do you think they end up? Lining your arteries. As we saw in Chapter 7, when lipoproteins deposit on the arterial lining, they attract white blood cells, and can cause blood clots and/or atherosclerotic plaques. A few cross-links on your white blood cells slow them down, making infections more likely and more serious. Debilitated white blood cells permit nascent cancer cells to grow under their noses, unchallenged. Are your joints creaky and stiff? AGEs can form in them, too. AGEs (primarily from high blood sugar) are one of two major biochemical phenomena that make us look and feel old (the other being free radicals, primarily from vegetable oils). To get a better idea of how AGEs impair normal body functions, let's take a closeup look.

HOW SUGAR AFFECTS YOUR
CIRCULATORY SYSTEM

Far from being a hollow tube where blood components randomly bump about, blood vessels are busy places where coordinated events take place in parallel with each other thousands of times per second. Guided only by the thermodynamics of their own design, the biologic materials in your blood perform acrobatics as perfectly choreographed as a Las Vegas circus act. This concerted effort between teams of biological micromachines is what makes a muscle contract, a sweat gland produce sweat, and your brain translate optic nerve input into a recognizable face. But when too much sugar creates cross-links between moving parts, *all* cellular activity is impaired. Let's take a look at just three cell types in your circulation—white blood cells, the blood vessel lining cells (called *endothelial* cells), and red blood cells—to see how sugar cross-links make it impossible for them to do their jobs.

Pushed by the currents of blood, circulating white blood cells travel over the lining of the blood vessels by rolling along like little tumbleweeds. When responding to the call of tissues in trouble, white blood cells must exit the bloodstream. How do they know where to go? Inflammatory chemical messages from the affected tissue seep through intercellular spaces to reach the endothelial cells lining the bloodstream. Those cells then put up little flags on their surface telling white blood cells to exit the blood vessel. The white blood cells magically transform from stiff, tumbling spheres into flowing, flat amoeba-like creatures, and wriggle through tiny spaces between endothelial cells into the troubled tissues below. All of this is basic physiology. But our knowledge of the biochemistry of sugar helps us understand how glycation reactions between sugar and protein can cross-link the endothelial cells, block those tiny spaces, and prevent white blood cells from getting to where they're needed. And it follows that the more cross-links you have, the more your immune function is impaired.

AGEs are a primary reason diabetics develop circulatory problems. Over the life of a red blood cell (three months or so), the protein-rich red cell sops up sugar like a sponge, growing stiff and bloated. One of the jobs of the spleen is to test the quality of red blood cells in active circulation. It does this by making them pass through a maze of gradually narrowing corridors. Any cell too puffed up with sugar gets destroyed. But when sugar levels are high all the

QUANTITY OVER QUALITY

Earlier in the book, we talked about the need to revise the way we think about food. Rather than "building blocks" made of carbs, fat, and protein, food is more akin to a language comprised of, and ultimately communicating with, complex dynamic living systems. That life-giving complexity is getting hard to come by.

As the remaining environment is polluted, used up, or replaced with human development, the unavoidable mathematics dictate a ratio of less complexity per capita. The more obvious outcome of this is the fact that it's becoming increasingly difficult for individuals to surround themselves with nature in their daily lives. Though less obvious, the very same process is taking place on our dinner plates.

A whole wild salmon, liver from a free-range, grass-fed calf, and a pint of unpasteurized cream from pastured cows all share in common the fact that they are highly complex living systems. And each communicates to our cells the conditions of the complex microecology from which those animals fed. What they also share is that they each require a large section of healthy earth or sea for their production. At the opposite end of the spectrum is carbohydrate. This relatively simple food, lacking in complexity, has the advantage of needing very little space to produce, and that space need not be pristine. Needless to say, it's cheap. As world resources shrink, economics increasingly necessitates that people consume more carbs, which is to say, sugar. The process represents a simple trade-off between human population size and individual health—quantity over quality. These days, much attention is devoted to access to healthcare. But the real health issue is access to nature, primarily by way of real, healthy food.

time, the spleen can't remove all the bloated cells quickly enough, so they wind up clogging tiny capillaries. This is why diabetics go blind and develop numbness and infections in their feet. What's true of white, red, and endothelial cells is true of every cell in your body. If sugar so drastically impairs the function of cells that are already fully formed, imagine what it might do to cells that are still developing.

HOW SUGAR CAUSES BIRTH DEFECTS

In Chapter 5, we discussed fetal alcohol syndrome, the term given for the constellation of congenital abnormalities attributable to maternal alcohol consumption. The more common version of this syndrome is called *fetal alcohol effects*. This describes the less profound effects of maternal consumption at (presumably) more moderate levels. Since most mothers would like to do all they can to avoid birth defects, they usually follow their doctors' advice to avoid alcohol altogether. I think doctors should apply the same kind of reasoning when it comes to the consumption of sugar.

It is an accepted medical reality that if you have diabetes you run up to ten times the risk of having a child with a major birth defect, including major facial anomalies like cleft palate. Uncontrolled diabetes has been shown to have "a profound effect on embryogenesis, organogenesis, and fetal and neonatal growth."[442] The most conscientious doctors, therefore, tell their diabetic patients hoping to get pregnant to get their diabetes under control first. But what about those women who are borderline diabetic, insulin resistant, and hyperglycemic?

In my opinion, just as doctors now prohibit even moderate drinking in pregnancy, I think it's time to take sugar consumption seriously as well. As we'll see below, tens of millions of Americans, including many expectant mothers, suffer from diabetic complications and don't know it. We know that *major* birth defects are more common in diabetics, but what about lesser growth anomalies like those of fetal alcohol effects or Sibling Symmetry Shifts? Could the cross-linking effects of a high-sugar, high-carb diet likewise impair the full development of facial features?

Given all we know about the disastrous effects of sugar on our cells, there's every reason to believe the answer is *yes*. A few cells sticking together at key points in embryologic development is very likely to disrupt and distort the development of a growing baby. This is why I counsel *all* my pregnant patients to reduce their sugar intake as much as possible. If they want something sweet, they'll have to wait for the perfect smile on their baby's face.

HOW EATING SUGAR CAUSES TYPE II DIABETES

Certain cells require a constant supply of glucose, so it must be readily available. The pancreas, a sock-shaped gland tucked behind the stomach, tries to keep sugar levels between about 70 and 85 mg/dl (in international units 4.2-4.4 mmol/ml) at all times by secreting multiple hormones including insulin—which helps to remove sugar from the bloodstream—and counterbalancing hormones like glucagon and somatostatin that all work together to keep glucose levels in that perfect Goldilocks zone. But a blast of sugar from a Big Gulp, a giant cookie, or a spongy soft piece of cake can overload the pancreatic control system and soak your tissues in sticky sugar long enough to form a mess of AGEs, which will need to be cleaned up. If the cleanup isn't finished before your next treat, cell membranes are so full of cross-links that they are slow to respond to insulin, and sugar levels rise higher. This enables more cross-links to form than before, and so the cells respond even more poorly to insulin. This is the downward spiral into which so many of us fall. Eventually, when fasting sugar levels rise above 90 (or 100, depending on the doctor), a person is diagnosed with elevated blood sugar levels (or prediabetes), and finally, as levels continue to rise, with diabetes.

Since so many people with blood sugar problems have parents with the same condition, they naturally assume it's hereditary, and therefore inevitable. But that's not the case. If anything is being passed from parent to child here, it's bad eating habits. If you can take control of your habits, you can escape the vicious cycle, normalize your blood sugar, and even cure diabetes.

Experts Recommend Treating Prediabetes as Diabetes

You may know that diabetes increases your risk of having a heart attack. What you may not have heard is that more moderate versions of elevated blood sugar are dangerous as well. A study done in 2007 showed that people whose fasting sugar was even the *slightest* bit above normal (currently defined as 100mg/dl) when admitted to the hospital with a heart attack were up to *five times more likely to die* in the next year than heart attack victims whose levels were normal.[443] These people with elevated blood sugar weren't given a diagnosis of diabetes. Instead, they were told they had "impaired fasting glucose." What that diagnosis too often translates to the patient's mind is that—since they don't have "diabetes"—they're in the clear.

But here's the truth: all the things that frighten us when we hear our doctor say the word *diabetes*—like kidney failure, blindness, stroke, amputation, heart attack, etc.—apply to impaired fasting glucose as well.[444] People with "impaired fasting glucose" or "glucose intolerance" or "insulin resistance" or "prediabetes" or even the slightest elevation of fasting blood sugar levels, should be warned that they are at risk for all the complications associated with diabetes. If it were up to me, we'd put all of it under the umbrella of diabetes. But whatever you call it, if your blood sugar is elevated, take that as a big red flag telling you that it's time to cut your sugar (and vegetable oil) intake dramatically.

So exactly how high is too high?

Two Numbers That May Save Your Life: 89 and 100

Many experts have suggested that the threshold at which we diagnose diabetes (a fasting blood sugar level of 125 mg/dl) should, in light of all this evidence, be revised down. I agree. When I first started practicing medicine, I used the cutoff that everyone else used: 125. But the longer I've been practicing medicine, the more I've noticed something remarkable: once people's fasting levels reach 89, they tend to start gaining weight. And because high blood sugar disrupts the lipid cycle, some even develop atherosclerosis. If you have a fasting level of 89 or higher, you may be on the threshold of being sucked into the downward spiral that leads to overt diabetes. In my practice, I check fasting sugar levels on anyone who has any kind of symptom attributable to diabetes or who is simply overweight. If the level is 89 or higher, I recommend that they permanently cut their total intake of carbohydrates (including sugars) down to 100 grams a day or less.

Maybe it seems as though I'm being overly strict about sugar. To put the issue into perspective, realize that two hundred years ago, refined sugar was a costly commodity traded in tiny portions, like pepper. As you'd expect, sugar-related health problems were confined to the wealthy.[445, 446] Today, thanks to cheap energy and labor—and sugar from beets and corn—diseases attributable to sugar have been made available to all.

Hypoglycemia is a commonly recognized problem of low blood sugar. But it may also be the earliest sign that a person is on their way to developing insulin resistance. The symptoms of hypoglycemia include feeling tired, hungry, shaky, or nauseated before lunch or dinner. These feelings come from adrenaline, which helps the liver pump out more sugar but also makes us shaky, nauseous, even panicky. Because sufferers often figure that their symptoms are due to low sugar levels, they often self-medicate by eating more sugar, which, as we'll see next, only makes the problem worse.

TRUE TALES OF SUGAR-HOLICS

Sugar-Induced "Spells"

Meet Mary, a nurse who worked in my office a few years ago. Always on top of her game, she double-checked the charts to make sure we doctors didn't overlook any records. To stay alert, she would eat something sweet several times a day. Not candy, mind you. Just "healthy" stuff, like fruit and energy bars. She was fit, exercised regularly, and kept her weight down. Over the years, however, she began to notice some shaking in her hands when she was hungry. She could make it stop by having another sweet snack, which she would keep stashed away in a special section of her purse. When she hit menopause, those hunger spells suddenly morphed into something more frightening. One day, when the surgeon she was assisting asked for a suture, Mary just stared into space, unresponsive and confused. She remained in a fog for about two minutes before snapping out of it. To make sure it would never happen again, she decided to eat something sweet a little more often. Later, when her blood was tested, the doctor told her everything was fine. If anything, he said, her fasting sugar levels were on the low side.

"It's my hypoglycemia," Mary told me. I told her that she was *causing* hypoglycemia by eating sweets and blunting her response to hormones so that the body produced more and more to get the same response. Neither of us was expecting what came next.

A few months later, Mary blacked out at the wheel and drove off the road into a ditch. Luckily, nobody was hurt. In the hospital, the neurologist said those spells she'd been having were seizures and put her on anti-seizure medication. But the medication made her drowsy and she didn't want to take it, so she came to me looking for an alternative.

As any menopausal woman knows, fluctuating hormone levels can cause irritability. This was part of Mary's problem. Rising and falling estrogen and progesterone were affecting her brain and causing anxiety. But that wasn't the only issue. The big problem was the foil-wrapped snack hiding in her purse. Years of the habit had soaked her tissues in extra glucose often enough to generate crosslinks too numerous to clean up. Since her cellular response to insulin was just a little delayed, her pancreas would keep releasing more. Of course, her response to glucagon—the hormone that tells the liver to release sugar—was sluggish as well. Imagine an airline pilot trying to fly a plane whose response to the controls is delayed by ten seconds or so. As her sugar levels dropped below 60, Mary's brain was deprived of glucose, triggering a stress response from the adrenal glands. They would in turn release *adrenaline*, which, like glucagon, instructs the liver to release stored glucose. Adrenaline also affects the nervous system, causing anxiety, shakiness, and even nausea. Rising and falling sugar, estrogen, and progesterone in combination with mixed signals from high levels of insulin, glucagon, and occasional bursts of adrenaline ultimately caused a short circuit in the brain that resulted in a seizure. Once a short circuit like this develops, it makes it easier to have another seizure. So taking her off the seizure medication, as she wanted me to do, could be risky.

I suggested a compromise. I recommended that she follow a strict low-carb diet, which we reviewed. I also lowered her medication a bit, monitoring her blood to ensure we were still in the therapeutic range. I cautioned that if she were ever to lapse from the diet she would need to raise the dose of medication again. After some initial difficulty taming her ferocious sweet tooth, Mary was able to follow the diet and has now been seizure-free on a low dose of medication for eight years.

Is this a happy ending? I suppose. She is, after all, less dependent on seizure medication than if she had continued her high-sugar diet. Had she continued, even the full dose of medication may not have been able to prevent the seizures completely. But here's the other side of the coin: from what I've learned about sugar and its effects on human health, it's not altogether unlikely that suffusing her bloodstream with toxic levels of glucose over a period of years may have been a sufficient cause of her seizure disorder. In other words, take the energy bar out of her purse ten years ago, and Mary might never have had any need for seizure medication, *ever*. Does this make me want to grab energy drinks, energy bars, and fruit juices out of people's hands? You bet. Not just because sugar causes illness, but because sugar-induced problems pull otherwise healthy people into a medical system that loses revenue when people are healthy. It needs them—meaning you—to be sick. That's why I'm giving you all the details. Hospitals, clinics, and much of the medical industry depend on keeping you in the dark. But your genes depend on you to learn the truth about what it takes to eat right.

"I Don't Want Heart Surgery"

Gary is a scuba instructor. His job requires him to be ready to take action whenever one of the tourists on his boat gets into trouble. When he started feeling a fluttering in his chest, he needed to nail down exactly what was happening and do something to stop it. Though he could navigate the Hawaiian currents with his eyes closed, he had no idea how to navigate the medical system. So like many people, instead of starting with a visit to his primary care doctor, he went straight to the emergency room.

The ER doctor couldn't diagnose the source of Gary's problem because when he went in everything was fine. The ER doctor ordered a few tests, including blood tests and an EKG, all of which turned out normal. Just to be thorough, the ER doc sent Gary to his primary care doctor to get a referral to a cardiologist, who did still more tests. All normal. Just to be sure, the cardiologist wanted an angiogram. If that test showed anything out of the ordinary, like a slight narrowing of an artery, the patient would be nudged into position as a candidate for a major procedure—a stent, or even heart surgery.

This is when Gary came in to see me. His regular doctor was on vacation, and he was too anxious to wait.

"I don't want heart surgery," he said. I told him that since I don't do heart surgery, he'd come to the right place. I looked over his records and only one element of his entire history caught my attention, his fasting sugar level. It was 92. Though generally considered normal, I see this number as high because, as I mentioned earlier, anything *over* 88 (89 or higher) seems to invite problems. I wasn't surprised to find his sugar was a bit high. I'd noticed that his heels were slightly calloused, and I've found that patients with high sugar levels often develop dry calluses on their heels.

The chest-fluttering Gary described is termed a *palpitation*. Palpitations are disturbances in the heart rhythm, which, in my experience, occur more often in people who eat lots of sugar. Just as with seizure disorders, sugar-induced surges in hormone and energy levels irritate the nerves. In Gary's case, the swings disturbed the nerves surrounding his heart. I asked Gary to tell me about his diet and discovered he was a classic sugar-holic. A sweet cereal for breakfast, a Snickers bar at 10:00 A.M. to buoy him through his morning lull, then a sandwich for lunch, followed by another Snickers. Oh, and don't forget the fruit juice and soda. It was a routine he'd followed for years, but now, at thirty-nine, it was catching up with him. Whenever his sugar levels dropped, the palpitations started.

I told him that if he wanted to avoid palpitations, he would need to cut his sugar in half, minimum. And to make clear the seriousness of his predicament, I also told him that his high fasting glucose was a bellwether sign that he was on the verge of losing his sensitivity to hormones—all hormones, including testosterone. Testosterone helps men (and women, by the way) maintain libido. But when you gum up testosterone receptors on the surface of cells, they don't respond to signals as readily. And when you're gumming up the cells lining the blood vessels, the vessels can't dilate and fill up with blood. What we have here is a recipe for erectile dysfunction (ED).

For Gary, this warning struck home. I explained that if he wanted to avoid diabetic complications, including ED, it would be best for him to cut sugar out altogether. And that's what he did. Within a couple weeks, he was seeing all kinds of improvements, and so was his girlfriend. He traded in sugar for something even sweeter, and sugar-induced palpitations for a better kind.

Gary didn't need heart surgery. He needed a "sugar-ectomy." Had he gotten his angiogram, there's a fair chance that the cardiologist would have found something of interest. A tiny anomaly, a narrow spot on the dye-shadow, something—anything—to convert this healthy, fit, life-loving person into a cardiac case. And once that happens, as the side effects and complications from pills and procedures begin to pile up, once you are dependent on one or more medications for the rest of your life, once a healthy heart is refashioned into a living carrying case for the latest piece of medical gadgetry, you've been absorbed into the system. And good luck finding the door. In Gary's case, as with millions of Americans, the passage into the medical labyrinth from which so many people never return is encrusted in sugar.

Cutting Cholesterol Medications by Cutting Sugar

Jane was a thin, suntanned, enthusiastic tennis player with a total cholesterol of 260 mg/dl and LDL of 170 mg/dl. A nurse, she was well indoctrinated with a fear of cholesterol. Because her father had had a heart attack, she kept her diet low in cholesterol, and she exercised fastidiously. Her cholesterol levels, she assumed, were "due to genetics." She also knew that cholesterol medications might cause muscle aches that would affect her tennis game. Still, she was so terrified of high cholesterol that she was willing to take the chance and came to me for a prescription.

Naturally, she was surprised when I said that first she needed to get a fasting blood sugar test. Now that you've read about the lipoprotein cycle in Chapter 7, you shouldn't be surprised that this is what I recommended. Blood sugar affects numerous physiologic functions, even those you might assume have nothing to do with sugar, like cholesterol.

Too much sugar makes LDL levels rise by several mechanisms. First, sugar elevates insulin. High insulin accelerates LDL production by turning on the enzyme HMGCoA-reductase—the very same enzyme statin drugs are engineered to turn off.[447] Sugar also glycates circulating LDL apoproteins, locking the affected LDL molecules in circulation by making their docking proteins unrecognizable (see Chapter 7), thus raising LDL higher. Then, over several years, sugar cross-linked capillaries grow stiff. Capillaries must remain flexible to allow the passage of LDL and other lipoproteins to underlying tissues. But once caked stiff, capillary channels cannot open fast enough, if at all; the blocked-off LDL is forced to stay in circulation longer, and LDL serum levels rise further still. Most of the cholesterol in circulation is manufactured by your body, so if your diet is high in sugar, it is nearly impossible to bring your serum cholesterol down—unless you get on a cholesterol-lowering drug.

Jane agreed to cut her sugar, and her LDL soon plummeted to 120, which, given her HDL of 85, was just fine. Jane's high LDL had nothing to do with family history and everything to do with her sugar intake. She didn't need a medication, she just needed to identify the hidden sources of sugar in her diet and avoid them.

The Sugar Headache

Susan's headaches were awful. As she described them, they felt like a hot blade had been plunged through her right eye. For twenty years, she'd been told that she had migraines and was given all kinds of migraine treatments, with little effect. Quite often, there was nothing she could do but wake her husband in the middle of the night to drive her to the ER for intravenous painkillers. Without warning, another agonizing series of headaches would materialize, tear her life apart for days or even weeks, and then just as suddenly disappear.

When I saw her, I told her a couple things she was surprised to hear. One was that these weren't migraines. They were cluster headaches, which would respond to an entirely different kind of therapy: breathing from an oxygen tank.

The second surprise was that she might be able to mitigate or even cure her headaches permanently by—you guessed it—cutting out sugar. I told her about sugar's effects on nerves and how adrenaline and other hormone fluctuations are so irritating to the brain that they can cause pain or, in extreme cases, seizures. Cluster headache sufferers are often addicted to sugar, eating sweets throughout the day. By the middle of the night, their blood sugar levels have bottomed out and hormones are swinging wildly to compensate. On some nights, this wakes them up with screaming pain. For any pain sufferer, cutting back on sugar is a great first move. Combined with a little exercise, cutting sugar could very well prevent Susan's headaches altogether.

Saying it is one thing. Doing it is another. "I don't eat that much sugar," Susan insisted. Very few people say otherwise. It could be true, or it could be the reflexive addict's denial. I remember responding the same way to my husband back when I was downing more than a quarter cup of sugar a day, which I admitted to Susan. We talked about her diet and, as it turned out, we both came to realize that she was in fact eating lots and lots of sugar. That's the good news. My advice to dump sugar, unfortunately, didn't take, and the habit won out. When the headaches came, she treated them successfully by reaching under her bed and breathing in the oxygen. When the oxygen wasn't enough, she headed to the ER for relief.

Whenever one of my patients goes to the ER, I receive a note. One day, it occurred to me that I hadn't received a note about Susan for a while. I thought maybe she'd moved, until she came in to see me for a physical. I asked her how her headaches were doing. She said she read somewhere that cutting sugar out of her diet might help her headaches and she hadn't had a single one since she'd changed her habits. She was very proud of the fact that she'd even resisted cake at her own birthday party.

Cutting sugar to treat headaches? Who would have thunk it? Sometimes people need to take ownership of information in their own way, and that's just fine with me. What matters is that she finally came around and decided to notify the cookie monster on her back that its free meal ticket had been revoked.

In all these medical cases, you may have noticed a theme emerging. Sugar wreaks havoc with the entire nervous system, so much so that one of the first things I ask about when someone comes in with a nervous disorder is their sugar intake. But it's not just nervous system disorders like anxiety, heart palpitations, and pain that make me think of sugar addiction. It's also recurring infections, joint problems, and allergic disorders like eczema, hives, runny noses, and more.

Susan's story, like mine, shows us that people can be in denial about their sugar intake even while suffering horribly from its effects. The forces of denial overwhelm the forces of reason, preventing us from seeing what we are doing to ourselves. And who among us is sober enough to break sugar addicts from their spell? We are a nation of sugar addicts, surrounded by fellow sugar addicts raising sugar-addicted kids, with constant access to cheap and powerfully addicting sugar. The addict's cravings go way beyond wanting the sweet taste. Long-term sugar abuse actually rewires the human brain, until we are all—in a very real sense—*cuckoo* for Cocoa Puffs.

THIS IS YOUR BRAIN ON SUGAR

Imagine you're a space alien doing research on the most potent drugs in the solar system. You've already written reports on cocaine, opium, alcohol, and nicotine. But on planet Earth, there's one more refined substance that seems to dwarf them all. There are few places where this substance isn't imported and included with almost everything the residents eat and drink. It's the first thing they ingest in the morning and the last they use at night. It's the centerpiece of celebration. Overweight children and elite athletes carry plastic receptacles filled with colorful, drinkable versions of the stuff as though they need it like air. And although, at some level, they know it's killing them, they just won't stop.

Your report will show that the acreage and energy dedicated to the extraction, refinement, and export of this drug rivals that of criminalized compounds. It takes 1,000 pounds of water to produce one pound of crude drug from cane and days of heating and refining to produce fine granules of sale-

STUDY SHOWS SUGAR MORE ADDICTING THAN COCAINE

Sugar has the edge over other addictive compounds thanks to the fact that it tastes better than most drugs. A study on rats entitled "Intense Sweetness Surpasses Cocaine Reward" found that between cocaine and sugar, sugar was more addicting. Their conclusion warns: "In most mammals, including rats and humans, sweet receptors evolved in ancestral environments poor in sugars and are thus not adapted to high concentrations of sweet [compounds]. The supranormal stimulation of these receptors by sugar-rich diets, such as those now widely available in modern societies, would generate a supranormal reward signal in the brain, with the potential to override self-control mechanisms and thus lead to addiction."

able product. A quick study of planetary history shows that this substance has been so highly prized that it has functioned as currency for trade, and its flavor—"sweet"—has earned it a greater presence in the lyrics of popular music than any other drug.

The subject of your report is, of course, sugar.

Sugar is the ultimate gateway drug. We now have research showing that exposure to sugar early in life has lasting effects on the brain that can make us more prone to developing chemical dependencies. When researchers gave young rats a steady supply of chocolate Ensure, they found that "daily consumption alters striatal enkephalin gene expression." In other words, the study rats had been programmed to consume substances that stimulate their opiate receptors.[448] Sugar acts as a powerful epigenetic instructor, telling your child's genes to construct a brain with a built-in hankering for drugs.

As Michael Pollan points out in *The Botany of Desire*, by producing chemistry desirable to humans, certain plants have domesticated us, turning people into pawns in their Darwinian battle to rule the landscape. Like THC in marijuana, the sugar in fruit and sugarcane entices humans and other animals to spread the plant's DNA. But this relationship is taken to dangerous extremes as refined sugar commands us to reorder the surface of the planet; millions of acres of tropical rainforest are burned every year to sustain the ongoing habit of a growing population.

We work for corn, too. Each step in the production of high-fructose corn syrup is a giant leap forward in corn's domination of the planet. Sugar-producing plants like corn, cane, beets, berries, and mangos give us a legal high every bit as addictive as a hit of crack cocaine, though less intoxicating. What I am arguing, however, is that sugar's hold on us is more dangerous than any illegal substance because its effects are subtler and more pervasive.

If a child were given a dose of heroin, the chemical would trigger a flurry of neural activity in the pleasure centers of his brain. Sugar, whether in juice, pureed pears, or infant formula, results in the very same kinds of responses "via the release of endogenous opiates triggered by sweet taste."[449] And if you regularly give kids sugar-rich commercial juices, sweet cereals, or daily cookies and candy, you're inadvertently playing the role of enabler. Though sugar doesn't actually contain opiates like heroin, it affects us in very much the same way because it makes us release our own endogenous opiates.

The effect is powerful enough for solutions of sugar to work as a pain reliever. In a common practice called sucrose analgesia, nurses give a sip of sugar water to infants to calm them during heel sticks, injections, and other painful procedures newborns routinely undergo. It works well and has the benefit of reducing fussiness for up to a week after the procedures.[450]

In 2002, a group of neonatal nurses at several intensive care units throughout hospitals in Montreal, Canada, wondered if there might be a downside to this common practice. Specifically, they worried about the effect on the babies' developing brains. In spite of the convenient benefits, the nurses were granted permission to give half the babies in their study plain water, while the other half got sugar water. They found that infants who got sugar in their first seven days of life suffered neurologic effects that were still measurable when the study ended, eleven weeks later. Higher number of doses of sucrose predicted lower scores on motor development and vigor, and alertness and orientation . . . and higher NBRS [NeuroBiological Risk Score, a reflection of processes deleterious to brain development]."[451] Essentially what this study indicates is that little nips of sugar water given to alleviate pain impair a baby's cognitive development.

How could sugar have such powerful effects? As I mentioned earlier, sugar induces endogenous opiate release. The study authors postulate that repeated artificially induced stimulation of the immature brain with endogenous opiates interferes with normal development of alertness and arousal systems, so much so that babies who got the most sugar became lethargic. Endogenous opiates normally play a role in making us feel okay *after* something bad happens to us. The authors suggest that using sugar to induce the brain to release endogenous opiates *during* trauma prevents the brain from developing strategies to deal with pain normally. Why is cognitive ability affected as well? That question has yet to be answered.

Life is full of stresses and trials. Normally, we deal with them and move on. But studies like this suggest that when we offer kids sweet treats as an incentive to settle down, we're rewiring their brains, potentially preventing them from learning normal, healthy, and more socially appropriate coping strategies than screaming for a box of juice. I have spoken with several child psychologists who feel that discipline among children is fast on the decline. For whatever reason, more and more adults seem unable to control their kids. My feeling is that if you start loading kids with sugar as a way of controlling behavior, you are not only training them to rely on external chemicals to feel good, you are training them to manipulate you to provide them with their fix. Sorry, Willy Wonka, but my patients who've taken their kids off sugar tell me they can't believe what a better, more balanced, healthier family life they now have.

Sugar Damages Brain Cells, Making It Harder to Learn

Those at the other end of life's journey should know that most research into the origin of Alzheimer's dementia implicates not genetic mutation, but sugar.

As we'll see in the next chapter, your body is constantly growing and responding to signals. And every part of you is swimming with chemicals directing growth and cellular change, including your brain. When a brain is overloaded with sugar, you can see the effects on its cells.

Normally, a single brain cell looks a lot like a tree, with thousands of bifurcating branches, called *dendrites*. Dendrites on one brain cell reach out to dendrites on other brain cells to exchange the chemicals that enable us to remember, think, and experience emotions. Not surprisingly, intelligence roughly

HIGH-SUGAR DIETS MAY LEAD TO DEMENTIA

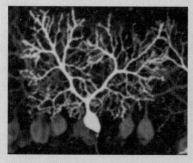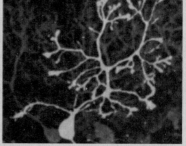

On the left is a normal brain cell, called a Purkinje cell. On the right, a Purkinje cell that exhibits the reduced branching seen in demented brains. Since insulin is necessary for normal brain cell health, insulin resistance (a result of high-sugar diets) may cause similar brain cell changes.

correlates with the number of branches in the brain's neural trees.

What makes the nerve cell grow more branches? It turns out that hormones do. The brain is constantly bathed in hormones that stimulate growth. Take away the hormones, and nerve cell branches die back.[452] In a way, growth factors act like dendritic Miracle Grow; the more growth factors you get, the more vigorous your brain cells can grow and the better you can think. One of the earliest stages of Alzheimer's dementia involves the loss of these branches, a process called *dendritic pruning*.[453] It's likely that sugar-induced cross-linking gumming up brain cell membranes is at least part of the problem. As with any cell membrane, cross-links reduce hormone sensitivity. Less receptivity means your brain cells can't respond to growth factors. Less response means fewer branches, which means fewer connections. It seems that sugar can act as a brain cell defoliant, changing the physical structure of your brain over the years and ultimately, for some, resulting in dementia. So if you've ever wondered why the Kool-Aid guy in the commercial is always busting through walls, consider how much sugar he's drinking. He probably forgot how to use a door.

Dulling Your Senses

A study done in Iraq on sweet taste habituation showed that the more sugar we eat, the less we taste it, and the less we taste it, the more we eat. In Iraq, sweetened tea accounts for the majority of sugar consumption in all age groups. Researchers offered people four cups of tea with increasing concentrations of sugar. In rural areas, where sugar was scarce, almost nobody wanted the sweetest tea, only 0.3 percent. But among those who had lived in the city for ten years or more, 100 percent preferred the sweetest tea on offer. The longer they'd lived in the city, the more sugar they wanted in their tea. The researchers asked everybody how much sugar they normally consumed, and then gave them another test to determine at what levels their taste buds could detect the presence of sugar. They found that the more sugar people tended to consume, the less they were able to taste it. Sugar had literally dulled their senses.[454]

I've done a similar experiment on my own. I researched the effects of sugar on an unwitting subject—myself. For nearly a decade, I poured homemade caramel sauce into my coffee, each dose containing a quarter cup of sugar. Luke (the experimental control) tried it once. After one taste, his eyes flew open wide, and he suggested I must be part insect. "You cannot possibly be drinking this every day," he insisted. I knew it was a lot of sugar, but no more than other people used. Like other junkies, I was rationalizing, and I ignored the advice to cut down. And that's what wore down my immune system so completely that a virus was able to take up residence in my knee. After a year or so of not being able to walk or get very much exercise, I decided maybe I should cut my sugar intake. Gradually, I cut back. First one-eighth cup, then half of that, and then just a teaspoon or two. As I did, over the course of months, I noticed my knee slowly getting better. But as an addict, I chalked it up to coincidence.

HOW I GOT OFF SUGAR AND CHANGED MY LIFE

Finally, I went on a trip and couldn't bring my caramel sauce, so I made do with just cream or milk in my coffee. To my surprise, it actually tasted fine. In fact, the cream tasted sweet. The next day, I noticed my knee was better than it had been in years. Recovering addicts often speak of moments of epiphany, or clarity, a moment when something finally clicks. Well, for me, the fact that I could enjoy the taste of coffee with milk and cream and *no sugar* meant that I really could do just fine without my little fix. And maybe, just maybe, my knee was improving because I was off the sugar. I'd had to step away from my habit, literally, to be removed enough from my daily routines and rituals in order to see the light. Now, as a recovered addict, I can better appreciate what my sugar-addicted patients are going through. I'm not just their doctor, I'm their sponsor.

From that day onward, I've never added sugar to my coffee. I've not had any soda or juice, and I don't eat candy or cookies. I eat very little fruit. And I've cut out most starchy foods (for reasons described below). Not only has my knee recovered, the extra fifteen pounds I had on my waist since college melted away. Now I have absolutely no desire for anything sweet—except chocolate (I *am* human). But the chocolate I choose, Dagoba, is 89 percent cacao, with hardly any sugar and no cheap fats. I have one-tenth of a bar three days a week, chopped fine and sprinkled over whipped cream (no sugar) as a topping for my coffee. I never thought I'd be the kind of person who passed on dessert. But now, not only am I freed of sugar cravings, my taste buds are rejuvenated. I can taste the natural sweetness in milk and cream. Even vegetables, like a raw carrot, now taste as sweet as candy. I eat as much as I ever did but weigh fifteen pounds less and spend less time feeling hungry. I wish I knew ten years ago how easy getting trim could be.

THE SUGAR SHELL GAME

Drug abusers say they don't have to look far to find their drug; the drug finds them. That's certainly true of sugar. The more people get wise about sugar and try to cut it out of their diets, the more manufacturers—the world's most successful drug pushers—sneak it into their products.

The problem is made all the worse by the fact that we've been taught to equate low-fat with healthy. But low-fat foods don't taste so great, so to make up for missing flavors from absent fat, manufacturers simply add sugar, and more sugar, and more. I'm looking at a can of Pediasure, which pediatricians frequently recommend over milk. The first ingredient is water. Guess what the second ingredient is. Sugar, accounting for 108 grams per liter.[455] Whole milk, by comparison, has 8 grams of sugar per liter.

Denying kids healthy fat often drives them to sugar. When Luke was growing up, he spent a lot of time with his grandparents who were, like many people, on a low-fat kick. Everything in their fridge was low-fat—skim milk, low-fat yogurt, no-fat dressing. By four o'clock, Luke and his siblings were tearing the place apart looking for fatty foods, anything with fat in it. And they found it, hidden in the cupboard in the form of Ding Dongs. On top of the fridge, in the Twinkies box. Out in the breezeway, on the wooden swing, behind the pillow, in the half-eaten package of Oreo cookies that Grandpa forgot to put back. Luke's grandparents were only trying to do the right thing, but they couldn't have set things up better to drive their grandkids not just to toxic, artificial fats, but also to massive doses of sugar. For this reason, weaning kids off sugar should be done in concert with providing plenty of healthy fats.

SUGAR'S PSEUDONYMS

Evaporated cane juice	Malt	Maple syrup
Corn syrup	Malt syrup	Brown rice syrup
Corn sweeteners	Barley malt syrup	Beet juice
High-fructose corn syrup	Barley malt extract	Muscovato
Crystalline fructose	Maltose	Succanat
Fructose	Maltodextrin	Turbinado sugar
Sucrose	Dextrose	Invert sugar

All of these are molecules of glucose and/or fructose and/or maltose and/or dextrose monosaccharides either alone, or bonded to one of the other two monosaccharides. All are converted to glucose or glycerine when you eat them. Glycerine can force your liver into fat-making mode the same way fructose does (see text).

Luke's experience happened a good thirty years ago. Since then, we've learned something about how too much sugar can be a real problem. Still, avoiding sugar can be harder than you think because of what I call the sugar shell game. You cut out Twinkies, but there's sugar in the salad dressing. You pass on the office cupcake, but there's sugar in the store-bought sushi. You decide to give up soda, but your "100 percent orange juice" is doped with corn syrup. (Some FDA officials suspect that many fruit juices claiming to be 100 percent natural juice are in fact sweetened with high-fructose corn syrup.[456] Fruit naturally contains fructose, so if manufacturers added more, how could anyone prove it?)

Sweeteners are some of the cheapest ingredients around. So as the American palate is desensitized to sugar, supermarket foods undergo a kind of sweetness inflation, a race between manufacturers to hide more sugar in their products than the competition. What do you think kids want more, plain milk or chocolate? Plain shredded wheat or the frosted kind? Ice water with a twist of lime or a liter of Mountain Dew? The inevitable product of this arms race is the "energy drink," a twelve-ounce atom bomb of sugar, carbohydrates, and caffeine—everything the addict needs but the syringe.

Another way of hiding sugar is by simply calling it something else. Let's take a peek at the label of a popular brand of Raisin Bran Crunch to see just how much extra sugar they sneak in the ingredients: "whole wheat, rice, sugar, raisins [mostly sugar], wheat bran, high-fructose corn syrup [more sugar], whole oats, glycerin, brown sugar [obviously sugar], corn syrup [still more sugar], salt, barley malt syrup [yes, that's sugar], partially hydrogenated soybean and/or cottonseed oil, almonds, modified corn starch, cinnamon, honey [full of sugar], nonfat dry

---

PACKING IN THE CALORIES: SUGAR VERSUS FAT

Dieters are typically encouraged to choose low-fat based on the idea that each spoonful of a low-fat product, say yogurt or a mocha cappuccino, will have fewer calories. This fails to consider the fact that manufacturers make low-fat taste more palatable by adding sugar. Far more sugar will dissolve into water than you might assume, and so the unsuspecting dieter often swallows a load of unexpected calories. Concentrated syrups like the kind used in low-fat foods contain more calories than cream or butter: while a dry teaspoon of granulated sugar has 16.8 calories, less than butter's 33.3, when dissolved into water, freely moving sugar molecules pack together to occupy one-fifth the space, so concentrated syrups can contain up to 95 calories per teaspoon.

milk, natural and artificial flavor, polyglycerol esters of mono- and diglycerides, niacinamide, zinc oxide, reduced iron, malt flavoring [also sugar], [and a few artificial vitamins]."[457] (See page 229 for alternative names for sugar.)

Calorie-wise, almost half of what's in the box is sugar. What makes up the other half? Carbohydrates. Remember, I said manufacturers play the sugar shell game. If they can't sell you sugar, they'll happily sell you the next best thing, dirt-cheap carbs. Pasta lovers aren't going to want to hear this but, *as far as your body is concerned*, carbohydrates *are* sugar. That's right, one of the most abundant sources of sugar doesn't even taste sweet.

Sugar, Sugar Everywhere

We live in a world of sugar. The single most common organic molecule on earth is *glucose*, a kind of sugar. But unlike the candy garden in Willy Wonka's factory, we can't just eat anything we see. To humans, most of the world's glucose is not edible. It's trapped in a structural carbohydrate called *cellulose*, which makes wood hard and leaves resilient. But another kind of carbohydrate called *starch* is digestible. Plants use starch to store energy and they reconvert it back to sugar when needed. The human digestive system can also convert starch into sugar, which is exactly what it does every time we eat starch. This is why, as far as your body is concerned, starch and sugar are almost the same.

Simple or Complex? Same Difference!

Everyone knows what a sugar high is. You eat a couple of pieces of cake, and the next thing you know you're bouncing off the walls. And what happens afterward? Your energy level plummets and you feel lethargic. If it's really bad, you feel like you're getting the shakes. The temptation is to treat these withdrawal symptoms with more sugar.

Sound familiar? Withdrawing from a sugar binge can feel a lot like withdrawing from a lot of other drugs, like alcohol. And we often treat it with the same homeopathic cure, a little hair of the dog. Of course, there are other options. To avoid hangovers, you could drink less or none at all. Or, alternatively, you could avoid the spikes and valleys by maintaining a more constant blood alcohol level. You could modulate your dose by drinking more often, starting first thing in the morning. It would really be convenient if you could find some kind of a "complex" form of alcohol, one that takes time for the intestine to break down so that four or five drinks, downed all at once, could provide a nice, steady buzz for the rest of the day. If there were such an alcohol, no doubt we'd call it the "good" alcohol, the one preferred by all health-conscious alcoholics to avoid ever waking up with a hangover again.

Sugar is a "simple" carb with a high glycene index. String a bunch of sugars together and you've got starch, a "complex" carb with a lower glycene index. There's much ado about complex carbs and low glycemic index foods being healthier than sugars, but nutritionally there's no difference whatsoever. The only differences between simple and complex carbs are how quickly they get into your bloodstream and how fast your insulin must respond to control the surge of sugar. So if you have diabetes or are just trying to avoid sugar swings, understand that when dietitians encourage choosing complex carbs for breakfast, it's very much as if they're telling a binge drinker to pace himself and get started first thing in the morning.

When you're eating pasta or a cracker, you don't feel as though you're doing anything naughty, because it doesn't taste sweet, like candy. But the molecules that make up starch *are* naughty; they're sugar. And once in your bloodstream, they'll be up to no good. Starch is like a chain gang that, when bound together in a long molecule (too long to fit into your taste buds), won't cause any harm. But if you let a cracker sit on your tongue long enough—or get broken down by digestion—the starch molecules turn into the very same sugar that you know is bad for your body. This means that if you've ever sat down and finished off a box of crackers you've essentially eaten a box of sugar. The take-home point is, whether you eat sugar or starch, your body winds up absorbing sugar.

When we're talking carbs and sugar, we need to define our terms clearly. All carbs are composed of individual sugar molecules, called *monosaccharides*. Table sugar is made from glucose and fructose monosaccharides bound together into a *di*saccharide called sucrose. Mono- and disaccharides are simple carbohydrates, aka sugars. If more monosaccharide units are added to the chain, the name changes to *oligo*saccharide, *oligo* meaning "few." Starches have hundreds of monosaccharide units connected together and are called *complex*.

Foods like bread, pasta, potatoes, and rice are little more than containers for sugar. A seven-ounce serving of cooked spaghetti is converted into the amount of sugar contained in four twelve-ounce cans of Pepsi. Unlike Pepsi, the pasta has been fortified with iron and a few vitamins. The starchy parts of plants also carry small amounts of protein and minerals, but white flour and white rice have had most of that removed. Whether the rice and bread are white or brown, whether the starch is in the form of breakfast cereal or tortilla chips, pasta or pancakes, complex or simple, you're mostly eating sugar.

As you'll see in the next chapter, traditional foods—foods that comprise the Four Pillars of World Cuisine—tend to have fewer carbs than their modernized counterparts. For instance, a slice of sprouted-grain bread has 70 calories. A same-size slice of regular wheat bread has 110. This is because during the process of sprouting, the seed converts its storage starch into nutrients. Seeds can do this easily. Our bodies can't.

WHY I'M NOT "ANTI-CARB"

I am not anti-carb. I'm pro-healthy carbohydrate proportioning.

What's happening on our plates is the inevitable consequence of what's happening on the planet: diverse ecosystems, both in the wild and in the form of small family farms, are being replaced by an ever expanding undifferentiated lawn of high carbohydrate monoculture crops like corn, rice, and wheat. And because high-carb foods are cheaper than more complex foods with higher nutrient content, these are the foods that are pushed in the grocery store and restaurants. Restaurants bring you free bread before a meal; I don't know any that bring free lobster.

Re-proportioning carbohydrates not only makes a dish more nourishing and less fattening, most of us instinctively find it more appetizing. In one of my favorite episodes of Chef Gordon Ramsey's *Kitchen Nightmares*, he instantly improves the presentation of a restaurant's signature dishes by cutting out a third of the carbs. This simple move makes for a more colorful, more professional looking dish.

In Chef Thomas Keller's beautiful *The French Laundry Cookbook*, you can find gorgeous photo after gorgeous photo of the kinds of dishes patrons pay upward of three hundred dollars per person (not counting wine) to enjoy. Almost every dish includes some starch—*but in the proper proportion!* Think of it this way: rather than a massive pile of mashed potatoes with a medallion of beef and sprig of green garnish, you would have that same beef medallion set atop an equal-size foundation of pureed potato, loaded with butter and cream, encircled with a moat of demi-glace reduction sauce all topped with a carefully arranged collection of colorful braised vegetables.

But you don't have to be a Michelin star chef to present your family with dishes that align with the same proportions we instinctively find appetizing. Whether it's Italian, Mexican, Southern, Chinese, or whatever, we're simply talking about holding back some of the beige and white so that the colorful flavor and nutrient-rich ingredients can dominate the composition.

I am not a big fan of breaking foods into carbs, protein, and all that. But because starchy, empty-calorie foods fill so many shelves in the store, it's one category we have to be aware of. I advise my patients with diabetes, or those who want to lose weight, to keep their *total* average carbohydrate intake under 100 grams per day. That allows for one small bowl of pasta, *or* four pieces of bread, *or* two apples, and that's it.

Fruit Sugar

Another big source of sugar that surprises many people is sweet, sugary fruit. We've heard time and again we should "eat fruits and vegetables," as though the two are equivalent. But they're not. Vegetables contain a higher nutrient-to-energy ratio than fruit. Even fruits with decent nutrient content—like wild blueberries—are *full* of sugar. When you eat citrus, you're getting a wallop of sugar with very little nutrient thrown in. That's why, for most people, eating one apple-sized portion of fruit per day is plenty. With all that sugar, fruit just doesn't make the grade as a health food. As I tell my patients, fruit is a more natural alternative to a candy bar. And fruit juice, which lacks fiber and many of the antioxidants, is little better than soda.

People often protest the idea that fruit should be consumed in limited amounts. "At least it's *natural* sugar!" they say. Sure, but all sugar is natural. Sugar cane is natural. So is the corn from which high-fructose corn syrup is made. The difference between sugar in fruit and sugar in high-fructose corn syrup (or confectioner's powder or granulated sugar) is that the former is still in its source material and the latter has been refined out of the source material and is devoid of other nutrients. And yes, that makes fruit a little better than sugar, but it's nothing to get worked up about. Though fruits do contain fiber, minerals, tannins, and other flavinoids, which can function as antioxidants, sweet fruit is mostly sugar.

What about honey? Same idea—mostly sugar and very little of anything else. Vitamin C happens to be a type of sugar we can't make and need to eat, and one orange a day gives us most of what we need. But then again, so does a green pepper (technically, a fruit), but without all the unneeded, damaging sugar.

To make matters worse for fruit lovers, fructose kicks your liver into fat-storage mode. Some believe the explosive growth of fructose consumption in the form of high-fructose corn syrup may be responsible for the increased incidence of a condition called *fatty liver*. So although nutritionists and doctors will still insist that fruit sugar is better than sucrose, others aren't so sure. But everyone agrees we're all eating a lot more sugar than we should.

IS HIGH-FRUCTOSE CORN SYRUP
WORSE THAN TABLE SUGAR?

What is high-fructose corn syrup? Is it really more likely to make you fat or give you diabetes than table sugar, honey, or any other sweetener?

Corn actually contains almost no fructose. It contains starch (a "complex" carb). Corn syrup manufacture begins with enzymatic breakdown of corn starch into its unit sugar molecule, glucose (this breakdown occurs in your GI tract during the digestion of any starch). Then, another enzyme converts glucose into fructose, to create high-fructose corn syrup (HFCS). The fructose in HFCS is identical to the fructose that occurs naturally. What's different is that the rest of the fruit (or grain) nutrients are missing.

Before the explosion of the HFCS industry in 1978, fruit and grain (wheat, rice, oat, barley, etc.) products were the primary source of fructose. Now, grain and fruit consumption is down, and though we consume far more HFCS, our total fructose consumption has only increased by one percent (from 8 percent to 9 percent of total intake[458, 459]). Fructose, therefore, cannot logically be blamed for today's obesity and diabetes epidemic. The root of today's obesity has more to do with the fact that total caloric intake has increased by 18 percent, and total carbohydrate intake has increased a whopping 41 percent over 1978 levels.

Can People Survive on Fruit?

Fruitarians, sometimes called fructarians, are a subset of vegetarians. Some people consider themselves fruitarians if at least half of their diet is fruit, while others go whole hog—if they'll forgive the expression—eating nothing but fruit. There are many explanations for choosing this lifestyle, from biblical references to anecdotal evidence of health benefits. The most popular seems to be that since we are related to monkeys and other fruit-eating primates, living on fruit is only natural.

It's important to remember that many primates, including monkeys, supplement their diet with other foods, like leaves, bark, bugs, nuts, and sometimes meat—even, on occasion, flesh of smaller primates. Some animals can get away with eating lots of sweet fruit because their big, rounded bellies contain digestive systems specifically designed for that purpose. The digestive tracts of orangutans, birds, and other fruit eaters are specialized to ferment the simple nutrients into more complex ones, enabling them to get far more nutrition from fruit than you could.

Animals that live on fruit or other sugary foods don't absorb very much sugar into their bloodstreams. The way their digestive tracts are organized enables these specialists to first ferment carbohydrates inside special chambers where bacteria, yeast, and other microbes grow, multiply, and manufacture vitamins, amino acids, and other nutrients (for their own use). These probiotic microbes ferment the sugar-rich fruits into a slurry teeming with life-supporting nutrients. By the time the slurry reaches a point along the digestive tract where absorption can take place, it has been transformed into something far more complex. The process is very similar to that employed by grass-eating animals to ferment high-cellulose foods into a more nutritious product. If our digestive tracts were designed like a gorilla's, we could eat a lot more fruit. But since we'd need a longer intestine to do it, we'd be carrying around gorilla-sized tummies as well.

EAT LIKE A GROWNUP!

When I was four or five, I thought of "kid foods" as things like cupcakes, peanut butter and jelly sandwiches on Wonder Bread, cereal—especially Cap'n Crunch!—and lots and lots of noodles. When the grownups went out to eat by themselves, I imagined they were eating things like liver, fish eggs, smelly cheese, and thick, meaty stews. In my imagination, they probably didn't even have dessert.

What I didn't know was that, since the 1980s, the U.S. Department of Agriculture has promoted practically nonstop consumption of sugar for everyone, recommending that 60 percent of our daily calories come from carbohydrate-rich foods. So, it turns out, most of the adults in my life were eating kid foods, too. Today, with all the finger foods, cookies, snacks, treats, and sugar everywhere, we might as well be having a non-stop birthday party. Little wonder, then, so many people are struggling with their weight.

So what does it mean to eat like a grownup? The first step is to reconsider the relationships between nature, your diet and your body. Rather than envisioning food in disconnected categories of often flavorless chemical compounds, I want you to understand it as your ancestors did, and to appreciate that nourishment captures the power of nature and carries it into your being. Once you learn about the Four Pillars of World Cuisine, and how to reproduce them, you will be well on your way to making your genes perform the way you want, releasing the power of your full genetic potential.

PART THREE

Living the Deep Nutrition Way

CHAPTER 10

The Four Pillars of the Human Diet

Foods That Program Your Body for Health, Brains, and Beauty

- There is one human diet that has the potential to provide optimal nutrition, no matter our race.

- The Human Diet is not defined using long lists of acceptable and forbidden foods, but rather by a set of strategies.

- Four strategies, which I define as the Four Pillars of the Human Diet, unify all traditional diets.

- The best chefs use all four strategies, which is why I say chefs are the original nutritionists.

- The modern American diet employs only one of these four strategies, the use of fresh foods.

If you've ever seen one of those museum exhibits of "ancient man," you might recall all sorts of arrowheads and spears. Or perhaps a diorama of hunters pointing weapons threateningly at a lumbering, large-tusked giant beast while, somewhere in the background, women smoke meat around a fire. With this masculine view of history, one could easily get the impression that sheer aggression enabled early humans to hunt down more animals than their competitors, outliving and outbreeding them to be the ones to venture from Africa to every corner of the globe. But this tells only half the story. The other half is what happens after the animal is killed and hauled back home. This chapter rotates our historical stage 180 degrees, so that the cooks are placed in front as the true heroes of our shared historical journey.

The astounding invention, creativity, and study human beings have honed into the craft of culinary art deserve more scientific appreciation. Other animals can hunt, but only humans have invented sophisticated techniques to extract every last bit of nutritional content from the edible world around us. That knowledge—inherited, improved upon, and passed down—was born of trial and error and plenty of inspiration. Armed with these skills, the Julia Childs of the ancient world could fold a greater diversity of nutrients into the narrative of human evolution than what would otherwise have been possible. In this chapter, we will examine regional cooking traditions from all over the world, not to identify which is best, but to describe what they all have in common. If you've read everything leading up to this, you've no doubt gotten the impression that I find the prerequisites of both health and sickness to be in no way mysterious. The rules of healthy living have been passed down freely from one generation to the next. Anyone with curiosity and common sense can recognize their logic.

Along the same vein, we needn't scratch our heads wondering which fad diet we should follow and which—because experts now say so—we're all supposed to reject. We need only return to those foods that have shepherded us through the toughest trials by which Mother Nature mercilessly tests and fine-tunes her creations. It is not just a happy coincidence we instinctively prefer the taste of those foods proved successful over millennia—not just in preventing cancer, protecting our hearts, and keeping our immune systems strong enough to ward off disease—those foods that have ensured the proper growth and health of our ancestors' offspring, their children, and their children, and theirs. Every fad diet is ornamented with claims of success. But only the Four Pillars, these four classes of foods—the nutritional foundation of the species *Homo sapiens*—can be said to have made us who we are.

THE FOUR PILLARS:
THE FOUNDATION OF THE HUMAN DIET

One way you could reproduce a healthy diet would be to simply pick a single region's traditional cuisine and copy it precisely. The problem is, we don't do that. When you get books on, say, the Mediterranean or Okinawan diets and use those recipes, rarely are you creating the same dishes as the people actually living in those regions. Why not? Typically, the recipes are inaccurate. The authors reinterpret them, replacing difficult-to-obtain or unfamiliar ingredients with substitutes you can find at any Costco. Traditional fats, like lard, are replaced by government-recommended vegetable oils. (Why is that a problem? See Chapter 7.) Variety cuts, unfamiliar and often unavailable, are replaced with boneless, skinless, low-fat alternatives. Any meal that takes more than an hour to prepare is deleted from the list of possibilities. And if the recipe originally required homemade components—like bone stock, fresh pasta, or fermented vegetables—the instructions are rewritten in the name of convenience and you wind up with instructions for making foods stripped of the very things that made them tasty, authentic, and *healthy* in the first place. You get American food with exotic spices.

I'm going to show you what all those cookbooks have been missing.

Those components of traditional cuisine removed from the typical diet or cookbook comprise the very components that every successful traditional diet has in common. I call these components the Four Pillars of World Cuisine. These fundamental foods provide healthy people all around the world the consistent stream of nutrition that, no matter the regional culinary peculiarities, adequately provides the nutritional input our bodies have been programmed to require. Though each local interpretation appears unique, as far as your body's cells are concerned, healthy diets are all essentially the same, resting on the same Four Pillars:

- **Meat on the bone**
- **Fermented and sprouted foods**
- **Organs and other "nasty bits"**
- **Fresh, unadulterated plant and animal products**

To our palates, the spectrum of regional cuisines is as diverse as the ecology of our planet. In Hawaii before Captain Cook's arrival, the staple food was *poi,* a paste made of roasted and dried taro (a tuberous root vegetable) that could be stored for months, rehydrated on demand, and then, as a final step, fermented. This staple was supplemented most often with fish, coconut, and banana. (Interestingly, the *alii,* or royal class, ate less *poi* and more high-nutrition foods like fish and they were also taller. I suspect that, as with any society, the cause-and-effect relationship between height and access to the choicest foods went in both directions: better foods made some people relatively tall; being taller offered access to better foods.) Until around 1940, the Netsilik Eskimo traditionally ate seal, fish, lichen, and not much else. In the Mongolian desert today, nomadic bands of camel breeders eat mainly dairy products, some grains, lots of tea, root vegetables, and meat. In the rain forest of Papua New Guinea, one of the last surviving hunter-gatherer groups, the Kombai, dine on fat grubs of giant flies, lizards, birds, pounded sago palm hearts, and—for special occasions—fattened pig. In West Africa, farmers known as the Mofu grow millet, beans, and peanuts, forage for insects, and raise goats and chickens, just as they have for thousands of years. While each of these seemingly diverse diets contains foods that may strike you as strange, the nutritional content they represent is as familiar to your body, and to your epigenome, as salt or water. As far as your body's cells are concerned, vegetable oil and massive doses of sugar are downright bizarre. If you've been eating a standard, food-pyramid-compliant American diet, any authentic regional diet, no matter how exotic, along with the abandonment of vegetable oil and sugar, would bring your body, your cells, and your genes a welcome and long-awaited relief. But you don't have to move to get the benefits of these traditions. Simply include foods from each of the Four Pillars in your diet. Start with eating something fresh once every day. And work your way up to using foods from two or more categories daily.

French Cuisine

Although no region has cornered the market on health, French cooking is special. Against the backdrop of international food, French cuisine stands out for its variety, depth, and indulgent sensuality. The French literally wrote the book on culinary arts, as every chef trained in the Western tradition owes his or her skills to Auguste Escoffier and the culinary pioneers who preceded him. Some would argue that China deserves equal billing with France as a culinary epicenter, as it is the original source of so many foods we now take for granted. But unlike Chinese, Italian, or Mexican food, French food served in the United States and around the world is often prepared using age-old techniques, allowing it to retain unparalleled flavor profiles and healthful character. You could say that French cuisine stands firmly on all of the Four Pillars.

Of all the cuisines in all the restaurants in all the world, why would French food enter the twenty-first century looking very much the same as it did in Napoleon's court?

In a word, snobbery. This famously French attribute definitely has its good side, because without it the universally celebrated gift of authentic epicurean expression would never have come to exist.

The early nineteenth-century middle classes wanted to prove that they had been elevated beyond "the mere physical needs of nourishment."[460] The result was a new brand of cooking that the upwardly mobile, who could now afford to hire chefs, would come to call *grande cuisine*. Grande cuisine was, and is, a style of cooking offered by high-class restaurants.

Chefs would seek out the best regional ingredients in season and perfect the techniques used to prepare them, not so much to maximize nutrition as to maximize flavor. "The grande cuisine attained its status because it emphasized the pleasure of eating rather than its purely nutritional status."[461] In spite of this new emphasis, grande cuisine originated at a time when real ingredients—as opposed to things like MSG and sugar—were the only edible materials available. So as these chefs concentrated real, quality ingredients to intensify flavor, they couldn't help but concentrate their nutrients at the same time.

The codification of grande cuisine in professional texts has encapsulated in amber centuries-old techniques for extracting flavor and nutrients from foods grown throughout Europe and Asia. By no coincidence, foods representing each of the Four Pillars appear again and again in classical French cooking. In Chapter 5, I told you about the "Hispanic Paradox," the fact that relatively less affluent, recently immigrated Hispanic women, eating traditional Hispanic foods, somehow still manage to have healthier children than the average American woman. As you know, the French have their own health paradox—relatively low rates of heart disease, despite a notoriously rich diet. Now that you understand that these traditional diets are actually far healthier than the typical American diet, you can see that there really never was any mystery at all. The answer is in healthy fats, very little sugar, and plenty of foods from each of the Four Pillars, starting with meat on the bone.

Pillar I
MEAT ON THE BONE

It's easy to enjoy well-prepared meat, but we're not born with the knowledge of how to make it taste good. That part, we have to learn. Though the art of making meat taste great can be as simple as it is rewarding, if you've never seen a person do it, you'd never know the trick.

The secret? Leave it on the bone. Thanksgiving dinner is, for many, the most memorable meal of the year which happens to be centered on a large bird, slow-cooked whole. When cooking meat, the more everything stays together—fat, bone, marrow, skin, and other connective tissue—the better. This section will introduce you to the simple techniques that primitive and haute cuisines use to make meat taste succulent, juicy, and complex. The better the material you start with, the better it tastes, and the better it is for you. For that reason, and more, animals raised humanely and pastured on mineral-rich soil are best. I'll show you the four rules you need to know to preserve and enhance the taste and nutrition of all our precious animal-derived items. And I'll show you the science that explains why mastering the art of cooking meat is the first step toward capturing the true power of food.

COOKING MEAT, RULE NUMBER ONE:
Don't Overcook It

There are two kinds of people, those who like their steak rare and those who don't. If you're the medium-rare type, you'll know which side you fall on by answering this question: What would upset you more: if the steak you just ordered came to your table undercooked or overcooked?

When I started eating meat again after experimenting with vegetarianism in graduate school, Luke's opinion that well-done meat is wasted meat was unconvincing. But after studying the chemistry of well-done versus rare, I recognized that, once again, his primal instinct was spot on. I can still recall the effort required to swallow my first bloody, glumpy, chewy bite when I crossed over to the other side of the culinary divide. Luke's delicious brown stock gravy helped my first time go much easier. Now, twelve years later and much the wiser, I find meat cooked as much as medium to be stringy, chewy, coarse, and devoid of savory flavor. I'll never go back.

When it comes to steak, it's not the size that matters; it's the consistency and texture. Overcooked meat is tough because its fat, protein, and sugar molecules have gotten tangled and fused together during a wild, heat-crazed chemical orgy. The result is a kind of tissue polymer that requires more work to cut with a knife and more chewing, as well as more time to digest. The worst part is that so many of the nutrients we need are ruined.

Ruined nutrients don't just politely disappear. Once ingested, your body won't be able to simply flush them down some metabolic drainpipe. When heat

HYDROLYTIC CLEAVAGE

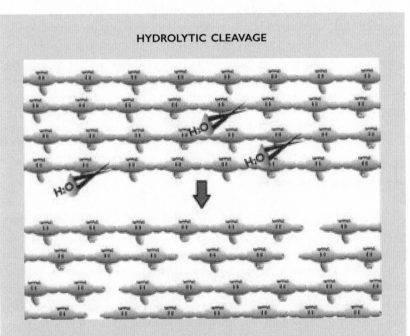

Perfectly done. Gentle, moist heating clips just enough peptide bonds to break long protein chains (upper half) into peptide segments (lower half). As long as the meat stays moist, the rows stay neatly aligned and separate. Trouble arises if the meat dries, or if the temperature rises above 170 degrees Fahrenheit. If the chef allows either to happen, hydrolysis stops, the chains themselves curl and bend around creating a tangle, and new, unbreakable bonds form between amino acids in distant chains, between amino acids and sugar, and between amino acids and fats. These undesired reactions create toxins, destroy nutrients, and make the meat tough to cut and chew.

kills nutrients, it does so by causing reactions *between* nutrients, forming new chemical compounds including known carcinogens (such as *aromatic hydrocarbons* and *cyclic amines*), as well as other molecular fusions that damage your kidneys and blood vessels.[462] When meat is cooked properly, fewer harmful reactions occur.[463] The nutrients and flavor compounds survive, and can now be gently released into the meat's juices where they are more bioavailable, and more readily tasted and absorbed.

So how much heat is too much heat? If, when you slice it, there's not even a trickle of juice, it's way overdone. Steak should be juicy and red. I recommend you work your way down to medium rare, and once you get used to that, go for rare. One last thought: if you're an Anthony Bourdain fan, you already know that restaurant patrons who order their steak well done get the oldest, least choice cuts. It's not that the chefs have it in for people who order their steaks brown; they have to save the freshest product for those palates that can taste the difference.

COOKING MEAT, RULE NUMBER TWO:
Use Moisture, Time, and Parts

Not long ago, at a party, I met a dark-eyed Peruvian woman with a sultry accent who had just discovered her slow cooker. She'd owned it for two years before a visiting friend released it from confinement in the back of the kitchen cabinet. That whole week they ate nothing but stews. After years of indifference toward it, my new friend had fallen in love with her slow cooker because "it giff so mush flavor!" When I told her that good, complex flavor means good nutrition, and that she should use it as often as she wants, she fell in love with me.

It is a little-known fact that when a chef talks about flavor, he's also talking about nutrients. When he says, "some flavors take time to develop," he's saying that sometimes you have to wait for certain nutrients to be released. Cooking meat slowly is the best way to turn an ordinary meal into something extraordinary—in terms of taste *and* nutrition. The potential flavor of meat, or any food, derives from its complexity. Depending on the cut, "meat" may include muscle, tendon, bone, fat, skin, blood, and glands—each a world of chemical diversity. When that diversity is released on your tongue you can taste it, and the rich, savory flavor means a world of nutrients are on their way.

You don't actually need a slow cooker to cook meat slowly and enjoy all the same benefits. All you need is moisture, time, and parts (as many different tissue types as possible: ligament, bone, fat, skin, etc.). Making soup, stewing, keeping a top on to trap the steam, basting often when cooking in the oven—all these techniques keep the moisture inside the meat, enabling water molecules to make magic happen.

Here's how. The transformation of, say, a cold and flavorless chicken leg into something delicious begins when heated moisture trapped in the meat creates the perfect conditions for *hydrolytic cleavage* (see figure on page 245). At gentle heating temperatures, water molecules act like miniature hacksaws, neatly chopping the long, tough strands of protein apart, gently tenderizing even the toughest tissue. And because water also prevents nearby strands from fusing together, keeping meat moist prevents the formation of the protein tangles that make overcooked meat so tough.

How does hydrolytic cleavage translate into taste? It's simple. Taste buds are small. The receptor site where chemicals bind to them is tiny. So things that impart taste (called flavor *ligands*) must be tiny, too. If you were to take a bite of a cold, raw leg of chicken, you wouldn't get much flavor from it. Cooking releases trapped flavor because, during the process of hydrolytic cleavage, some proteins are chopped into very small segments, creating short strings of amino acids called *peptides*. Peptides are tiny enough to fit into receptors in our taste buds. When they do, we get the sensation of savoriness food manufacturers call the "fifth flavor," or *umami*. (Sour, bitter, salty, and sweet are the other four major flavors.)

How does having additional parts (skin, ligaments, etc.) create additional nutrition? Water molecules tug apart the connective tissue in skin, ligaments, cartilage, and even bone, releasing a special family of molecules called *glycosaminoglycans*. You will find the three most famous members of this family in nutritional supplements for joints: glucosamine, chondroitin sulfate, and hyaluronic acid. But these processed supplements don't hold a candle to gelatinous stews, rich with the entire extended family of joint-building molecules. What is more, cartilage and other connective tissues are nearly flavorless before slow-cooking because (just as with muscle protein) the huge glycosaminoglycan molecules are too big to fit into taste bud receptors. After slow-cooking, many amino acids and sugars are cleaved away from the parent molecule. Once released, we can taste them.

Slow-cooked meat and parts are more nutritious than their mistreated cousins for still another reason: minerals. Mineral salts are released from bone and cartilage during stewing, as well as from the meat itself. These tissues are mineral warehouses, rich in calcium, potassium, iron, sulfate, phosphate, and, of course, sodium and chloride. It turns out our taste buds can detect more of these ions than previously suspected, including calcium, magnesium, potassium, and possibly iron and sulfate, in addition to the sodium and chloride ions that make up table salt.[464] Overcooking traps these flavorful materials in an indigestible matrix of polymerized flesh that forms when meat begins to dry out. You can only taste, and your body can only make use of, minerals that remain free and available.

A word about flavor complexity. Although we've been told that some taste buds taste only salty, others sour, others bitter, and others sweet, studies have revealed that though taste buds may taste one kind of flavor predominately, one bud can in fact detect different flavor ligands simultaneously. It turns out, the more different kinds of flavors there are, the more we taste each one. When peptides *and* salt ions bind at the same taste bud, the result is not a doubling of flavor, but a powerful thousand-fold magnification in the signal going to your brain.[465] In this way, our taste buds are engineered to help us identify and enjoy (nutritional) complexity. (This is why hot dogs, for instance—or better yet, actual sausages—taste better with *sauer*kraut and *bittersweet* mustard.)

Now, some of you might still pine for your Arby's or your Big Mac. But keep in mind, the MSG and free amino acids in fast foods are tricking your tongue. The artificial flavoring MSG (the sodium salt of an amino acid called *glutamate*) binds taste receptors just as peptides in slow-cooked meat would. MSG and other hydrolyzed proteins are manufactured by taking hydrolytic cleavage to its completion, fully breaking down plant or animal protein products into individual amino acids while refining them away from other cellular components. Health food stores sell these taste-enhancers in the form of Bragg's Aminos, which is no better for you than hydrolyzed soy sauces. The problem with these products is that certain amino acids have neurostimulatory effects that can lead to nerve damage (amino acids glutamate and aspartate are the most potent). When consumed in small amounts as part of a meal containing a diversity of nutrients, amino acids are actually good for us. But when consumed in large quantity without their normal complement of nutrients (most notably, without calcium or magnesium),[466] neurostimulatory amino acids can cause temporary memory loss, migraines, dizziness, and more. This is why the concept of whole foods must be applied to animal products as well as plants. Simply refining the protein away from its source turns normal, healthy amino acids into potentially harmful compounds. (By the way, traditionally brewed brands of soy sauce derive flavor from peptides, which do not overstimulate nerve cells.)

COOKING MEAT, RULE NUMBER THREE:
Use the Fat

We need to eat animal fat, just as we always have. Many people believe that the animals we eat today are unusually fat, but that's not true. While grain-fed animals do contain unhealthy fat (see section "Why Organic, Pasture-Raised Meat Is Worth the Price," later in the chapter) and lots of it where it's bad for the animal (like within the muscle), the animals humans historically ate were relatively chunky too because, whenever possible, people picked them at the peak of plumpness. Free-range deer, for instance, are only 15 percent fat (by weight) in summer.[467] But by the time hunting season rolls around they've stuffed themselves for winter fasting and tip the scales at 30 to 40 percent body fat.[468] According to early American explorers like Samuel Hearne and Cabeza de Vaca, North American natives preferred the fattest animals, and valued their fattiest parts most of all. When hunting was especially good, they'd leave the lean muscle meat behind for the wolves.[469, 470]

What are the nutritional benefits of our appetite for fat? For one thing, fat is a source of energy, like sugar. Unlike sugar, however, fat is a major building material for our cells, comprising 30 to 80 percent (dry weight) of our cell membranes. And unlike sugar, fat doesn't trigger the release of insulin, which promotes weight gain. Furthermore, a high-sugar meal damages our tissues, but a high (natural) fat meal doesn't (see chapters 7 and 9). And this is something I was tested on in med school but forgot right after the test: we need fat to be able to absorb most fat-soluble nutrients, including vitamins A, D, E, and K. The fact that the presence of fat in meat also helps protect it during cooking—let's just call that a happy coincidence.

To be honest, though, it's not always just a coincidence. Since, to keep meat moist, fat must be located on the outside of a cut of meat, good butchers strive to produce cuts encased inside a neat layer of rich, tasty fat. In smaller, leaner animals like birds, most of the fat sits right under the skin, naturally in the perfect location to keep meat moist during cooking. If you want a flavorful, juicy bird, for goodness' sake don't peel off the skin!

One of the latest new trends in the food world falls squarely in the category of everything-old-is-new-again: grass-fed beef. Pasture-raised beef has all kinds of advantages, both for you and for the animals. You may have heard that grass-fed is good for you because of its higher omega-3 content. That's true. It's also a source of bone-building vitamin K2 and anti-inflammatory conjugated linoleic acid (CLA). But to get that omega-3, K2, and CLA, you have to get meat with an exterior layer of fat (or the liver or the bone marrow or other "nasty bits"—see below). Compared to most grocery store beef, which comes from grain-fed cows and is heavily marbled with heat-resistant saturated fat, the muscle in pastured cows is relatively lean. So when you buy a grass-fed steak, know that it will require a more gentle cooking technique than does the typical grocery store steak you might be used to.

More Than Flavor:
Fat's Synergistic Effects

Have you ever wondered why fat tastes so good? We have five well-known flavor receptors:

1. Sweet, which detects carbohydrate
2. Sour, which detects acid (acid plays a role in making nutrients more available)
3. Bitter, which detects antioxidants, some of which are also poisons
4. Salty, which detects sodium and other minerals
5. Umami, the amino-acid detector described above

If we have no receptor for fat, why do we like it so much? It's not just your imagination that fat-free cookies don't taste as good as the real thing. Fat was long thought to impart flavor by way of the nose. But in 2005, French researchers blocking off study subjects' ability to smell using—you guessed it—clothespins on their noses found evidence of a receptor in the mouth that does detect fat, called CD38.[471] The subjects proved they could detect a variety of long-chain fatty acids, from saturated, to monounsaturated, to polyunsaturated, as well as potentially harmful oxidized fat. They could even discriminate between fatty acid types.[472, 473] Just as Ayurvedic culinary masters indicated thousands of years ago, there may be six major flavor groups our tongue can detect.

Not only can we detect fat, but just as with other flavor ligands, there is also a synergistic effect. When fatty acids bind to their receptors, it affects other taste buds such that their ability to detect sour, salt, and bitter flavors is enhanced. This makes sense because many of the compounds that taste sour and bitter are fat-soluble, and fat would be expected to enhance their absorption into our bodies as well. So it appears our tongues are wired to guide us toward nutritionally complex foods. Unless a food has been "doped" with MSG, other artificial flavor agents, or sugar, or if our senses are dulled by chronic sugar ingestion, if something 100 percent natural tastes delicious, it is almost guaranteed to be good for you.

Why Organic, Pasture-Raised Meat Is Worth the Price

If you have a limited budget and you want to get organic, skip the fruits and vegetables and head over to the butcher aisle. Organic animal products give you more bang for your buck because they benefit from *bioconcentration*. Concentration refers to the percent of a substance present in something. *Bioconcentration* is a process that results in a living organism having a higher concentration of a substance than its surrounding media.

Bioconcentration is usually used in reference to pollutants. When you spray plants with herbicides and pesticides, some gets taken up into their tissues. When animals eat these plants, they also eat the pesticides and herbicides. The majority of these chemicals are fat-soluble and will accumulate in fat. Since vegetables are naturally low in fat, when you buy organic vegetables, you are only avoiding a little bit of poison. When you buy organic meat, especially the fatty cuts, you're avoiding a lot.

Bioconcentration has a good side, too. After all, it's what eating is all about, getting lots of good information from what you eat. Plants bioconcentrate nutrients from the soil, so that a pound of grass, for instance, has more potassium than a pound of the dirt in which it grows. Animals carry this process one step further. Their tissues bioconcentrate the minerals that grass has taken from the soil and the vitamins that grass manufactures.

Research has shown that caribou can see which blades of grass are the most nutrient-rich and preferentially graze on those. Presumably, other herbivores also have the same ability. This suggests that organically raised animals kept in confinement will not be as healthy as those raised on large pastures. And a creature living freely in the wild should be healthiest of all. So if you hunt, or if you know a hunter who has extra, don't let this amazing resource go to waste: eat as much of the animal as you know how!

There's one more factor making organic meat worth the price. Organically grown animals cannot (yet) legally be given antibiotics or other drugs except in case of illness. This means the farmer has to keep them healthier, which means they're healthier to eat. Nor can organically grown animals legally (at this point) be fed or injected with growth hormones. Growth hormones have been proven capable of surviving the cooking and digestion processes. And some believe growth hormones in animal products used to increase the "feed conversion efficiency" are adding to the problems of obesity and cancer.[474] Unfortunately, as the mega-industries grow stronger, they are changing the rules to make it easier to put the word *organic* on the label. The best bet is to get friendly with your local farmers.

COOKING MEAT, RULE NUMBER FOUR:
Make Bone Stock

More than anything else, the health of your joints depends upon the health of the collagen in your ligaments, tendons, and on the ends of your bones. Collagens are a large family of biomolecules, which include the *glycosaminoglycans*, very special molecules that help keep our joints healthy. People used to eat soup and stock made from bones all the time, and doing so supplied their bodies with the whole family of glycosaminoglycans, which used to protect people's joints. Now that few people make bone stock anymore, many of us are limping into doctors' offices for prescriptions, surgeries, and, lately, recommendations to buy over-the-counter joint supplements containing glucosamine. And what is glucosamine? One of the members of the glycosaminoglycan family of joint-building molecules.

Veterinarians have been using glucosamine supplements to treat arthritic pets for decades. But physicians dismissed the practice as a waste of time, assuming that, since glucosamine is a huge molecule, the digestive system would break it down. Nobody can explain how, but studies have shown that glucosamine is somehow able to resist digestion and pass through the intestinal wall intact.[475] Once it gets into your bloodstream, *glucosamine has a special tropism for cartilage.*[476] (That's technospeak for "somehow, it knows just where to go.") Even more amazing, glucosamine can actually stimulate the growth of new, healthy collagen and help repair damaged joints.[477]

And collagen isn't just in your joints; it's in bone and skin and arteries, and your hair, and just about everywhere in between. This means that glucosamine-rich broth is a kind of youth serum, capable of rejuvenating your body, no matter what your age. After decades of skepticism, orthopedists and rheumatologists are now embracing its use in people with arthritis, recommending it to "overcome or possibly reverse some of the degradation that occurs with injuries or disease."[478] Given these facts, it hardly seems far-fetched to suggest that eating this stuff in soups and sauces from childhood makes joints stronger in the first place.

One of Luke's golfing buddies, local Kauai born and bred, didn't need convincing. As a child of a Filipino household, he ate lots of meat on the bone growing up. One day, chopping a goat leg to stir into stew, he asked his mother about the white, shiny stuff on the ends of the bones. She told him that he had the very same kind of material in his own joints. Instantly, he decided that eating that shiny cartilage would be good for his shiny cartilage. He has eaten meat on the bone ever since, making sure to chew on the ends. Now his friends are on arthritis meds, while he's surfing and golfing twice a week.

Not only do bone broths build healthy joints, the calcium and other minerals help to grow your bones. One of my patients is a charming young boy whose father is a chef. The chef is five-foot-ten and his wife five-foot-five. Both parents are lactose intolerant, and so for years his dad, the chef, made bone stocks and used them as a base for making rice, mashed potatoes, soups, and reduction sauce gravies. He did this so that he and his lactose-intolerant wife would get plenty of dietary calcium. Aside from calcium, bone broth also contains glycosaminoglycans, as well as magnesium and other bone-building minerals—basically a total bone- and joint-building package—most of which the chef didn't know about. However, his son's DNA did. This child of average-height parents started life at normal size, but his growth chart illustrates that, over the years, he's gotten progressively taller than average. Now, at age ten, his height and muscle mass are already off the chart. By the way, his teeth are straight, he doesn't need glasses, and he is the number-one swimmer on his team.

Coincidence? Misleading anecdotal data? I don't think so. We all know that vitamin D and calcium are good for a child's growing bones. And as we saw in Chapter 5, it takes a whole array of vitamins and minerals to build a healthy skeleton. Cooking meat on the bone extracts all those well-known vitamins and minerals, plus the glycosaminoglycan growth factors. To have tall, strong, well-proportioned children, we're often told to get them to drink milk. And if we're talking about organic whole milk—especially raw!—I'm all for it. But if it were my kids, I'd also make sure they were getting regular helpings of homemade soups and sauces, and anything else I could think of to get them to eat more stock.

The benefits of broth consumption far outweigh the benefits of taking a pill for a couple of reasons: first, the low heat used to slowly simmer the nutrient material from bone and joint is far gentler than the destructive heat and pressure involved in the production of glucosamine tablets. Second, instead of extracting only one or two factors, broth gives you the entire complex of cartilage components—some of which have yet to be identified in the lab—plus minerals and vitamins. Broth's nutritional complexity makes it a nearly perfect bone-building, joint-health-supporting package. And it's no coincidence that it tastes great. Rich, satisfying flavors convinced the father of modern French culinary science, Auguste Escoffier, that stock was an absolute kitchen essential. "Without it, nothing can be done."

Our ancestors probably discovered the magic in bones a very long time ago. In the Pacific Northwest, archeologic digs have uncovered evidence that, centuries before Escoffier, early Native Americans supplemented their winter diet of dried fish by deliberately fracturing herbivorous animal bones prior to stewing them. Not only did this release bone nutrients, it released the marrow fat and vitamins into the simmering soup. And anthropologists studying hunter-gatherers from Canada to the Kalahari find that this practice of exploiting bone and marrow nutrients was and is "almost ubiquitous."[479, 480] While visiting a farm in New Zealand, I met a spry and engaging eighty-something woman who told me about the Scottish tradition of "passing the bone." In the little village where she grew up, nothing went to waste. Cartilaginous knee joints and bony shanks were especially prized, and passed from house to house. Each family would put the bones into a pot over the stove to simmer for a night before passing them on to their neighbor until the bone was "spent." As she hiked with us over the rolling green hills of her estate, she explained that the bones were shared because she and her neighbors were convinced that "something in them was sustaining." Indeed there is. So skip the pharmacy aisle and head straight to your local butcher for bones to make your own homemade stock.

For thousands of years, people all over the world made full use of the animals they consumed, every last bit right down to the marrow and joints. You might suppose that, over all that time and all those generations, our bodies, including our joints, might grow so accustomed to those nutrients that they wouldn't grow, repair, and function normally without them. You'd be right. And what is true of bones is true of other animal parts. Over time, our genes have been programmed with the need and expectation of a steady input of familiar nutrients, some of which can only be derived from the variety meats, which include bones, joints, and *organs*.

Pillar 2
ORGAN MEAT, OFFALLY GOOD FOR YOU

Long ago, when a deer was killed and lifted on a hook to be dismembered, the hunter began by inserting a knife just below the xiphoid process at the lower end of the sternum and briskly drawing it down to the pubic bone. When properly done, the guts spilled out of the belly and naturally fell to the ground—*off fall*. In modern usage, the term *offal* encompasses every part of an animal except ordinary muscle meat.

If you've ever seen one of those travel shows hosted by a snarky gourmand eating strange foods in exotic locales, you might recall watching scenes of street vendors in Calcutta frying brains on a skillet, or sweetmeats served in a dusty open-air eatery in Uzbekistan, and thinking, *How can they eat that?* It's all a matter of what you've grown up with. Had you been born elsewhere, you might drool at the sight of lungs on a stick just as you might now go gaga over a greasy corn dog. In fact, until recently, those offal meats were a big part of American dining, integrated into our diets through a wide range of dishes. Turn the cookbook pages back just a few generations and you'll find Halloweenish recipes calling for organ meats and other variety cuts alongside familiar casseroles and crumb cakes. My 1953 edition of *Joy of Cooking* lists Calf Brain Fritters and ten other brainy recipes, as well as instructions for making meals from liver, kidney, tongue, heart, head, and thymus.

If you dig further back to cookbooks printed before the Industrial Revolution, you'll find ghastly instructions requiring a witch's arsenal of implements, from large cauldrons to bone-splicing hatchets. From *The Ladies New Book of Cookery*, published in 1852, listed under preparation of beef, we learn the private housewife was to "take a green tongue, stick it with cloves, and boil it gently for three hours." Also included are practical tips on how to estimate internal temperature without a meat thermometer: "When the eyes drop out, the pig is half done."[481]

Our founding fathers' wives followed recipes that made extensive use of offal meats, especially in the fall when many animals would be killed to conserve precious grass and hay for the best breeders that could repopulate the pastures again in spring. Since offal goes bad quickly, they needed to be consumed or preserved as soon as possible. The prudent housewives of the seventeenth, eighteenth, and early nineteenth centuries would want to make use of every last scrap and, nutritionally speaking, nothing would better prepare their families for the long winter ahead. Offal meats are rich in vitamins, especially fat-soluble vitamins, which can be stored in our own fat reserves for months. As winter wore on and root cellars emptied, those larders of nutrients built up internally by feasting in the fall sometimes made the difference between life and death, or a successful pregnancy and one fraught with complications.

WHY YOU SHOULD EAT THAT LIVER PATÉ

One of offal meat's most famous proponents was Adelle Davis, a biochemist who pioneered the fledgling field of nutrition in the mid-twentieth century. A patient of mine, who was taken to see Davis in the 1940s on the advice of his pediatrician for help with his disabling asthma, was not simply treated. He was *cured*. Back then, there were no handheld inhalers. Every time he developed a cold or the weather changed, his mother would have to rush him to the hospi-

ORGAN MEATS VERSUS FRUITS AND VEGETABLES

100 gram portion			
vitamin A	7*	10.602	261*
vitamin B1	0.02	0.2	0.063
vitamin B2	0.02	4.1	0.13
vitamin B6	0.07	0.91	0.2
folate	4	217	108
vitamin C	8	23	64.9
niacin	0.1	10.7	0.553
pantothenic acid	0.08	4.57	0.616
magnesium	6	20	21

Pound for pound there's no comparison. In Chapter 5, we saw how terribly undernourished most American women are today. One big factor is the near complete elimination of organ meats from our diets. Without these most nutrient dense of foods, it's nearly impossible to get adequate vitamins and minerals.

*Retinol equivalents. Only animal products contain true vitamin A; fruits and vegetables contain carotenoids and retinoids, which must be converted in the digestive tract. The conversion factor used has overestimated the value of fruits and vegetables by a factor of four. These data have been revised to reflect the current knowledge, but the nutrition tables on grocery store goods have not and thus exaggerate the true amount of vitamin A.

tal for shots of adrenaline. Davis advised his mother to send him off to school with a thermos of pureed raw cow's liver every day, which he managed to drink primarily because he wanted to avoid the emergency room. The raw cow's liver provided a spectrum of missing nutrients to calm the inflammation that triggered his asthma attacks. But it may also have done much more, ensuring his entire nervous system was wired correctly. Today, in his seventies, his reflexes are still so fast that he can trounce Luke on the tennis court.

I don't recommend you eat raw liver unless you are familiar with the source and have taken proper measures to prevent parasites.[482] But a quick glance at the nutrition tables for liver and other variety cuts reveals why nutrition-oriented physicians might use these parts as cure-alls like Davis did; they're the *real* vitamin supplements. As she explains in her book *Let's Cook It Right*, "The liver is the storage place or the 'savings bank' of the body. If there is an excess of protein, sugar, vitamins, and any mineral except calcium and phosphorus, part of the excess is stored in the liver until it is needed. . . . Liver is, therefore, nutritionally the most outstanding meat which can be purchased."[483] Of course, if the cow is sickly, or raised on depleted soil, the savings bank of the liver is likely depleted as well.

The following are just a few examples of the benefits of eating different variety meats:

The Latin name for the retina of the eye is *macula lutea*. (*Lutea* is Latin for *yellow*.) This thick, membranous yellow layer of the eyeball is a rich source of the nutrient *lutein*, a member of the retinoid family of vitamin A precursors. Lutein supplements are now promoted as being good for prostate health and for preventing macular degeneration. The fat behind the eyeball is a rich source of vitamin A and lutein. (If you think you'd rather swallow a supplement than pop an eyeball after breakfast, remember that vitamins are heat-, light-, and oxygen-sensitive and unlikely to survive processing.) And while you're digesting the idea of eating eyeball fat, consider that the gooey juice in the eye is primarily hyaluronic acid, rich in glycosaminoglycans. You can get hyaluronic acid injected into your lips (to fill them out), your knee (as a treatment for osteoarthritis), and even your own eye (to treat certain ocular diseases) for $200 a dose (twenty one-thousandths of a gram). It's called Restylane. But you can get this useful nutrient into your body just by eating the eyes you find in fish head soup, and the glycosaminoglycans will find their way to the parts of the body that need them most.

Brain and nervous tissues are fantastic sources of omega-3 and other brain-building fatty acids and phospholipids, and with more than 1.2 grams per 100-gram portion, they are a richer source of this vital nutrient than almost anything else.[484] Even windpipes contain stuff we don't get enough of these days—those glycosaminoglycans again. Many of my patients spend upward of a hundred dollars a month buying supplemental nutrients that are far less potent than what our ancestors enjoyed daily, simply by including variety meats in their diet.

You may have noticed a pattern here: eating eyes is good for your eyes. Eating joints is good for your joints. The idea that the consumption of a part of an animal's body is good for the same part of your own is an interpretation of homeopathy—meaning *like cures like*. Unfortunately, today most of these powerful "supplements" are going to waste as meat producers wash these rich sources of nutrition down drains in the slaughterhouse floor, or pass them off to rendering plants where heaps of rotting tissue are reprocessed into animal feeds, yellow fat, and something called "recycled meat." The good news is, since our society values them so little, if your butcher can save them for you, he'll likely sell them to you cheap. The bad news is, once we've got them, making them taste good isn't especially easy to do; it takes a little time and know-how. (Chapters 13 and 14 have tips and recipes that will get you started.) For adults, the reward is a powerful resistance to disease. For children, the awakening of their genetic (growth) potential brings rewards that are indescribably greater.

Pillar 3
BETTER THAN FRESH: FERMENTATION AND SPROUTING

> Egytians set aside their dough until it decayed,
> and observed with pleasure the process that
> took place. —*Herodotus, fifth century B.C.*[485]

On a recent trip to the Bay Area where I was giving a talk on nutrition, a good friend took us out for lunch. "You're into healthy food," she said. "There's a hip new vegan restaurant we've got to try." Opening the menu felt like cracking open a textbook to do your assigned reading; nothing looked appetizing. Though the menu was peppered with pop-nutrition vernacular—"living," "dynamic," "enzyme," the selections were simply awkward interpretations of familiar foods: the raw pizza, the cold burrito. Luke ordered the burrito, a compressed disc of rancid seeds laureled with a splash of fresh greens. I ordered the pizza, an identical compressed disc with a different kind of dressing on the greens. The greens were good. The disc was not. Truly living food is more dynamic than salad leaves, and more potent than a plate of compressed seeds; it's food that's been *awakened* by the process of fermentation (a kind of controlled rotting), sprouting (germination of a seed), or both.

Vegetarians in particular will benefit from these two potent methodologies for enhancing nutrition because getting adequate protein is more challenging on a plant-based diet since even the most protein-rich plants also contain a good deal of blood-sugar–elevating carbohydrate, whereas most high-protein animal foods are zero carb. How do the processes of fermentation and sprouting reduce carbohydrate content? During the sprouting process, enzymes convert energy-rich storage starch into the many nutrients a seedling requires. During fermentation, multiplying microbes seek out simple sugars and convert them into a wide variety of nutrients they use for their own growth.

Fermentation and sprouting are also crucial for another, very simple reason: plants didn't evolve with the idea that they should be good to eat. In fact, plants spend a great deal of energy thwarting overzealous grazers and other creatures that would gladly eat them into oblivion. Not as helpless as they may seem, plants protect their foliage, stems, seeds, roots, and to a lesser degree even their fruits, with natural insecticides and bitter toxins that make some plants unsafe for human consumption. Unless your species has evolved the physiologic means to neutralize them, a plant's various hemagglutinins, enzyme inhibitors, cyanogens, anti-vitamins, carcinogens, neurotoxins, and allergens say, "Eat at your own risk." Although I disagree, some investigators have gone so far as to suggest that "nearly all the carcinogens in the diet are of natural rather than—as widely perceived—industrial origin."[486] Sprouting and fermenting effectively deactivate many of these irritants, which explains why sprouted grains and lacto-fermented vegetables are known to be easier to digest.

Many of today's best foods were originally fermented, sprouted, or both. Take away fermentation and there's no such thing as wine. Or beer. You can forget bread, yogurt, and cheese. Chocolate's out, since cacao nibs must sit in the sun for a week or so to let the fruit ferment around the nibs and develop the full symphony of flavor. And the same goes for coffee berries. The list of fermented foods grows surprisingly long when you throw in things like sauerkraut, pickles, ketchup, and other condiments that—though now industrially mass-produced by steeping in vinegar and salt—traditionally generated their own acid preservatives during fermentation. In *The Story of Wine*, writer Hugh Johnson celebrates fermentation as a central driving force of civilization. The oldest recipe known to exist, written in cuneiform, is for a kind of beer bread. If we'd never allowed cereal grains to sprout, we would never have invented bread nourishing enough to sustain a population; for the first ten thousand years of wheat and grain cultivation, the technology to crush open the kernels did not exist.[487] And so, for the majority of human history, life-giving bread was made not with flour, but with partially germinated seeds. Unfortunately, even in places like France, people often fail to appreciate their own wild, indigenous microbes. And so many foods (cheeses, breads, wines, etc.) have had their flavors tamed by way of pasteurization, by the use of faster-acting cultures that are easier to work with, or both.

In the next two sections, we'll take a look at the battle of wills between human and vegetable, and see why traditional, low-tech methods for neutralizing plant toxins and maximizing nutrition are far more effective at producing healthy products than contemporary methods.

FERMENTATION, PART I:
Single-Cell Vitamin Factories

The human digestive system is a chimera. It's one part *us*, one trillion parts *them*. We supply the long, hollow tube that begins at our mouth and coils for a dozen meters or so inside our abdominal cavity until it terminates at what we physicians call the rear end. The microbial world populates the tube with enough bacteria and fungi to outnumber our own cells ten to one.[488] The average human colon contains over 800 species of microbiota and at least 7,000 different strains.[489] Sixty percent of the fecal matter you produce consists of microbial bodies. Are all these microbes just freeloaders, or do we somehow benefit from their presence?

To answer that, we need to understand something about a process called *fermentation*. My Webster's dictionary describes fermentation as an "enzymatically controlled transformation of an organic product." The key term is *transformation*. Bacteria are capable of transforming indigestible, bland, and even toxic compounds into nourishing and delicious foods. Without them, multi-celled organisms, from flies to frogs to mammals, would be unable to digest their food. With an arsenal of enzymes, microbes can break down toxins that might otherwise sicken or kill us outright, turn simple sugars into complex nutrients, make vitamins our diets might otherwise lack (such as K2 and B12), and wage chemical warfare on would-be pathogens. All we do for them is provide a warm place to work and plenty of water. From their perspective, we are the freeloaders living off their hard labor.

The obliging microbe isn't especially particular about where it lives. Requiring little more than a consistent temperature, water, and a few organic materials, bacteria and fungi are equally happy whether inside our digestive tract, a warm clay pot in the sun, an oak casket in a cave, a leather sack, or even an egg buried underground. Thousands of years ago, people learned to harness the power of these invisible "factors," which developed predictably under a certain set of conditions. That skill opened up a world of possibility, enabling us to preserve our food and create a whole new set of flavors. Fermentation would ultimately be put to use by people around the globe, and form one of the foundational pillars of all traditional cuisine.

Though today we tend to think of bacteria and fungi in our food as unwanted enemies, usually calling them "germs," civilization owes much to these contaminants. Without yeast naturally present in the air, we never would have been able to leaven our bread. In the 1960s, doctors discovered a dramatic example of the value of leavening. Poor Turkish families were having children with a type of dwarfism initially thought to be due to genetic mutation. When no defective gene could be identified, researchers looked to nutritional problems. It turned out that the mothers of affected children, as well as the children themselves, had low levels of zinc and other minerals. Further investigation revealed the cause of the mineral deficiency to be unleavened bread consumption.[490] Wheat, like all seeds, contains mineral-binding compounds called phytates, which hold minerals in stasis until conditions are right for germination. Yeast and other microbes (such as those in sourdough) contain enzymes (called phytases) that break down phytates in the seed, freeing the zinc, calcium, magnesium, and other minerals from their chemical cages. The parents of dwarfed children were buying cheaper, unleavened bread and were also unable to afford much meat, a good source of zinc and magnesium. The unleavened bread was the last straw. Bound to phytates, the zinc and magnesium in the bread passed through undigested, leading to mineral deficiencies that prevented proper expression of the children's bone-building genes.[491] This is just one example of what happens when people buy food based on price rather than on its nutritional value. Because few people appreciate the difference between authentic food that costs more, and similar substitutes that cost less, manufacturers skip the labor-intensive fermentation steps whenever they can.

Which is why I want to tell you the truth about soy.

Some of my patients speak so proudly about how they've started eating tofu and drinking soymilk, obviously presuming that I think these things are healthy. I can hardly bear to burst their bubbles. Soybeans contain chemicals called *goitrogens* and *phytoestrogens*, which disrupt thyroid and sex hormone function. The Chinese and Japanese who traditionally ate soy would soak, rinse, and then ferment the beans for extended periods, neutralizing the harmful compounds and using the fat- and protein-rich beans as a substrate for microbial action. Traditional tofu, natto, miso, and other cultured soy products are incredibly nutritious. Commercially made soymilk, tofu, and soy-based infant formulas, on the other hand, are not. Loaded with goitrogens and phytoestrogens, overconsumption of these foods is known to cause hypo- and hyperthyroidism, thyroid cancer, and—particularly during infancy or pregnancy—male and female reproductive disorders.[492, 493] I have helped several patients with abnormal thyroid hormone levels and menstrual irregularities return their lab results and their bodies back to normal simply by advising them to stop eating so much soy.

Pound for pound, fermented material will have more nutrition packed into it than the raw material it came from because, aside from acting like miniature detoxification machines, microbes add heaps of nutrients to whatever it is they're growing in. Using enzyme power, single-celled bacteria and fungi manufacture all the vitamins, amino acids, nucleic acids, fatty acids, and so on that they need from simple starting materials like sugar, starch, and cellulose. They can thrive on foods that would leave us horribly malnourished. But we are bigger than they are. When we eat yogurt, real pickles, real sauerkraut—or any food containing living cultures—our digestive juices attack and destroy many of the little critters, exploding their fragile bodies. Many survive (and protect us, see below), but those that are digested donate all their nutritious parts to us. Though after the fermentation process is finished, foods like wine and cheese no longer contain living organisms, they have been enriched by the life-forms they once housed: wine has more antioxidants than grape juice, and cheese more protein than milk.[494] The little critters can actually make all the vitamins we need except D, and all the essential amino acids. And they have one more trick up their sleeve. As if it's not enough that they can free up minerals, preserve our food, manufacture vitamins, and clean up the nasty plant chemicals our bodies can't handle, once inside your body they will literally fight for your life.

FERMENTATION, PART II:
Boost Your Immune System With Probiotics

In 1993, E. coli hamburgers from Jack in the Box restaurants sickened hundreds of children, killing several. Around the same time, E. coli outbreaks in the apple industry led to the requirement that apple juice be pasteurized. In 2006, spinach laced with manure made more people ill. In 2008, Salmonella-tainted tomatoes were blamed for another outbreak—until it was determined that jalapeño peppers were the true culprits. It seems as though there's always something yucky in our food ready to make us sick. No doubt, there are nasty microbial agents in the general food supply all the time. The question is, *Why do they make some people deathly ill while leaving the rest of us alone?*

Turns out, it has to do with our social lives. I'm not talking about the people we go to parties with, but our bacterial bosom buddies. Microbiologist Dr. Bonnie Bassler discovered that microbes have social lives, too.[495] Far from behaving like mindless, pre-programmed specks, they form gangs, share information, and even scheme against other groups of bacteria. In fact, the turbulent world of microorganisms displays all the violence and drama of a spaghetti Western. And the microbial world operates under the same binary rubric. As far as your body's concerned, when it comes to bacteria and fungi, there really are just two kinds: good and bad.

The first group, often referred to with the umbrella term *probiotics*, is comprised of the same beneficial bacteria that preserve, detoxify, and enrich our food. These microbes are friendly and very well-behaved. After all, we feed and house them, so it is in their best interest to keep us healthy. To that end, they secrete hormones that help coordinate the muscular contractions of intestinal peristalsis, while keeping a sharp lookout for bad guys: the *pathogens*. Probiotics work with our immune system. If pathogens hope to gain a foothold, they have to get past the phalanx of probiotics first. While you're watching *Survivor* or *Top Chef,* microbes in your gut are making alliances and scheming against each other for control of your internal real estate.[496] Not only does the outcome of their battles determine whether or not a deadly strain of E. coli in your manure-tainted spinach kills you, studies have shown that live-cultured foods containing probiotics help to prevent a whole range of allergic, auto-immune, and inflammatory diseases.[497, 498, 499]

The people who originally mastered the art of fermenting fruits, vegetables, meats, and so on were probably seeking ways to preserve their food. Crops tend to ripen all at once. Fish swim in schools. Many game animals travel in large herds. These periodic abundances necessitated the development of effective food-preservation methods. The microbial world is so obliging that a little salt, a container, and some know-how are all you—I should say the microbes—need. Today we have simpler options for preserving our food, including canning, refrigeration, freezing, pickling (steeping in vinegar), and drying. But in terms of nutrient conservation, each pales in comparison to fermentation, which often adds new nutrients. Even your refrigerator can't keep fresh fruits and vegetables from declining in nutrient content. For instance, refrigerated green beans lose 77 percent of their vitamin C content after only seven days off the vine.[500]

If you've never fermented anything, you should give it a try. (See chapters 13 and 14 for recipes and tips.) With a little instruction and practice, you can make yourself the best sauerkraut you've ever tasted. And it's ridiculously easy: shred a whole, large cabbage in the food processor or thin-slice by hand. Mix with a full tablespoon of salt and a little liquid from a jar of pickles (or other fermented vegetable product) and pack into a lightproof container with something heavy, like a jar full of water, sitting on top to keep the cabbage under the liquid. Cover with a towel to keep the bugs off. Wait a week or so, and eat.

Not simple enough? Okay, here's something even easier. With sprouting, you just let nature take its course.

SEEDS OF CHANGE:
Why Sprouted Grain Bread Is Better Than Whole Wheat

A lot of my patients tell me that they feel better when they cut wheat from their diet, and more kids than ever are developing celiac disease and other allergies to wheat and products made from wheat. After 10,000 years of cultivation, why the sudden change? There are plenty of potential causes, from GMOs to pesticides to the fact that flour is often heavily contaminated with mold toxins and allergenic proteins (insect parts and rat feces).[501] Even when organically grown, manufacturers treat wheat flour like a construction material, extruding it into geometric shapes and puffing it into crunchy cereal cushions, fusing molecules into unnatural configurations that confuse the immune system.[502] Whether you suffer from wheat allergies or you just want to buy the healthiest bread available, bread made from sprouted wheat (or other grains) is your best bet.

Wheat seeds are called wheat berries. Like all seeds, wheat berries can be sprouted. These days, the only exposure most of us get to sprouts is at the salad bar. People used to eat sprouted stuff all the time, only they didn't let the sprouts develop as fully as those in a salad bar. Our ancestors who didn't have mills were able to acquire more nutrition from their harvests of grain than we do today with all our technological advancements simply by adding water and waiting for the germination process to begin.

Why does germinating a seed first make it more nutritious? Seeds are designed to greedily hang on to their stored proteins, fats, and minerals over extended periods of time. To that end, the plant sheaths them in a hard, nearly impenetrable carapace and locks down nutrients with chemical binders that digestive enzymes can't loosen. Moistening the seeds for a few days activates the plant's own enzymes—including phytase, which digests phytates—to soften the seed, free up bound nutrients, and even create new ones by converting stored starch and fatty acids into proteins and vitamins.

Today's bread is nothing like the bread described in the Bible. The crust of a Domino's pizza and bread made by indigenous people around the world are, nutritionally speaking, as alike as a packet of chicken-flavored powder and wild grouse. Modern bread is made of flour, while ancient breads were made of ground, germinated seeds. Although some of the stone artifacts found in places like Peru, the Nile Delta, or North America may look like something you could use to grind wheat berries into dry flour, I suspect the berries were partly germinated first. Wheat berries are as hard as ball bearings. It's far easier to use seeds softened by germination. I know because I've conducted a study.

In grade school, a friend of mine returned from a visit to a Native American reservation with a set of milling stones around which we just *had* to build an afternoon's drama. We both plaited our hair in what we understood to be proper Native American fashion and walked out into her backyard to figure out how to make "genuine" Indian bread. It was 1973, when every East Coast mother walked in step with hippy trends, so naturally my friend's kitchen had plenty of wheat berries with which to experiment. Enthusiastic as we were, those tiny brown pebbles tested our patience to the breaking point, shooting laterally off the grinding stone and onto the ground until we were convinced that this methodology would fail to generate oven-ready dough by the time my mom was to pick me up. We decided to take a shortcut. Back in the kitchen, her mother had a jar of lentils soaking in water, softened but not yet fully sprouted. They were smushy enough to hold still under the rolling stone. In no time, we had ourselves a small pile of greenish-yellow lentil "dough." (More of a paste, really, since lentils have no gluten.) Ever since, I've been skeptical of anthropologists' claims that similar stones were used to grind wheat or other hard seeds into flour. More likely, seeds used for making bread were pre-softened by letting nature take its course.

You can sprout any kind of seed you want, from kidney beans to wheat berries and more. Simply put some into a jar, cover with water, then cover with a bug-proof cloth and, in anywhere from one to four days, the seeds will start to germinate. On day two, drain and rinse the seeds to be sure to wash any mold spores away. You'll need to rinse the seeds once or twice a day depending on local humidity. You can tell once they've awakened because you'll see a tiny white rootlet begin to take form. That's the point at which it's ready to be used as a vitamin-rich version of an ordinary kidney bean or wheat berry. Or even easier than doing it yourself, you can buy breads made with sprouted grain in health food stores. Usually, you have to look in the freezer section because, without artificial preservatives, these breads mold quickly.

If you can't find sprouted grain breads, the next best thing is sourdough. When shopping for any sort of bread, be aware of a savvy marketing trick. The label on brown bread can say *wheat flour* even though they used white flour because, yes, even white flour originally came from a wheat field. The addition of caramel coloring turns the dough dark, completing the illusion that you've bought healthier whole wheat bread. What should you do? If you want whole wheat look for the words *whole wheat flour*. Or better yet, grind up wheat berries in a coffee grinder and use them to bake your own bread.

Pillar 4
FRESH: THE BENEFITS OF RAW

Every time I give a talk about nutrition, someone in the audience will raise a hand to ask my opinion of the latest antioxidant miracle being said to have otherworldly curative properties. Maybe it's bearberry, or bee pollen, or goji, or ginseng. It could be a liquid extract, or a powder, or a pill—it doesn't really matter. The idea behind *all* antioxidant supplements on the market is the same: to give the consumer a blend of electron-trapping chemicals that help prevent the two most common causes of tissue inflammation and degenerative disease: lipid oxidation and advanced-glycation-end-product formation (see chapters 7, 8, and 9). And every time, my answer is, "If you want antioxidants, skip the latest fad products and use that money to buy fresh food."

FRESH GREENS:
Potency That Can't Be Bottled

There are so many antioxidant miracles on the market now that, if you were so inclined, you could spend an entire paycheck and barely scratch the surface. But it would be a waste of good money. What the nutraceutical industry doesn't want you to know is that there's nothing unique about any of their "unique" formulations; *all fresh fruits and vegetables* contain antioxidants, flavinoids, and other categories of chemicals used as selling points on nutraceutical packages. In fact, as they will tell you, they make their products from fresh fruits and vegetables. It's just that they use fruits and vegetables with more exotic-sounding names.

The truth is, you'll get a better blend of antioxidants simply by eating a variety of familiar greens, along with fresh herbs and spices: sprinkle your marinara with basil and thyme, or make your own salad dressing with garlic and dill. Because supplements have been processed and certain chemicals may concentrate, supplements can have side effects. Fresh, whole foods (including raw meat and fish) universally contain a safe, balanced blend of antioxidants because all living organisms—plant and animal—use them to prevent oxygen damage. Plants are capable of manufacturing so many different kinds of antioxidants that we'll probably never catalogue even a tenth of them. Family names for some of the more common antioxidants include flavinoids, terpenes, phenolics, coumarins, and retinoids (vitamin A precursors). Since antioxidants must work as a team to be effective, where you find one, you find a lot—*but only when they're fresh.* If you want a power pack of antioxidants, you can get them cheap if you follow writer Michael Pollan's advice and grow a tray of fresh herbs out on the balcony. They tend to taste a whole lot better than a capsule of sterile dust.

Why is freshness so important when it comes to antioxidants? Oxygen spoils antioxidants. Antioxidants protect our tissues against oxygen damage by acting like selfless chemical heroes, throwing themselves in the line of fire to protect other chemicals from free radical and oxygen damage. Not only do antioxidants gradually lose their ability to do this over time, as oxidation inevitably occurs during storage, their potency can be neutralized through the drying and/or heating of processing. This is why a lot of foods deliver the most antioxidant punch when eaten raw.

You can taste how much nutritional power a given plant is packing: more intense flavor means more intense nutrition. Both nutrient density and flavor intensity result from a bioconcentration of vitamins, minerals, and other nutrient systems. Pungent vegetables like celery, peppers, broccoli, arugula, and garlic contain more antioxidants, vitamins, and minerals per bite than starchy vegetables like potatoes and turnips. Remember, cooking burns up antioxidants and damages many vitamins. So the more you eat cooked foods, the more you need to balance your diet by eating fresh, uncooked, pungent-tasting herbs and vegetables.

But be aware that raw isn't always better, thanks to cellulose, the material that gives plants their stiffness and their crispy crunch. Locked within cellulose-rich cell walls, vitamins and minerals in high-cellulose plant products pass right through our omnivore's digestive system. Without heat or caustic chemicals, cellulose can only be broken down using specialized bacteria and extended gut-fermentation—something humans lack the intestinal yardage to accomplish (though they can replicate it via fermentation, as we've seen). Studies show that a mere one percent of the retinoids (vitamin A precursors) in raw carrots, for instance, get absorbed.[503] But cooking (which hydrolyzes cellulose in much the same way it hydrolyzes proteins) increases that percentage to 30.[504]

However we eat our veggies, raw or gently cooked, freshness is paramount. As Mrs. A. P. Hill wrote in her 1867 cookbook, "It cannot be questioned that articles originally good and wholesome derive a poisonous character from changes taking place in their own composition." Therefore, "a few only can be kept twelve hours without detriment."[505] This was before refrigeration, of course. But even so, the precipitous drop in nutrition and flavor after picking—and the fact that most grocery store vegetables are grown in poor soil, picked before they're ripe, and then travel the world in cold storage, reducing nutrition and flavor further still—helps explain why so many kids won't eat their veggies.

While gaining access to many of the nutrients in plants often requires (judicious) use of heat, many animal products are so abundant in nutrients that adding thermal energy risks fusing them together. This is why we need to cook our meat so gently, and why raw meat and seafood dishes comprise a valuable part of many international diets, from *sashimi* in Japan to *ceviche* in Spain and South America to steak tartare, popular around the world. But there's one animal product we think of as fresh even though the vast majority of what we find in most grocery stores is, in reality, anything but: milk.

FRESH DAIRY:
Why Mess With Udder Perfection?

Milk may be the single most historically important food to human health. Not just any milk, mind you, but raw milk from healthy, free-to-roam, grass-fed cows. The difference between the milk you buy in the store and the milk your great-great-grandparents enjoyed is, unfortunately, enormous. If we lived in a country where raw milk from healthy, pastured cows were still a legal product and available as readily as, say, soda or a handgun, we'd all be taller and healthier, and I'd see fewer elderly patients with hunched backs and broken hips. If you're lucky enough to live in a state where raw milk is available in stores and you don't buy it, you are passing up a huge opportunity to improve your health immediately. If you have kids, raw milk will not only help them grow, but will also boost their immune systems so they get sick less often. And, since the cream in raw milk is an important source of brain-building fats, whole milk and other raw dairy products will also help them to learn.

It's a common misperception that milk drinking is a relatively new practice, one limited to Europeans. The reality is that our cultural—and now, our epigenetic—dependence on milk most likely originated somewhere in Africa. It is highly likely that milk consumption gave those who practiced animal husbandry such an advantage that it rapidly spread across the continent and then into Europe and Asia. With such widespread use, it's likely that to allow for optimal expression, many of our genes now require it. In those countries where people's stature most benefited from the consumption of raw milk, when raw milk is replaced with a processed alternative, their bones take the hardest hit. It's a case of the bigger they are the harder they fall. In places like Norway, Sweden, and Denmark, people now suffer from particularly high rates of osteoporosis and degenerative arthritis.[506]

Our genes have been infused with real dairy products for tens of thousands of years. Recent geologic and climatologic research reveals that from 100,000 to 10,000 years ago, the Sahara Desert was a lush paradise of grassland. During that window of abundance, the human population exploded. To deal with the consequential depletion of wild resources, people began experiments in "proto-farming," a term coined by biologist and historian Colin Tudge to describe humanity's slow-motion leap from living in harmony with the land as hunter-gatherers to adopting the now-familiar program of altering the ecology to suit our interests. Author Thom Hartmann explains in his book *The Last Hours of Ancient Sunlight*:

> Something important happened around 40,000 years ago: humans figured out a way to change the patterns of nature so we could get more sunlight/food than other species did. The human food supply was determined by how many deer or rabbits the local forest could support. . . . But in areas where the soil was too poor for farming or forest, supporting only scrub brush and grasses, humans discovered that ruminants (grazing animals like goats, sheep, and cows) could eat those plants that we couldn't, and could therefore convert the daily sunlight captured by the scrub and wild plants on that "useless" land into animal flesh, which we could eat.[507]

Or drink, as the case may be.

For millennia, much of the world's population has depended largely on milk for nutritional sustenance. However, the medical world has been ignorant of milk's nearly ubiquitous use, confused by the issue of lactose intolerance. Because Europeans have lower rates of lactose intolerance, most Western physicians presume that only European populations have historically practiced dairying. But this confusion arises in part because most Western physicians don't know very much about fermentation.

LACTOSE INTOLERANCE

Lactose is the major type of sugar in milk. Nearly everyone can digest it while we're babies and dependent on our mother's milk, but many people lose the lactase enzyme in the lining of the intestine, growing lactose intolerant as they get older. Fermentation breaks down lactose, so you don't need that enzyme as long as you only eat fermented dairy products, such as yogurt and cheese. The reason people living in warmer climates tend to be lactose intolerant more often than Europeans stems from the fact that fermentation progresses rapidly in warmer climates. Once fermented, the potentially irritating lactose sugars are gone. A child living in a warmer climate would, after weaning, have such infrequent need for the lactase enzyme that the epigenetic librarian would simply switch the gene off. In cooler European climates, fresh milk stays fresh for hours or days, and was presumably consumed that way often enough to keep the lactase enzyme epigenetically activated throughout a person's life. If you have true lactose intolerance, as opposed to a protein allergy, you should be able to tolerate plain (unflavored) yogurt, cheese, and cream (dairy fat contains little to no lactose—and minimal protein).

WHY MOST MILK IS PASTEURIZED TODAY

Most of us also have heard that milk needs to be pasteurized to be safe. But we haven't heard the whole story. For perhaps thousands of years, people who gave their animals the humane care they deserved survived and thrived drinking completely fresh, raw milk. The need for pasteurization became a reality when in-city dairies housed diseased cows whose hindquarters ran with rivulets of manure. (Pasteurization is a process that significantly reduces foodborne microbes, both good and bad, most often using high heat.) Tainting milk's reputation even further, around the same time, dairymen were often infected with diphtheria, spreading the deadly bacteria through the medium of warm, protein-rich milk. But no epidemics have *ever* been traced to raw milk consumption when the cows were healthy and the humans milking them were disease free.[508] If the animal is sickly—as they invariably are when they are raised in crowded, nightmarish conditions—its milk should probably not be consumed at all. When that's your only choice, then yes, it ought to be cooked first to reduce the risk of potentially lethal infections including undulant fever, hemolytic uremia, sepsis, and more. But it's not your only choice.

If you erase any ethical entanglement, impulse of social responsibility, nagging moral prohibition, and investment in human health, you could call milk

AFRICAN PETROGLYPH

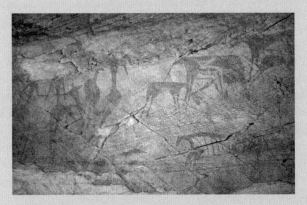

Unpasteurized milk is not a new idea. This depiction of a woman milking a cow can be found in the same "Cave of Swimmers" featured in the movie *The English Patient.* It is located in an area of Egypt known as the Gilf Kabir and believed to have been painted around 10,000 years ago, when the Sahara was a lush grassland. The woman on her knees appears to be collecting milk in a gourd with her left hand while holding off the calf with her right.

pasteurization a good thing. In terms of volume of product output per production unit, pasteurization plays a crucial role in converting small family farms into perfectly efficient milk producers for the national brands: cheaper feed (silage and grain instead of fresh grass and hay), more cows per square foot, more "milk" per cow. That explains why big agribusiness roots for pasteurization. But how did the rest of us get convinced?

Our fear of fresh milk can be traced to the energetic campaigning of a man named Charles North, who patented the first batch-processing pasteurization machine in 1907.[509] A skilled orator and savvy businessman, he visited small towns throughout the country creating publicity and interest in his machines by claiming to have come directly from another small town, just like theirs, where people were dying from drinking unpasteurized milk.[510] Of course, his claims were total fiction and doctors were staunchly opposed to pasteurization.[511] The facts were on their side. Unfortunately, North had something better—fear. And he milked that fear right into a small fortune. The pasteurization industry mushroomed from nonexistence to a major political presence. Today, at the University of Pennsylvania, where medical professors once protested that pasteurization "should never be had recourse to," [512] medical students are given lessons on the many health benefits of pasteurization.

Whenever I have a patient who was raised on a farm, who looks tough and boasts how rarely he gets sick, I ask him if he drank raw milk as a child. Nine times out of ten, he says yes. Every family dairyman I've talked to keeps raw milk around for their own families and happily testifies to its health benefits. Unlike meat, or fruit, or really any other food, milk is unique in that its one and only purpose is to nourish something else. Not only is it loaded with nutrients, it is engineered with an intricate micro-architecture that is key to enhancing digestive function while preventing the nourishing compounds from reacting with one another. Processing fundamentally alters this micro-architecture and diminishes nutritive value significantly. How much of a difference does this make? Enough that, based on their health and bone structure, I can guess with a high degree of accuracy which of my patients had access to raw milk as a child and which did not.

Since 1948, when states began passing mandatory pasteurization laws, raw milk fans have waged a bitter battle against government intervention. During hearings in which laws requiring pasteurization have been challenged, pasteurization proponents deny any nutritional difference between pasteurized, homogenized milk, and raw. But as dairy scientists point out, heat denatures proteins, and homogenization explodes the fat droplets in milk. This is significant. Even to the naked eye, there's a difference: unlike processed milk, the fresh product has a layer of cream floating at the top. But to fully understand how these two products differ, we need to bring out the microscope.

THE DIFFERENCE BETWEEN FRESH AND PROCESSED

If we put a drop of fresh milk on a slide, we see thousands of lipid droplets of varying size streaming under the cover slip and maybe a living lactobacilli or two wiggling from edge to edge. These come from the cow's udders, which, when well cared for, are colonized with beneficial bacteria, as is human skin. We want good bacteria in our milk. These probiotics protect both the milk and the milk consumer from pathogens. Good bacteria accomplish this by using the same bacterial communication techniques we read about in the section on fermentation.

Using the powerful electron microscope, we can magnify milk 10,000,000 times. Now we can see casein micelles, which are amazingly complex. Imagine a mound of spaghetti and meatballs formed into a big round ball. The strands of spaghetti are made of protein (casein), and the meatballs are made of the most digestible form of calcium phosphate, called colloidal calcium phosphate, which holds the spaghetti strands together in a clump with its tiny magnetic charge. This clumping prevents sugar from reacting with and destroying milk's essential amino acids.

Each tiny globe of fat in the milk is enclosed inside a phospholipid membrane very similar to the membranes surrounding every cell in your body. The mammary gland cell that produced the fat droplet donated some of its membrane when the droplet exited the cell. This coating performs several tasks, starting in the milk duct, where it prevents fat droplets from coalescing and clogging up mom's mammary passageways. The milk fat globule's lipid bilayer is studded with a variety of specialized proteins, just like the living cells in your body. Some proteins protect the globule from bacterial infection while others are tagged with short chains of sugars that may function as a signal to the intestinal cell that the contents are to be accepted without immune inspection, streamlining digestion. Still others may act as intestinal cell growth factors, encouraging and directing intestinal cells' growth and function. As long as the coating surrounds the milk fat globule, the fat is easily digested, the gallbladder doesn't have to squeeze out any bile for the fat to be absorbed, the fatty acids inside the blob are isolated from the calcium in the casein micelles, and everything goes smoothly. But if calcium and fats come into contact with one another, as we'll see in a moment, milk loses much of its capacity to deliver nutrients into your body.

Let's go back to the light microscope to take a look at pasteurized, homogenized milk and identify what distinguishes it from raw. One striking difference will be the homogeneity of fat globule sizes and the absence of living bacteria. But the real damage is hiding behind all this homogeneity and is only revealed under the electron microscope. Now we see that these fat blobs lack the sophisticated bilayer wrapping and are instead caked with minerals and tangled remnants of casein micelles. Why does it look like this? The heat of pasteurization forces the sugar to react with amino acids, denaturing the proteins and knocking the fragile colloidal calcium phosphate out of the spaghetti-and-meatballs matrix, while the denatured spaghetti strands tangle into a tight, hard knot. Homogenization squeezes the milk through tiny holes under intense pressure, destroying the architecture of the fat globules. Once the two processing steps have destroyed the natural architecture of milk, valuable nutrients react with each other with health-damaging consequences.

Processing can render milk highly irritating to the intestinal tract, and such a wide variety of chemical changes may occur that processed milk can lead to diarrhea or constipation. During processing, the nice, soft meatball of colloidal calcium phosphate fuses with the fatty acids to form a kind of milk-fat soap. This reaction, called *saponification*, irritates many people's GI tracts and makes the calcium and phosphate much less bio-available and more difficult to absorb.[513] How difficult? Studies comparing fresh to pasteurized skim cow's milk and human breast milk show processing leads to a dramatic six-fold drop in mineral bioavailability.[514, 515] When fresh, the milk fat globule carries signal molecules on the surface, which help your body recognize milk as a helpful substance as opposed to, say, an invasive bacteria. Processing demolishes those handy signals, and so, instead of getting a free pass into the intestinal cell, the curiously distorted signals slow the process of digestion down so much that it can lead to constipation.[516] Heat destroys amino acids, especially the fragile essential amino acids, and so pasteurized milk contains less protein than fresh.[517] But the damaged amino acids don't just disappear; they have been *glycated*, oxidized, and transformed into stuff like N-carboxymethyl-lysine, malonaldehyde, and 4-hydroxynonanal—potential allergens and pro-inflammatory irritants.[518]

Proponents of pasteurization like to point out that there's no measurable difference in the protein or mineral content of fresh versus processed milk, as if that means these two products have identical effects on the body. Of course, if you buy into the idea that food is more than fuel—it's information—and once you learn how processing garbles the chemical information nature intends for milk to impart, you might suspect the two products would have very different abilities to direct child growth, and you'd be right. In the 1920s and 1930s, doctors compared the effects of raw versus pasteurized milk growth by dividing 1,500 institutionalized orphan children into raw-milk and pasteurized-milk feeding groups. Their findings, published in the *Lancet* and other reputable journals, revealed as much as 40 percent improvement in bone growth on the raw milk, along with improved moods, disease resistance, and more.[519, 520]

And there's more. Many of the active enzymes in fresh milk designed to help streamline the digestive process have also been destroyed. Other enzymes, such as xanthine oxidase, which ordinarily protect the milk (but cause damage inside our arteries), can play stowaway within the artificially formed fat blobs and be absorbed. Normally, our digestive system would chop up this enzyme and digest it. But hidden inside fat, it can be ingested whole, and may retain some of its original activity. Once in the body, xanthine oxidase can generate free radicals and lead to atherosclerosis and asthma. One more thing that makes raw milk special is the surface molecules on milk fat globule membranes, called *gangliosides*. Gangliosides inhibit harmful bacteria in the intestine. Once digested, they've been shown to stimulate neural development.[521] Homogenization strips these benefits away.

What does all this scientific data mean to you? It means that the processed milk you buy in the store is not milk. Not really. If you can't find a good source of fresh, unprocessed milk, what can you do? Get the next best thing: yogurt made from organic, whole milk. The fermentation process rejuvenates damaged proteins and makes minerals more bioavailable. A breakfast of yogurt, fresh fruit slices, and nuts is nutritionally far superior to cold cereal and processed milk. But if you aren't ready to give up milk for breakfast, then get organic whole milk (not low fat), preferably from cows raised on pasture—not grain! Non-organic dairy may seem cheaper, but in reality you get far less nutrition for the dollar than you do with organic because at least organically raised cows produce milk. The stuff that comes out of malnourished cows living in cement milk factories hardly qualifies as such. Whatever you do, avoid soymilk. The primary difference between Yoo-hoo, a junk food beverage snack sold in your local 7-Eleven, and the soymilk sold in the health food stores is that Yoo-hoo is flavored with chocolate.

FRESH MEAT

Here in the United States, white-gloved health department officials encourage us to cook our meat to death. Not because overcooked meat is tastier or more nutritious but because our meat has generally been slaughtered days or weeks before we buy it, let alone eat it, in filthy conditions that enable pathogenic bacteria to proliferate all over the surface. Those, we must destroy with plenty of heat in order to be "safe." If you are lucky enough to travel to Asia, Africa, or India, you might want to stop at one of those restaurants that keep chickens out back. Why do they do this? Because fresh meat is part of every world cuisine and fresh meat can, when the animals are known to be healthy, safely be cooked rare. Juicy pinkness indicates the presence of far more nutrients than you can get when meat is overcooked.

In the 1930s and 1940s, Dr. Frances Marion Pottenger conducted a ten-year experiment that gives us valuable insights into the potential long-term consequences of overcooking. Pottenger fed one group of cats raw meat and milk, and another group cooked meat and pasteurized milk. The all-raw cats produced ten generations of healthy and well-adjusted kittens. Not so, the cats on the cooked diet. By the end of the first generation, they started to develop degenerative diseases and became "quite lazy." The second generation developed degenerative diseases earlier in life and started losing their coordination. By the third generation, the cats had developed degenerative disease very early in life, and some were born blind and weak and died prematurely. There was an abundance of parasites and vermin in this group, and skin disease and allergies increased from an incidence of 5 percent in normal cats to over 90 percent in the third generation. Males became docile and females aggressive. By the fourth generation, litters were stillborn or so sickly they didn't live to reach adulthood. This research prompted pet food manufacturers to add back some of the vitamins lost during heating. Still, dried and canned pet food is nothing like the diets cats thrive on.

Pottenger's research highlights the importance of eating vitamin-rich, *fresh* meat. But if you don't have access to the quality of meat that can safely be cooked rare, then it's all the more important for you to make sure to get the freshest greens you can and eat them raw or gently cooked.

HOW THE FOUR PILLARS WILL MAKE YOU HEALTHIER

Whatever your age, whatever illnesses run in your family, whatever your "risk factors," however many times you've tried to lose weight or build muscle, eating the foods I've described in this chapter will transform your body. And if you are planning a baby, eating Four Pillar foods before, during, and after conception, and then feeding them to your child as he or she grows up, will allow the genes in his or her body to express in ways yours may not have.

Meat on the bone will bring enough of the glycosaminoglycan growth factors and bone-building minerals to make a child's joints strong and their bones tough, enabling them to grow tall and excel in sports. In adulthood, these same factors will keep your joints well-lubricated and prevent aging bones from crumbling. No combination of supplements has the right balance of bioavailable minerals and collagen-derived growth factors to fortify your body as effectively as meat on the bone.

Organ meats bring the vitamins and brain-building fats that can ensure children will have mental stability and an aptitude for learning, and continued consumption of these foods is the best way to guarantee that your brain cells and nerves stay healthy for the rest of your life. Because these nutrients deteriorate so rapidly, no pills can effectively encapsulate them.

Fermented foods, full of probiotics, protect the intestinal tract from invading pathogens. Since a healthier intestine is more able to take in nutrients, probiotics may prevent infections and allergic disorders from developing elsewhere in the body, reducing the need for repeated doses of antibiotics. Probiotics living in our intestine also produce all sorts of vitamins, which help to round out a diet that might otherwise be deficient. Sprouted foods enable you to enjoy your breads and breakfast porridges without consuming the empty calories that cause obesity and diabetes.

And finally, fresh foods are naturally loaded with more antioxidants than can possibly survive the processes of drying, overcooking, or being stuffed into a capsule and bottled.

This is just a brief look at the benefits imparted by the Four Pillars. People who aren't connected to any culinary tradition don't consume any of the Four Pillars as often as they should. If you build your diet on the foundation of the Four Pillars, and get regular exercise and plenty of sleep, you will immediately notice vast improvements in how you feel. Those differences will compound over the years to keep you looking young.

TWO STEPS TO PERFECT HEALTH

Up to this point in the book, I have provided information that has, I hope, convinced you that the source of incredible health and vitality is no mystery. Rather than leaving your health in the hands of fate, you can take control of your genetic destiny by feeding your body the same nutrients your ancestors depended on. There are only two steps to doing that: (1) Find the best ingredients grown on the richest soil in the most wholesome, sustainable manner; and (2) Ensure that your body can use those nutrients most efficiently by preparing the raw materials according to the foundational principles of the Human Diet: the Four Pillars of World Cuisine.

When I say genetic destiny, I'm talking about your future and your children's as well. As you remember from previous chapters, the building of a whole body from a single fertilized cell requires an optimum nutritional environment. Every event during the nine and a half months in utero is a minor miracle requiring a wholesome, rich environment. No physiologic event is as dramatic as the transcription of epigenetic data from gametes to zygote. And therefore none is as dependent on good nutrients, or more vulnerable to the interference of toxins.

Nutrition's powerful influence upon every aspect of cellular growth and behavior—from assigning cellular identity to cell growth and maturation—is a process that continues throughout our entire lives. What scientists have learned about epigenetics and the protean nature of cells tells us that, just like a baby developing inside the womb, our bodies continue to be a work in progress throughout our lives, every cell in our body guided by what our diet is telling us about the outside environment. And because the message food carries is every bit as complex and nuanced as the environment from which it came, the re-

SIX BUILDING BLOCKS FOR A BETTER BRAIN,
AND WHERE TO GET THEM

We live in the age of the "super food." On TV shows, podcasts, and websites, health experts are more than happy to tell you what specific pungent root vegetable or little-known tropical fruit or what ugly-looking nut from the deep forest of the Himalayas is the one and only food guaranteed to prevent colon cancer or protect your heart or permanently stave off the ravages of dementia and memory loss.

The truth is almost any food grown in a healthy environment and eaten in the right proportion can play a role in supporting some function of the body. But given that the main threat to the health of your brain comes from oxidative stress, it is useful to identify the groups of nutrients most capable of preventing oxidative stress in the fragile PUFAs that compose so much of your brain. That's why I pack my brain food list not with specific foods but with groups that provide PUFA protection, either by serving as a source of healthy, unoxidized PUFAs, or by protecting PUFAs from oxidative damage.

1. **Omega-3 brain builder:** 15 percent of the (dry) weight of the brain is composed of docosahexanoic acid (DHA), and roughly 4 milligrams a day meets the brain's needs. Sources: cream and butter (better if raw) from grass-fed cows, oysters, oily fish like sardines, mackerel, salmon (also better raw, gently cooked, smoked, or if canned, packed in water or olive oil), and fish roe. Plant sources include raw flax, chia seeds, and walnuts. Keep in mind, if you expose omega-3s to high heat, as in baking walnuts into muffins, the omega-3 may mutate from a healthy PUFA into not-so-healthy distorted MegaTrans molecules.

2. **Omega-6 brain builder:** 15 percent of the (dry) weight of the brain is arachidonic acid, and roughly 4 milligrams a day meets the brain's needs. Sources: egg yolk (poached or sunny side up), cheese, butter (whether grass-fed or not), raw or sprouted sunflower seeds, walnuts, edamame. Keep in mind, though omega-6 is less reactive than omega-3, it's still highly reactive and, when exposed to high heat, often transforms into MegaTrans.

3. **Antioxidant rainbow:** to protect the PUFAs from oxidation during digestion. Sources: colorful fresh vegetables eaten raw, fermented, or gently steamed, baby greens, celery, bell peppers, carrots, red and green cabbage, onions, garlic, cilantro, parsley and other fresh herbs, vegetable condiments like kimchee, pickles, sauerkraut, and pickled vegetables.

4. **Vitamin E:** to protect the PUFAs in your nerve cell membranes and in your lipoproteins as they travel to your brain. Sources: raw or sprouted

sunflower seeds, wheat germ, spinach, almonds, pistachios, avocado, soybeans, broccoli, shrimp, and herring.

5. **The amino acid cysteine:** the limiting ingredient for building the antioxidant glutathione, which plays a role in repairing vitamin E after it is oxidized. Sources: beef, lamb, chicken, pork, clams, tuna, mussels, cheese, eggs, soybeans, kamut, split peas.

6. **Vitamin C:** to repair glutathione. Sources: bell peppers, guava, kale, kiwi, broccoli, oranges, strawberries, peas, papaya, tomatoes.

ductionist "a calorie is a calorie" view undermines the true complexity of food's chemical message.

As you're about to discover, a far more realistic and useful way to think about food is as *information*, the chemical language with which nature speaks directly to our bodies.

CHAPTER 11

Beyond Calories
Using Food as a Language to Achieve Ideal Body Weight

■ There is more to losing weight than counting calories.

■ Food is more than fuel; it is chemical information.

■ Unhealthy foods instruct the body to build fat cells.

■ Exercise generates the signal to convert fat into muscle and other lean tissues.

■ The Human Diet provides the raw materials required for the body to respond to exercise signals.

In medical school I was taught a simple formula: calories consumed minus calories burned equals weight gained or lost. Then, as a resident treating my own patients, I'd sit down with people who wanted to lose weight and lay out the formula for their benefit.

Then things got complicated. Time and time again I'd hear, "*I don't understand it, Doc. I don't eat anything all day. I work out. But I'm still gaining! There must be something wrong with me. Can you check my thyroid hormones?*" I would, but the results were always normal. I'd try suggesting that they might have been consuming more calories than they realized, pointing out that eating on the go—while driving home, for instance—is still eating. But many times, patients really seemed to defy the formula. They'd eat little, go to the gym and take walks around the block, and yet the pudge refused to budge. Was it just their metabolism? Or could the energy-balance formula be flawed?

Turns out, weight gain and loss isn't so much about energy as it is about *information*. As you've read in the preceding chapters, food is far more than fuel; it's a language that programs every function of your cells. If you've been gaining weight, it's because you are eating foods and doing activities that, in essence, tell your body to pack on the pounds. You know how a few clever words can convince you to do things that, in retrospect, seem foolish? Our bodies can be convinced to do things we wish they wouldn't, too. It all depends on what we eat, and the kind of *messages* our food contains. Foods with the right messages immediately start making us healthy because our bodies are continually responding to what we do—and foods with the wrong messages can act immediately, too. The foods that constitute the Human Diet instruct your body to do its very best, and once you start eating them, better health will come automatically.

To see just how powerfully the chemicals in our food—and not their caloric content—influence our cellular decisions, let's take a look at two different kinds of fats. Essential fatty acids omega-3 and omega-6 are nearly identical to the chemists who draw them on their chalkboards. But to our cells, they are as opposite as night and day.

ENERGY VERSUS INFORMATION: WHY CALORIES DON'T ALWAYS COUNT

In 1995, a journalist named Jo Robinson struck up a chance conversation with a friendly Ph.D. candidate who was examining a biologic process called *apoptosis*, a kind of cell suicide in which a damaged cell recognizes that it is more likely to be harmful than useful and dutifully takes itself apart. Using catheter tubes to directly feed cancerous tumors growing in rats, he discovered that while injecting omega-3 slowed and even reversed the mice's cancer growth, injecting omega-6 accelerated that growth four-fold. These fatty acids contain essentially equivalent caloric energy, so why should one make cells divide and another bring cell division to a grinding halt?

Clearly, the process of growth is regulated by something other than calories. To Robinson, whom I interviewed in 2006, this research suggested something startling—not about growth in general but about the underlying cause of cancer: *a fatty acid imbalance might set us up for cancer.* Robinson asked the scientist what kinds of foods contain omega-6 and omega-3. He replied, "Omega-3 comes from things like eggs, cold-water fatty fish, and plants people don't eat anymore, like flax." The growth-promoting omega-6 fatty acids, on the other hand, are hard to avoid, as they are prevalent in corn, soy, animals fed these grains, and the vegetable oils in just about every package on the food store shelves.

Robinson relived that moment with me as we sat together in her home overlooking the Puget Sound in the state of Washington, and a mix of inspiration and determination came over her face. "I knew what I had to do," she said. Together with Artemis Simopolous, who ran the lab where she'd met the young scientist, she went on to write the best-selling book *The Omega Diet,* which introduced the world to essential fats and filled a huge gap in conventional nutrition education. Her book explains that in the Paleolithic era we ate roughly ten times more omega-3 than we do now, and far less omega-6. That shift in consumption has created a nationwide dietary imbalance that exacerbates numerous inflammatory diseases, including cancer, arthritis, and obesity.

Dozens of researchers have since built careers describing how omega-3 helps prevent all manner of disease. Incorporating just a little more of this one essential fat into your diet can help every cell in your body function better. That's great news. But while so much attention has been focused on specific benefits of omega-3, an even more promising underlying fact is being overlooked.

Imagine you work in a zoo. At feeding time you're considering whether to feed the ducks their usual birdseed or birdseed mixed with popcorn. By chance, you wonder out loud, "What do you think of the popcorn?" And the ducks answer in unison, "We love it!" The next morning, the headline in the *Weekly Zoo Report* reads, "Ducks Prefer Birdseed With Popcorn!" But there's a bigger story here, isn't there? Namely, that ducks can listen to what we're saying, and respond in English! Of course, it's very interesting that they like popcorn. But more amazing is the fact that not only are they capable of communicating with us, they may have been understanding us all along, perhaps even doing their best to comply with our every request.

Similarly, our discoveries about omega-3 and omega-6 point to a more powerful biologic truth than the fact that we could use more omega-3.

Our cells are extremely sensitive to the specific nature of the chemical messages we send them every time we eat. By altering the blends of nutrients (or toxins) in our food, we can actually control whether our cells function normally, or convert to fat, or turn cancerous. The nutrients and chemicals we consume in effect *tell* our cells what to do—when to divide, which protein to manufacture, and even what type of cell to become.[522]

Our omega-3 and omega-6 ratio problem is just one of many dietary imbalances that send a barrage of mixed-up signals to our cells, telling our bodies to store fat and lose muscle and bone—all the stuff we don't want them to do. What's key to being healthy, then, is eating foods that send the right messages. Once we appreciate how common foods convince our cells to behave in ways that make us sick, we can understand why so many of us struggle with something as fundamental as maintaining optimum bodyweight. So the *Deep Nutrition* formula for weight loss is simple: *Get rid of inflammation that blocks cellular communication, and eat foods that enable you to convert fat cells into healthier tissues.*

Of course, there's more to health than a healthy diet. Sleep and physical activity generate other chemicals that help your body know what you are expecting of it. So in order to reshape your body and achieve maximum health, your regimen *must* include eating real food, resting properly, reducing stress, and doing the right kinds of exercise. The rest of this chapter will take you step-by-step through what you need to do to make the most of your body's amazing potential for change.

STEP 1: APPRECIATE WHAT FAT DOES FOR YOU

You'll never get on *Baywatch* without body fat, and I'm not just talking about Pamela Anderson's most obvious assets. A twenty-year-old's face has far more fat around the eyes, lips, and chin than that of a seventy-year-old. Well-placed fat makes people look young. And, truth is, we can't be healthy without it. Aside from acting as simple mechanical insulation and cushioning, body fat (known medically as *adipose tissue*) generates chemicals required for sexual development and reproduction, immune defense, blood clotting, circadian rhythm, and even mood and concentration.[523, 524, 525] Life without any adipose tissue would be very difficult indeed. Paradoxically, not enough and too much fat can cause many of the same problems: "Fatless mice are prone to insulin insensitivity, glucose intolerance, hyperphagia, weight gain, fatty liver, and high triglyceride [levels]."[526] Just like fat mice.

Most of us, of course, are trying to slim down. If you've gone on a diet without achieving the body-changing results you had hoped for, chances are you've never been given the full story on fat, its function, and the steps you can take to control it. The more we understand the reasons our bodies create and retain fat, the better we can understand how to turn unwanted fat into something better.

The wonderful news is that fat cells, like all cells, are always ready to follow our instructions on what to do next. Those instructions come primarily from physical activity and the foods we eat. Contrary to popular belief, fat cells are *not* forever. But the strategy is not to "melt the pounds away" by starving, or sweating them out. As with the tumor cells that killed themselves when omega-3 was added, you can command your fat cells, by way of certain chemical signals, to do what you want.

Why Supplements Won't Work

So what are those chemical signals? That's the question that a multi-billion-dollar industry has been obsessing over for decades.

In 1995, researchers working with a breed of grossly overweight mice discovered that the breed lacked a chemical called *leptin*. Biotech companies immediately saw dollar signs, investing heavily in leptin research. They even patented the gene. Shortly after its discovery, leptin was found to suppress appetite and fat cell division. Leptin researchers thought they'd stumbled onto a goldmine.

They had, but it was fool's gold. Obesity isn't a simple matter of leptin deficiency; it's a complex problem of multiple imbalances. It soon became clear that overweight people are not only leptin deficient but also leptin *resistant*. Their bodies are unable to hear the signal leptin sends, so giving them more leptin will not help. Worse, one potential side effect of leptin supplementation includes breast cancer.[527]

And so, as quickly as it came, the leptin gold rush was over. The rise and fall of leptin is emblematic of our misplaced faith in technological fixes for biological problems. The real solution will come not from technology, but biology—in the form of healthy food.

After learning that obese people were leptin resistant, the researchers missed an opportunity. If they'd recognized that leptin resistance might indicate that signals were being blocked, they might have asked a crucial question: *What might be blocking them?* We've already hinted at it in earlier chapters: a kind of chemical static that interferes with normal metabolic processes called *inflammation*.

STEP 2: RID YOUR BODY OF INFLAMMATION

Pro-Inflammatory Foods: What Not to Eat

Inflammation is a huge buzzword in the nutrition world these days. Plenty of books, articles, and apps offer inflammation indices, lists of anti-inflammatory and pro-inflammatory foods, and anti-inflammation menu plans. And there are plenty of supplements claiming to be anti-inflammatory. Why is inflammation so bad?

Inflammation is disruptive. It can block chemical signals required for normal, healthy cellular growth. Inflammation also tends to generate its own signals that tell our bodies to store fat. You could say that healthy foods will educate your cells so they'll grow up to be useful members of your physiology, while pro-inflammatory foods trick individual cells into doing things that are dangerous for the body as a whole. The tendency for processed foods to cause inflammation is one big reason we have to go beyond the calorie content listed on a package to understand how the foods we eat will make us gain or lose weight. Instead of focusing on calories, if we look at the *signals* different meals generate, we can readily understand why processed foods make us build fat and why the Human Diet helps us to lose it.

Distorted Fats Damage Enzymes and Lead to Cellular Death

If you've read chapters 7, 8, and 9, you know that heating vegetable oils leads to the formation of oxidized and distorted fats called MegaTrans, and that these two groups of fats can generate free radicals, which are pro-inflammatory. You also know that saturated fat helps you resist free radical damage, and therefore resist inflammation. So you already know two factors other than calories that influence how fats affect your health. As we'll see, distorted fats like Mega-Trans can also make you gain weight.

Distorted fats are pro-inflammatory because of their unnatural shapes; they act like a booby trap for your enzymes. An enzyme called delta-9 desaturase mistakes trans fat for saturated fat and picks it up. The delta-9 desaturase enzyme enables us to metabolize certain fatty acids. But once the delta-9 desaturase has picked up trans fat, its fat-metabolizing days are over. There's a kink in the trans molecule that acts like a barb on a hook, so that once trans slips into the enzyme, it won't come out. Another enzyme called delta-6 desaturase thinks trans fat looks like an omega-3 or omega-6 fatty acid, so it picks it up and runs into the same problem: once the enzymes touch trans, they can't let go. Trans fat in your diet effectively deactivates many of your delta-6 and delta-9 fat-metabolizing enzymes.[528] With enough of these enzymes shut down, your cells can no longer metabolize normal, healthy fatty acids fast enough.[529] Not only does that block your body's ability to convert fat into energy, it can lead to abnormal free fatty acid accumulations inside the cells of your body's organs, including brain, heart, and adipose tissue. This excess of free fatty acid can prevent the affected organ from performing its duty.[530, 531]

One of the most widely recognized complications of toxic free fatty acid accumulation is a condition called *fatty liver*, which can be diagnosed with an ultrasound test.[532] Fatty liver used to be associated exclusively with alcoholics, diabetics, and severe obesity. Now, fatty liver is being identified in nondrinkers and nondiabetics who are close to normal weight.[533] Fatty liver turns on fat-building enzymes in the liver and elsewhere, which can lead to toxic levels of free fatty acids inside a cell.[534] Even in the early stages of fatty liver, people lose control of their weight as so many of their body tissues are forced (by

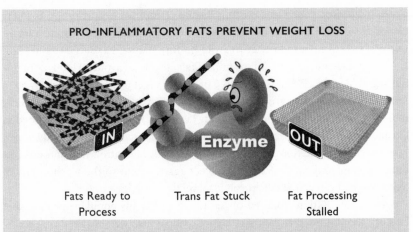

PRO-INFLAMMATORY FATS PREVENT WEIGHT LOSS

| Fats Ready to Process | Trans Fat Stuck | Fat Processing Stalled |

This poor enzyme has picked up a molecule of trans fat and now he can't let go. Abnormally shaped fatty acids knock key enzymes out of action. Without these enzymes, the body cannot act on the message to burn fat or build muscle—no matter how much you exercise.

malfunctioning enzymes) to convert sugar (and carbs) into fat.[535] Low-calorie diets don't reliably cure fatty liver. What a person with fatty liver needs to do is rehabilitate their liver, and the Human Diet can do that.

Free fatty acids within liver and other cells may become toxic simply because too many can get "underfoot" (like kids' toys) and end up disturbing normal cellular activity. In muscle cells, for example, free fatty acids can interfere with the assembly of internal supports, called *microtubules*, which enable muscle cells to contract.[536] With too much free fatty acid polluting a muscle cell, the microtubules cannot be properly constructed. And so they break apart. As fat continues to build up and internal supports break down, the cell enters a state of decay called *lipoapoptosis*.[537] Lipoapoptosis kills healthy cells, and leads to inflammation, immune disorders, and the buildup of additional fat.[538]

The more distorted fat you eat, the more inflammation you're fighting against. Trans fat reduces your ability to metabolize the saturated *and* essential fatty acids that you need to be healthy, so eating trans fat can initiate a vicious cycle. The Nurses' Health Study, the largest, longest-running study of women's health, showed that a mere *2* percent increase in trans fat consumption correlated with a *40* percent increase in insulin resistance and diabetes.[539] Once you develop diabetes, your metabolism is deeply committed to converting as many calories as it can into fat. Given the power of unnatural fats to disturb metabolism, it's no wonder the advice to avoid healthy, natural fats sets us up to fail.

To successfully avoid eating oxidized fats, you must avoid all foods containing vegetable oils. As I described in Chapter 7, vegetable oils are high in *polyunsaturated* fats, which are particularly prone to oxidation and readily deform into the collection of distorted fatty acids I call MegaTrans. And, as explained in Chapter 7, saturated fat resists oxidation—so much so that, in the body, it can help check inflammation before it gets too far out of control. Eating foods like butter, cream, and coconut oil can protect against some of the worst effects of oxidation and can actually help you lose weight.

Dr. Robert Atkins focused on saturated fat for his popular low-carb diet because he noticed that eating it helped people lose weight. He didn't know about the anti-inflammatory effects of saturated fat. He just knew what worked. But without knowing exactly *why* it worked, he couldn't go so far as to advise people to avoid pro-inflammatory vegetable oils. Because of the prevailing view that saturated fat is harmful and vegetable oils beneficial, physicians and nutritionists running weight-loss organizations—from South Beach, to Lindora, to Weight Watchers—wrongly advise people to avoid saturated fat and encourage the consumption of unhealthy vegetable oils. Without the full story, people who try these kinds of weight-loss programs may enjoy temporary success but in the long term are likely to run aground.

To Avoid Inflammation, Keep Total Daily Sugar Intake Under 100 Grams

High fructose corn syrup can make it practically impossible for you to normalize your weight. We've all heard that when bears need to fatten up for winter, they eat berries. It turns out that fructose sugar (in fruit, fruit juice, soda, and more) sends especially powerful fat-building signals by switching on liver enzymes for converting sugars to fat.[540] Since most of the food you eat gets sent to the liver first, eating fructose effectively traps dietary carbohydrates in your liver and converts them to fat, preventing them from ever making it to muscle tissue, where they could be burned during exercise.

So fructose-containing foods can make you pack on the pounds, but there's really no sugar that's *good* for you. As we saw in Chapter 9, sugar sticks to things. A sugar coating on your cells (in the form of AGEs) blocks hormone signals. This blocking ability is *disruptive*, and so sugar itself (when consumed in high levels) is pro-inflammatory. For example, excess dietary sugar disrupts hormonal signals for building muscle. You'll see below that the process of converting fat to muscle involves all kinds of hormone signals, and sugar-induced AGEs can block them all.

Because carbohydrates in your food are converted into sugars, a diet high in pastas, breads, and so on is inherently pro-inflammatory as well. Worse, these starchy foods are so bereft of vitamins and other antioxidants that building a diet around them can make it hard for your body to control oxidation reactions once they start. This puts you deeper into a pro-inflammatory state.

For all these reasons, I tell my patients who are having difficulty shedding the pounds to keep their total carbohydrate intake to less than 100 grams per day (this total includes sugars and "complex" carbs like starches). Of course calories do play some role in all this. That's why it's good to be aware that sugar dissolves in water so well that a teaspoon of sugary syrup can contain *up to four times* the calories as a teaspoon of granulated sugar. This means fat-free cookies can pack more fat-producing power than regular cookies. It also explains why those who have the toughest time losing weight often have kitchens full of fat-free products.

STEP 3: LEARN WHERE FAT COMES FROM—AND WHERE IT GOES

Fat Grows from Stem Cells

You've probably heard of *stem cells*, immature cells derived from embryos with the potential to grow replacement parts for any organ. These are the cells you've seen researchers use to grow ears on the backs of mice. Many believe stem cells hold the cure for Alzheimer's, Parkinson's, and a host of other currently incurable diseases—and some day they may. But if you want to reshape your body, harnessing stem cell versatility can help you achieve that goal today.

One of the most frustrating things about fat is its ability to seemingly appear from nowhere. It's really coming from stem cells.[541] When you eat sugar, starch, and trans fat without exercising, your body will churn out new fat cells like a termite queen producing eggs. When stem cells turn into fat cells and grow plumper, you grow plumper, too.

One reason diets fail is that cutting back on calories without changing any other habits sends precisely the wrong message. The body presumes that the meager food intake, in combination with little activity, must mean food has become so scarce that you've given up looking for more. If it has the slightest chance to store surplus energy as fat, the panicked body reasons it had better do so. Under these circumstances, stem cells stand at the ready to convert themselves into more energy-storing fat cells. Frightening our stem cells into turning into fat cells is exactly the wrong thing to do. Instead, we should capitalize on the stem cell's protean nature and convince it to turn into a kind of cell we want.

Like what, you ask? Like muscle, blood vessel, nerve, and bone. This is, we now know exactly what happens when a person optimizes their body composition. Draining fat cells requires building new nerves to blood vessels that will assist in more efficient export of the fat.[542] New muscle and reinforced bone and tendon to support the more intense force generation all require new infrastructure, too. And the technology to build all this is encapsulated in every stem cell in our bodies. What's even more remarkable than stem cell versatility is the fact that grown-up fat cells seem capable of changing their identity almost as readily as stem cells can. That means you don't need to starve to get rid of all that flab; it can be *transformed* into the healthy tissues of a brand-new beautiful you.

Fat Can Transform Back into Stem Cells and Other Types of Cells

You might find this hard to believe, but fat cells require constant attention to maintain their girth. Many people who have tried to improve their looks by having fat injected into their lips and cheeks have seen their enhancement melt away when the transplanted fat cells refused to flourish in their new locations. When researchers investigated this phenomenon, they found that not only had the once-plump cells slimmed down to mere slivers, some had changed into an entirely different type of cell, called a *fibrocyte*, the type of cell most prevalent in the tissues into which the fat cells had been injected.[543] Apparently, fibrocytes surrounding the transplanted fat cells refused to make the introduced cells feel at home (by producing the necessary fat-sustaining hormones). Without these hormones, the receptors and enzymes that enable fat cells to do their thing—ingest sugar and fat and grow pudgy—began to shut down. Shrinking under the peer pressure of a hormonally cold shoulder, the unwelcome guests simply conformed to the rules of the neighborhood and reinvented themselves as fibrocytes.

You may be able to coerce fat cells into becoming just about anything you want. Fat tissue belongs to a class of body material called connective tissue, which collectively includes collagen, bone, muscle, blood, and associated cells. Some cell biologists now believe that one type of connective tissue cell permanently retains its ability to transform into another cell type whenever chemical signals instruct it to do so. So muscle cells can become fat cells; fat

THE RIGHT SIGNALS CAN TURN FAT CELLS INTO MUSCLE, BONE, OR NERVE

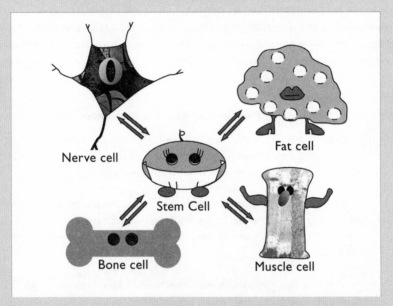

A metabolic process called transdifferentiation can make fat cells leave your adipose tissue and migrate to become new muscle, bone, and even brain cells. You can control stem cell growth by eating right and exercising, and that includes exercising your brain. (See text for supporting references.)

can become bone; and then a bone cell can change back to a fat cell again. This process is termed *transdifferentiation* (see illustration). As I'll discuss later, there is evidence that the potential for transdifferentiation may even extend across *all* tissue types.[544, 545, 546, 547]

Although this kind of cell transformation has so far only been observed in a laboratory setting, the research opens the door to the possibility that a fat cell on your thigh today might once have been a muscle, bone, or skin cell, living some place else in your body. But why, you may wonder, would any cell decide to pack its bags and head to an entirely new location? It would if it received a chemical memo saying that its service in its current tissue is no longer required, and that it should head to its new assignment in the fat department.

So if some fat cells were once cells in preferable kinds of tissues, how can we order them to go back? One of the most effective ways to send that kind of message is with exercise. According to Dr. Robert Lustig, Professor of Pediatric Endocrinology at University of California, San Francisco, the reason exercise treats obesity *is not* because it "burns" calories. "That's ridiculous," he says. "Twenty minutes of jogging is one chocolate chip cookie. I mean, you can't do it. One Big Mac requires three hours of vigorous exercise to burn off. That's not the reason exercise is important."[548] Exercise is important because it generates signals to

---

EXERCISE WORKS AT LEAST THREE WAYS

1. It increases insulin sensitivity, so you need less insulin to get sugar out of your bloodstream. This allows your insulin levels to drop, which tells your fat cells to slow the conversion of sugar into more fat.

2. It reduces the stress hormone cortisol. Cortisol packs fat around organs (as opposed to under the skin), where it produces lots of pro-inflammatory chemicals, which in turn tell the body to produce still more fat.

3. It builds new blood vessels through muscle and adipose tissues, which enables your body to more readily burn fat.[549]

---

build muscle—or bone or other lean tissues—instead of unwanted fat.

Once fat cells store energy, they guard it jealously, reluctant to give it up. But when you exercise enough to trigger new muscle growth, that process of building muscle burns fat, draining fat cells of some of their energy-rich contents. What's more, fat cells can be convinced to undergo the same kind of cellular suicide that tumor cells can, a process called *apoptosis*.

This discovery that so many cellular transformations are occurring has unsettled the medical community, which must now abandon the old notion of a cell as something created to be a lifelong member of one particular cellular species. This model grossly underestimates the cell's protean nature. Just as genes change in reaction to what we eat, think, and do, cells change their construction, too. When a fat cell, for instance, reverts to a stem cell, in a process called *redifferentiation*, that cell is once again *pluripotent*, meaning it can once again redifferentiate—that is, specialize into whatever cell type is needed by the body tissue into which the cell has been recruited. The culture medium scientists use for inducing all those cellular transformations is not an alien brew of unnatural chemicals, but rather a full complement of vitamins, amino acids, and sugar, plus different mixtures of naturally occurring growth factors and hormones that a healthy, young body normally manufactures. The readiness and completeness with which cells respond to such instructions suggest that these conversions are an integral aspect of healthy physiologic function.[550]

How Fat Cells Change

Nearly every step of the fat cell self-improvement program has been replicated in the lab. Though no one knows exactly how it functions in the body, the lab tests indicate that it probably goes something like this: first, an individual fat cell loses much, or all, of its lipid stores. Then the shriveled fat cell gets a signal to *de*differentiate into either a preadipocyte,[551] a baby fat cell containing no fat, or even an entirely different, more mobile cell type, one that is indistinguishable from a stem cell.[552] The baby fat cell can then readily undergo the process of apoptosis, whereas adult fat cells resist this process and may not even be able to delete themselves without becoming a baby fat cell first.

You can think of the different abilities and levels of mobility of cells as something like chess pieces on a chess board. The adult fat cell, like the king, is very limited; it cannot leave the fat tissue and—just as the king cannot offer himself up (because it would end the game)—cannot eliminate itself through apoptosis. The baby fat cell, like a pawn, has the same mobility constraints but can, however, take itself out of the game. The stem cell would be the queen of the cell types, as it can delete itself at will as well as travel freely out of the fat tissue and, riding the currents of the bloodstream throughout the body, take its new place among whatever group of cells has requested a new, additional member. If muscle tissue issued the request, then the pluripotent stem cell simply adheres to the wall of a tiny blood vessel in the muscle and then waits for the stimulus to migrate into that tissue. Once it gets the right signal, it moves inside the matrix of the new tissue and *re*differentiates to match the other cell types in its new location. Whatever the exact sequence of cell reassignment, the abilities of the magical morphing cell suggest that our body is composed not of cellular specialists, but of generalists, ready to be retrained and reassigned at a moment's notice. And that's encouraging news, because it tells us that if we know what we're doing, our best health may still be ahead of us.

Why Moderation, Small Portions, and Starvation Diets Fail

Moderation, as a program for healthy eating, made perfect sense 200

OVERWEIGHT AND PREGNANCY

If you're overweight, your body is almost certainly suffering under a constant state of low-level inflammation. This inflammatory chemical static is so powerfully disruptive that it can interfere with some of the most important signals in the biological world, those that the next generation depends on. In Chapter 5, we learned that the baby's placenta sends signals to the mother's body, demanding her tissue relinquish nutrients for the benefit of her fetus. But when mom is significantly overweight, the message can't get across. As a result, blood vessels supplying baby with nutrients become thin and shriveled, leading to "major placental growth restriction" when compared to normal-weight moms. So if you're planning on getting pregnant, it's essential to get yourself to a healthy weight first. This will not only facilitate a happy pregnancy, but also help with fertility so that you can get pregnant in the first place.

years ago when crops were grown organically on healthy topsoil, and the worst chemical monstrosities of the food industry were yet to be invented. Back then, there were no such things as Twinkies, curly fries, high-fructose corn syrup, or trans fat. Today, few places remain on this planet where people flavor food with homemade broths instead of with MSG, where they still ferment vegetables and meats instead of storing them in the fridge, where they eat every part of the animal instead of just a few cuts. In places like this, "everything in moderation" would actually work. But in the world of modern, processed foods, "everything in moderation" is a recipe for a moderate level of health, which these days is hardly something you want to aim for.

Another kind of "moderation" is moderating the volume of food consumed, i.e., calorie restriction. You might think that calorie restriction could convince fat cells that they're no longer needed, and lead to apoptosis. On calorie restriction diets, fat cells shrink but they rarely disappear. For the most part, as soon as the calories return, so does the fat inside the cells. Why? It appears the body is cautious, and like any good manager, resists taking drastic action—like firing a cell permanently—until it has darn good reason.

The reluctance of your body to permit fat cells to undergo apoptosis means that if you never exercise *properly* (see below), though you restrict your calories, your fat tissues never receive the chemical memo that more cells are needed in another department, and so the fat cells stay put. As long as fat cells are fat cells, they have no choice but to try to pack on more fat and will do so at any opportunity. What's more, as the body converts fat cells into muscle cells, there's little net loss of mass, which would explain why people who start exercise programs don't notice weight loss right away.

Many doctors and diet gurus argue that calorie restriction works. Just look at prisoners who've been starved for months or even years. Their energy expenditure was higher than their energy intake so, *ipso facto*, the coal furnace model of physiology (the one I condemned at the opening of this chapter) holds. It's basic thermodynamics, they argue. And to an extent, they're right; there's no cheating physics. But if you're trying to reshape your body simply by reducing portion size of unhealthy, low-nutrient foods, then realize that you're basing your dietary program on what you've seen the human body do under extreme, long-term, incredibly unhealthy conditions.

Earlier, we talked about how calorie restriction without exercise tells your body to convert stem cells into fat cells as soon as you start eating again. And the body doesn't just wait patiently. It cranks up your appetite to prod you into increasing your food-seeking efforts while readying fat cells you already have to receive any forthcoming bounty. When you finally do eat a full meal, your body rushes the energy into storage—hence the typical yo-yo cycle of weight loss and rapid gain with small-portion diets.

As long as you manage to deal with your hunger, your body is forced to start using up fat cells—just as you'd hoped—but will also mine other tissues for vitamins, minerals, protein, and essential fats. These tissues can include brain, connective tissue, and muscle. Of course, since muscle burns calories all by itself, once you start losing muscle it becomes harder to lose weight. The lesson here is that hunger is not the way to reshape your body. In Hawaii, the surfers have a saying: "Never fight the ocean." If you want an athletic, svelte, attractive figure, then don't fight your body. Call a truce by eating according to the Human Diet, exercising, cutting stress, and getting a full night's sleep.

Inflammation Makes Fat Invasive, Like Cancer

Now that you know all kinds of body tissues can interconvert, let's take a look at how this process can work against us to make us not just too heavy but also unhealthy.

On a pro-inflammatory diet, our physiology starts making fat cells so fast you'd think it were some kind of nervous habit. In the same way that so many of us deal with stress by heading straight for the Häagen-Dazs, so too do our physiologies: a pro-inflammatory diet stresses our cells, and, as I've described, transdifferentiation converts all kinds of cells into fat.

In patients with age-related dementia, gray matter gets replaced by

FACTORS THAT MAKE YOU BUILD FAT	
Omega-6 fatty acids	Enzymes in your body can convert these into arachidonic acid (AA), which can make fat cells divide. Stress, sleep deprivation, and obesity can lead to an excess of these enzymes. Excessive consumption of omega-6 fats can also generate too much AA.
Insulin	Increases fat cell numbers. Signs that you may have abnormal levels of insulin are dark patches of skin in creases and under your arms, and central obesity—fat that tends to collect around the waist and under the chin. Irregular periods may also indicate abnormal insulin levels.
Sugars	Sugar drives insulin production, and insulin turns on enzymes in the liver and in fat cells that convert sugar into its storage form: triglyceride fat.
Thiazolidinediones (a common type of diabetes medication)	Stimulates fat cell division and increases fat storage. These were originally thought to be weight-loss pills based on a ridiculously optimistic analysis of their effects on cell metabolism. Now we realize they so powerfully promote fat storage that bone cells start storing fat. These pills can cause weight gain, bone fractures, and heart failure. If you are on this medication, ask your doctor if there is an alternative.
Glucocorticoids	Stimulate fat cell division. The body makes glucocorticoids all the time, but levels rise during stress and sleep deprivation.
MegaTrans fats (omega-3 and omega-6 breakdown products)	Promote free radical formation, cell membrane damage, and inflammation—all of which lead to the deposition of omental (belly) and submandibular (neck) fat while intercepting healthy cell-building signals.

cells containing excessive amounts of fat.[553] Osteoporotic bones have had bone-forming cells replaced by fat cells.[554] And fatty liver, a common cause of chronic indigestion and gastro esophageal reflux disease (GERD) symptoms (like heartburn), is caused by fat cell formation at the expense of normal, functioning liver cells. To put all this in terms of the larger regulatory picture, when muscle, bone, gland, and nerve cells are denied a full complement of vitamins, amino acids, minerals, and so on, they seem to take that denial as a signal to dedifferentiate and start storing fat. With so many cells abandoning their posts in healthy tissues to join the growing ranks of fat cells, you can imagine how poorly these tissues function. This whole degenerative process can be expedited in the presence of cortisol from stress and lack of sleep, or from the many inflammatory factors that build up from a lack of exercise. An imbalanced diet, which releases still more inflammatory signals, makes things even worse.

FACTORS THAT ELIMINATE FAT	
Exercise	Reduces insulin and corticosteroid levels as well as levels of many other less well-known pro-inflammatory and fat-promoting chemicals.
Sleep	Reduces corticosteroid levels, and increases levels of immune system chemicals that reduce inflammation and fat cell number.
Conjugated linoleic acid (CLA)	Reduces fat cell numbers and reduces appetite.
Retinoids	These include vitamin A from animal fat and organ meats, and vitamin A precursors (called carotenoids) from vegetables.
Leptin	Reduces fat cell numbers.
Cholesterols (Cholesterol actually represents a whole family of molecules.)	Reduce appetite. Studies have shown that plant sterols and stanols effectively reduce appetite. What are plant sterols and stanols? Cholesterol that plants make. Bile acids also contain cholesterol. When secreted into the small intestine after a meal, they signal the body that you've had enough to eat. Unfortunately, nobody can get funding to study any potential benefit of cholesterol. But you can try this simple experiment yourself: Day one: eat two eggs cooked in 2 tablespoons of butter for breakfast and see if you're hungry by lunch. Day Two: eat one cup of granola in one cup of skim milk and see if you're hungry by lunch. Both have about 500 calories.

Fat-making may seem like the body's default reaction, but really it's just the default reaction in periods of stress and nutrient deprivation. When the body gets all the real food, exercise, and rest that it needs, the default reaction is to convert unwanted fat cells into something better. Which physiologic directive your body follows is ultimately up to you.

Some nutrient deficiencies and stress levels are so severe, however, that it becomes increasingly difficult to ship nutrients throughout the body effectively. If sugar and fatty acids can't make the journey from wherever they were (usually your digestive system) into a proper fat-storage cell, then they end up lining your arteries, seeping into your tendons, and polluting your body. Now, instead of building fat, you just get sick. White blood cells will have to enter these polluted segments of artery, joint, or any other compromised tissue and try to clean up the mess. But white blood cells cause inflammation, which damages tissues (including arterial walls), makes your joints hurt, and clots your blood. This is why a diet that makes you fat also makes you feel bad, raises your blood pressure, and causes diabetes, heart disease, kidney problems, and so many other diseases. It's also why white blood cells filled with fat are found in so many degenerated organs.

Cancer is a consequence of unhealthy cell communication: the cell mutates because it receives abnormal chemical instructions. When these mutants divide rapidly and invade other tissues, they are called *metastases*. Many cancer cells produce hormones to maintain a state of constant growth, unrestrained by the body's instructions. Like cancer, fat produces pro-inflammatory factors that stimulate its own growth.[555] More fat sends a louder signal to the body to create still more fat. And fat cells invade other tissues, just as cancer does. Even thin people can, through poor diet, encourage fat to infiltrate healthy tissues. When fat invades, we develop cellulite, weakened bones, and brain and muscle atrophy. Finally, like cancer, obesity is associated with blood clots, fatigue, and premature death. Obesity behaves like a self-sustaining tumor, and anyone who is overweight can feel trapped in its vicious cycle. I see people whose losing battle against their weight has them as frightened as someone with cancer, willing to pay anything for a cure.

Fortunately, fat cells *can* be retrained.

And that's the word I want you to keep in mind, *retraining*. People are often amazed how amenable their pets are to training—once they learn to communicate with them effectively. The same goes for our cells. A key point of my message is that our cells react to the signals we send them through diet and activity, and they do their best to comply. Once you've cleared your body of inflammation, exercise helps your body know what to do with the food it gets. It's like sending a wish list to your cells: *I'd like more muscle in the pectorals, less flab on my thighs, and—oh yes, I've been clumsy lately—I'd like more proprioceptive neural tissue coordinating motion of my ankles and my lower spine.* For most of us, the wish list includes a trimmer waistline, more energy, and a sexier physique. To accomplish that, we need an exercise program that will send that message, which means—since each sends a distinct set of signals—one that includes both aerobic *and* anaerobic activity.

STEP 4: EXERCISE

Aerobic Exercise—Make Sure to *Feel* It

Ah . . . the eighties. Purple spandex and hot pink leg warmers. In Syracuse, New York, during the long gray winters, I'd drive through the slush to my local YMCA to avoid freezing my lungs while running outside. I would sweat buckets into my rather unfashionable T-shirt-and-shorts ensemble, grasping the handles of my treadmill to keep from falling over the edge, shifting posture, and creating more commotion than the women in matching outfits over on the stationary bikes sedately reading romance novels and listening to their Walkmans while their legs rotated in tiny circles beneath them.

Given the kinds of lousy foods I was eating in those days, my extreme exercise regimen might have been doing me more harm than good. Without adequate nutrition, all that full-throttle effort may very well have been breaking down my tissues. In terms of sending the message to build muscle, I was perhaps overdoing it, while the ladies on the bikes might as well have been window-shopping. Exercise, rest, and eating right all work together to give you the kind of body you want. But in order for exercise to contribute as much as it can, you have to know how to get the most out of your workout.

Don't let anyone tell you that just because you're dressed to work out, you're in a gym, and you're using a fancy new machine, that you are doing aerobic (oxygen-requiring) exercise. Don't get me wrong. Even strolling along at a tra-la-la pace on an elliptical station beats sitting on the couch eating fruit roll-ups. But unless your workout makes your lungs work harder and makes you break a sweat, you aren't doing aerobic exercise; you're just breathing.

This level of workout demands your concentration. Yoga instructors call it *mindfulness*. Weight lifters who argue for the benefits of free weights over universal machines believe they get faster results when they have to concentrate on things like balancing a heavy barbell above their chests. The more aware we are of the act of exercising, the more we engage our muscles. Concentration level influences how nerve and muscle cells respond, so whether for an intense run or just walking up the stairs, you'll see more results if you *focus* on every motion—the swinging of your arms, your calves lifting your spine, your hip rotation. If you're running, focus on really filling your lungs. If going up the stairs at work, focus on working the calves for one flight, then try to engage the butt muscles the next. Focus on the contra-body motion— different parts of your body rhythmically moving in opposing directions. Dancing, swimming, golf—each involves contra-body motion, which helps you to involve the whole body. Mindfulness of motion applies to all forms of exercise and is a prerequisite to improving performance.

A good walk, as with any exercise, works out more than your legs, and you get a better workout if you are conscious of your body's balanced involvement in contra-body action. Opposing motions across the fulcrum of your hips and spine allow you to take advantage of a physiologic "spring" built into your muscles, which cardiologists first recognized as the means by which heart failure patients survive. It's called the *Starling* effect. When a muscle is stretched before it contracts, it magnifies the force of the contraction automatically, without any additional input from the nerves. In a failing heart, the muscle needs the extra energy generated by the Starling effect to pump blood effectively. In a dance move, a happy walk, or a properly executed golf swing, extending your limbs to the edge of the swing allows your muscles to stretch and then rebound effortlessly. Paying attention to how your muscles react helps you to hone the technique of whatever it is you're trying to accomplish. That's thinking like an athlete, and it really does make any exercise more fun.

I let all my patients suffering from depression in on a little secret: studies show that exercise is at least as effective as the best antidepressant medications.[556] Aerobic exercise releases *endorphins*—chemicals your body makes that activate the reward centers of your brain. Not only do these natural feel-good chemicals regulate and improve mood, they act directly on muscles to help them burn more energy and contract with more power.[557] Exercise also cleans the bloodstream of a chemical that makes us feel bad, something called tumor necrosis factor (TNF). TNF is a powerful, pro-inflammatory signal that increases sensitivity to pain. (It also inhibits muscle growth and makes blood clots form more easily.)[558, 559] So aerobic exercise doesn't just pump up your muscle, it pumps up your mood.

It can also pump up your brain—literally. These days, aging baby boomers who forget where they left their car keys jokingly call it "early Alzheimer's." But if you've had personal experience with this progressive disease, you know it's no laughing matter. In search of ways to combat this terrifying illness, scientists put thirty sedentary older adults (ages sixty to seventy-nine) to work. Over a six-month period, test subjects exercised for an hour a day, three days per week, doing aerobic muscle toning and stretching exercises. Amazingly, brain MRIs showed "significant increases in brain volume, in both gray and white matter" in four areas of the brain, several of which are related to making new memories.[560] As I alluded to earlier, the life of a cell is far more unpredictable than we thought, and even nerve cells can grow and divide throughout our lives.[561]

If you want your brain to work better, take it for a hike.

Anaerobic Exercise—Why Intensity Matters

The main thing that distinguishes aerobic and *an*aerobic exercise is the level of intensity. Aerobic exercise is easier to do while daydreaming about something else, like the scenery you're jogging through or where to go on your next vacation. Anaerobic exercise requires single-minded focus, a higher level of concentration, as you would need to do while sprinting or pulling a loaded wheelbarrow up a steep hill. But the payoff is a whole new level of muscular coordination and capability. Anaerobic exercise generates a flood of body-sculpting signals so that you become stronger, faster, and more athletic.

When you work so hard that your oxygen demand exceeds the capacity of the body to deliver blood to the tissue (which is why it's called anaerobic, as in "without air"), you have entered that higher realm of exercise called the *anaerobic threshold*. It burns. That burn means you have only seconds or minutes before your muscles begin to fail. The time limit has to do with the fact that the metabolism of sugar to energy occurs in two stages.

The first stage, called glycolysis, doesn't require oxygen and is therefore an anaerobic process. It produces the starting material (pyruvic acid) for the second stage, along with some energy for your cells, called adenosine triphosphate (ATP). The second stage uses oxygen to burn the products of the first reaction, and is therefore an aerobic process. The aerobic stage of sugar metabolism produces lots and lots of ATP.

If the muscles don't get enough oxygen to burn all that pyruvic acid, the acids start building up and you feel the burn, telling you your muscles are about to fail. And that's a useful signal. If you were being chased by a lion, for example, the burning signal would warn you that your muscles were on the verge of seizing up. Time to start looking for a tree!

Once the anaerobic activity is over, your metabolic management team furiously takes notes on the physiologic event that just took place, taking record of which muscles worked the hardest and will need to be tweaked for better performance in the future. From the crucible of intense activity emerges a stronger form of muscle that will last longer than it did before. On the savannah, this would make you a more elusive prey and a better hunter, enabling you to run a little faster and chase your quarry a little farther the next time. Anaerobic exercise is *the* classic example of "no pain, no gain." In the modern world, anaerobic exercise can help transport a dedicated athlete into the zone of superstardom. For the rest of us, however, it's a really great way to burn fat because it flips the body's muscle-generating switch to overdrive, and you start converting flab into firmness like nobody's business.

How much of this kind of intense exercise do you need to do any good? Less than you might think: *Try eight minutes a week!*

For years muscle-bound men and women have encouraged us to *feel the burn*. But nobody suggested that fairly sporadic activity would do the job. Doctors at the Exercise Metabolism Research Group in Ontario suspected that chronic fatigue induced by *daily* training could actually hamper athletic improvement. They investigated how a *minimum* of super-intense exercise affects muscle work capacity. The test subjects started with four intervals and gradually increased to seven over a two-week period of training performed on Mondays, Wednesdays, and Fridays. The intervals consisted of thirty seconds of all-out cycling with four-minute rest periods, totaling just fifteen minutes over the two weeks. The subjects improved their exercise capacity by 100 percent. You read that right. Over a two-week period a *total* of fifteen minutes of cycling as if their lives depended on it *doubled* their muscle power! Incredibly, the body is so ready and able to respond to signals that the most urgent signal of all—*run for your life*—produces astonishing gains in performance.[562]

How? Our physiology is our patient and faithful servant. And it is logical—you could say intelligent—in the way it responds. When stimulated to build more muscle, the body does exactly what a smart city planner might do in an expanding metropolitan center: it increases enzyme activity in the muscle to handle the increased workload (the equivalent of hiring more policemen, firemen, and so on), it increases blood flow to handle more nutrient and oxygen traffic, and produces more mitochondria to generate plenty of energy. We call this synchronized set of responses *increased metabolism*.[563]

All this infrastructural development—making more of these complex tissues—can't be accomplished with exercise alone. You need more nutrients to manufacture new enzymes, build more cell organelles, grow larger cells, reproduce more cells, pave more blood vessels, and then maintain all this new equipment. Without a healthy diet, anaerobic exercise can't build these tissues, and can actually break your body down. Healthy diet, along with a balance of aerobic and anaerobic exercise, helps generate the perfect internal environment to clear away the fat-building signals and replace them with a new message: *Get fast. Get tough. Get strong.*

These benefits exist for persons of every age. As we get older, we gradually lose the growth factors that help maintain our fat where we want it and keep our muscles, bones, and joints strong. But during and immediately after exercise, growth factors and hormone levels spike, so you get an infusion of youth serum every time you work out.[564]

Three Habits of Successful Exercisers

1. Mindfulness. Use your body consciously. The best exercises involve the entire body. I don't care if you are thumb wrestling; think about your stance, your balance, your breathing, and you'll fake-twitch faster, grab harder, jive better, and bring the opposing thumb to its knees. Never forget that exercise should be fun. Don't allow yourself to do anything that causes a pinch or a dull ache.

Listen to your body. If it's objecting, take time off or change what you're doing. Keep in mind that exercise builds more than just muscle, it builds practically all functional tissues; it increases their investment with nerve endings and blood vessels, builds bone, strengthens ligaments, and so much more. Many exercise physiologists firmly believe that conscious intention during and after exercise—visualizing what you are doing *and what you hope to accomplish*—is key to getting the most from a workout.

2. Time management. Aerobic exercise takes time. The more time you give it, the more it gives you. (Up to a point. A reasonable cap is an average of thirty to forty minutes per day.) Want to detox? Aerobic exercise cleanses your system of inflammatory debris. If you're new to exercise, start with ten minutes a day and increase by 10 percent each week. And don't forget to get plenty of sleep. If your bed's uncomfortable, get another one. And nice pillows and sheets—it's all money well spent. It's mostly during sleep that our bodies heal and rebuild tissue, so sleep is crucial.

3. Push yourself. Anaerobic exercise demands more concentration than aerobic exercise. If your doctor says you're healthy enough for intensive exercise, then you should get to the point where you feel a burn and then keep going for another minute or two. Do that ten times per week and you will see improvement. Make sure you can distinguish a healthy anaerobic burn from the pain of an overstressed muscle. Keep in mind, even an aerobic workout can include elements of anaerobic strain, which helps you build healthy tissues faster.

Preventing Physiologic Chaos

As we've seen, fat storage is a kind of default action the body performs during periods of nutritional imbalance. When too much fat invades healthy tissues, it weakens them and impairs function. If you want to be healthy, if you want to build bone and muscle and reduce your stores of malignant fat, you must send your cells the clearest possible message. If you fill your metabolic airways with static, the message won't arrive, keeping you from getting the results you want.

The bad news is, the battle between clarity and static isn't a fair fight. In a universe that tends toward disorder, there are all kinds of weird food products and distorted chemicals that can disrupt our physiologies, but only one class of foods—the natural kind—that can maintain internal order. Makes sense, right? Painting the *Mona Lisa* takes more energy and talent than shooting at it with a pistol. Dietary imbalances rapidly generate inflammation and static that can take weeks or months to clear. So when someone tells me they only eat junk food "occasionally," I try to help them realize that they're setting up a competition in their body that they're bound to lose. If you are struggling with weight, or have any chronic medical issue, you can't afford to ship fresh ammunition across the front lines to the enemy. That means no junk food, period.

Here's the good news: for every junk food you love, there's a healthier, and tastier, alternative. Seriously! If you like McDonald's french fries, you'll get even better flavors using traditional ingredients at home. You can make fries using peanut oil or animal fat (lard, tallow, duck fat, etc.), or make home fries seasoned with spices and baked in pan drippings. If you like sitting down with a sack of chips, you'll get similar, but far more intense, flavors from a few slices of quality, aged raw milk cheese—so satisfying you *can* have just one. While junk food flavorings make you hungrier, naturally flavor-rich foods contain appetite suppressants like cholesterol and saturated fat.

In this chapter, I've focused on the problem of weight. But the same signal disruption (from inflammation and trans fat) that leads to the generation of excess fat also leads to the *de*generation of bone, nerve, and organs. It even causes immune system dysfunction. In fact, because pro-inflammatory foods disrupt normal cell development, the same foods that make us fat also lead to problems we typically associate with aging, from heart disease to Alzheimer's to cancer. What this means is that following the Human Diet will do more than make weight loss automatic. It will keep you from developing all these diseases of aging. In other words, it will help keep you young.

But while all the cells described in this chapter can be born anew at any stage of life, there's one type of tissue that depends—more than anything else—on being built right in the first place. I'm talking about connective tissue. *Feeling* old comes primarily from having connective tissues that break down prematurely. If your connective tissue was built as well as possible, your joints will stand up to incredible abuse, both physical and nutritional. In the next chapter, you'll learn how to gauge your connective tissue health and what you can do (even if it wasn't built as well as it could be) to prevent your body from aging faster than it should.

CHAPTER 12

Forever Young
Collagen Health and Life Span

- Strong, flexible, healthy collagen is key to youthfulness.

- Bone broth is a missing food group collagen tissues crave.

- Inflammation damages collagen in ways that make us feel older than our age.

- Food allergies are a warning sign of collagen-damaging inflammation.

- Three key practices will keep your collagen healthy.

One morning, several years ago when I was still practicing in Hawaii, a woman ran into our office shouting, "My baby! My baby!" and disappeared back out into the parking lot. The nurse on duty raced out front to find a panicked mother struggling with a car seat where a baby lay listless, strawberry red and covered in blotchy hives, his lips purple and swollen. The infant was having a severe allergic reaction and was struggling just to breathe.

Baby Kyle, a mostly formula-fed toddler, was in the throes of an anaphylactic reaction, triggered by a few spoonfuls of low-fat, high-sugar blueberry yogurt. Anaphylaxis is an allergic reaction involving inflammation of the blood vessels throughout the body, and it can be fatal. In the last chapter, we saw how inflammation interferes with cell communication and leads to weight gain. Anaphylaxis is a classic case of inflammation gone completely out of control. Fortunately, the pediatrician on call administered powerful anti-inflammatory medications, which saved little Kyle's life.

Anaphylactic reactions like this are the most extreme example of an allergic reaction, which is what happens when a person's immune system, disoriented by the noise of low-grade inflammatory signals, makes a serious mistake. Allergies are a more common manifestation of such immune system malfunctions than is anaphylaxis. Whether allergic reactions are triggered by pets or molds or foods, the underlying issue is the same: the immune system confuses a harmless protein for an invading bacteria, and launches an attack.

Serious food allergies are on the rise.[565] According to the CDC, the number of children hospitalized for food allergies rose 300 percent between 1996 and 2006.[566] This and other disturbing medical trends are mysteries to researchers and sources of frustration for parents. But now that you know sugar and vegetable oil (the main ingredients in infant formulas, the mainstay of Kyle's diet) combined with nutrient-deficient foods make up the perfect pro-inflammatory diet, you already know what was wrong with Kyle and what might have been done to make him healthy.

Kyle's severe reaction was too dramatic to casually brush away as one of the normal, or at least common, experiences of childhood. But many parents do view less severe allergic reactions in that light. I would like to change that, because I see *any* allergy as an indication that someone is very likely to develop other inflammatory issues down the road, problems that can break down what I call the youth tissue, collagen, and make their bodies age far more rapidly than they should.

PRO-INFLAMMATORY FATS AND SUGAR CAN DAMAGE COLLAGEN

You hear all the time about supernutritious foods touted as anti-aging miracles. The combination of sugar and vegetable oil, and its effects on the tissue whose integrity is most related to your physiologic age—collagen—might rightly be called the miracle foods of age acceleration. Because when it comes to staying young and feeling young, collagen is a big deal. If your parents aged well or lived a long time, you can be sure they had good, strong collagen.

Unfortunately, however, you can't count on inheriting collagen of the same quality. The quality of a person's collagen is not written in genetic stone. (As you now know, there's no such thing as "genetic stone," since your genes are always changing.) Like other tissue types, collagen is made from raw materials you must eat. Unlike other tissues, however, collagen is uniquely sensitive to metabolic imbalances. When your body is making collagen, it's performing a physiologic high-wire act, a feat of extraordinary timing and mechanical precision. This level of complexity makes collagen more dependent on good nutrition and more vulnerable to the effects of pro-inflammatory foods than other tissue types.

FEEDING YOUR SKIN WITH BEAUTY CREAM

The highest quality skin products contain the collagen-building nutrients your skin needs to restore itself. Even skeptical doctors admit that regular use of these expensive products can have impressive results. However, skin care expert Dennis Gross, M.D., warns that it's not an overnight solution. "It takes time, molecule by molecule, to build collagen fibers." Dermatologists advise patience and regular application to get anti-wrinkle creams in contact with skin as much as possible. Why not also feed your skin from the inside?

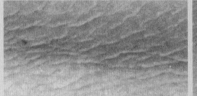 

Left: Fine wrinkling on an eighty-four-year-old woman's arm. *Right:* Her skin after just three months of applying a vitamin A cream.

FEED YOUR SKIN SOUP

If a cream containing two or three collagen-building nutrients can help your skin, imagine how effectively you could nourish and rebuild your dermal collagen if you ate a meal containing dozens of growth factors. The nutrients in bone stocks switch the genes for collagen manufacture to "on." This effect is magnified by vitamins A, D, E, and C, and a few common minerals. Whether in a skin cream or your soup bowl, the same natural ingredients help you look young. But when you ingest them, you infuse all the layers of your skin, and all the other tissues of your body, with rejuvenating nutrients.

When we talk about people who have aged well, one of the first things we think about is healthy skin. But if you've read any beauty magazines in the past decade, you know that skin health depends on collagen health. Michelle Pfeiffer is one of the most beautiful actresses working today, but whether she retains that beauty as the years wear on depends not so much on the superficial layers of her skin but on what lies beneath.

ANATOMY OF SKIN

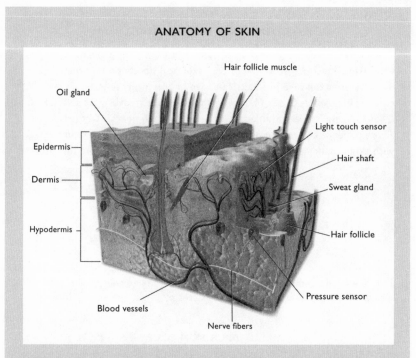

Epidermis, dermis, and subcutaneous fat. The outer layer, called the epidermis, is a husk of dead cells that are filled with waterproofing material and pigment. The middle layer, called the dermis, is the support system of your skin, containing blood vessels, nerves, sweat and oil glands, and the muscles controlling hair follicles, all held in place by strong and elastic fibers made of collagen. The innermost layer is called the subcutaneous fat. It's where the bulk of our body fat is stored.

Collagens: Molecules That Make Us Strong

Collagens are a family of extra-cellular proteins that give skin its ability to move, stretch, and rebound into shape. Thin wisps of tough, elastic collagen molecules run between adjacent cells in the outermost layer of skin, called the *epidermis*. And larger bundles of collagen form strips that weave together in a continuous layer beneath the epidermis, in a part of the skin called the *dermis*.

Collagens aren't just in skin; they're everywhere, imparting strength to all your tissues. Just as strands of collagen running between skin cells hold our outermost layer of skin together, collagens unite adjacent cells in all your glands and

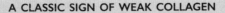

A CLASSIC SIGN OF WEAK COLLAGEN

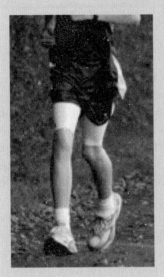

This child has a mild case of intoeing, which is associated with abnormal collagen growth and lax ligaments. Were he to play soccer or ski, this child would be at higher than normal risk for joint injuries (like ligament tears). Today, more children than ever need joint reconstruction after sports injuries. Unlike my medical colleagues, who believe the problem is increased physical activity, I believe the root of the problem is decreased collagen strength. To protect their joints, children must expose their tissues to the stimulus of exercise and give their bodies the collagen-building foods needed for growth and repair. (See Chapter 10.)[567]

organs, from collagen-rich robust tissues like bone and heart valves to squishy soft lower collagen-content organs like brain, liver, and lungs. Bundles of collagen form extended strips and sheets in the sturdier tissues like ligaments and tendons that surround your joints and hold your skeleton together. Collagen is the most prevalent kind of protein in your body; about 15 percent of your dry weight is pure collagen (dry weight is your body weight without water, which composes about 60 percent of a normal adult male's total mass). Without it, we wouldn't just fall apart at the joints; we would literally disintegrate into small piles of individual cells. While it may seem like an obvious connection, doctors are only now beginning to appreciate the relationship between collagen strength and sports and, for those with jobs that involve lifting or physical labor, work performance. Research now reveals that people with weak collagen experience more injuries throughout their lives.[568, 569, 570]

The reason collagen health is so dependent on a healthy diet has to do with the complexity of the individual collagen molecules. You can get some idea of how hard collagen is to manufacture from the wound-healing process. If you've ever cut yourself so deep that you needed stitches, you may have noticed how long the scar takes to heal—sometimes a full year. When new collagen is formed in a wound, it's composed of shorter, less organized strands than the original. By six weeks, the collagen fibers have become far more organized and they've grown longer, but they're still only back to about 70 percent of their original strength.[571] As the supporting collagen becomes gradually more organized, the scar on the surface fades. In about a year, the skin strength is just about what it was before the injury, though a small scar may remain if the collagen fibers below could never quite iron out smooth.

All collagens are made from chains of amino acids coiled around each other in sets of three to form a triple helix. The longer they are, the more strength they give to the tissue they're in. But the longest, strongest collagens are also the hardest to make. All collagens carry special molecules called *glycosaminoglycans* (which you might recall from the bone stock section in Chapter 10) attached like bangles on a necklace to the triple helix backbone. Each class of collagen varies in length and amount of attached glycosaminoglycan bangles, allowing for all sorts of variation in strength, flexibility, water retention, and lubrication. Once manufactured, collagen molecules get anchored to the exterior of the cell and unfurl throughout the extra-cellular matrix where molecules from adjacent cells can intertwine. The structural biology of collagen is incredibly complex; it is unquestionably a masterpiece of extra-cellular engineering. If you are one of the lucky people to be endowed with good quality collagen, not only will your skin resist wrinkling, you will have a better chance of avoiding joint and circulatory problems down the road.

If any one of the thousands of steps involved in making collagen goes haywire—which is likely to happen if your diet was poor during critical growth periods (meaning your diet was low in nutrient-rich foods and high in sugar and vegetable oils)—the integrity of the finished product is compromised and may break down prematurely. You might imagine that with lesser quality collagen holding us together, our tissues would start pulling apart and separating after a certain number of years. That's exactly what causes wrinkling,[572] arthritis,[573] and even circulatory problems.[574]

No matter the strength of your collagen today, how good you feel tomorrow depends a lot on your diet. People who eat pro-inflammatory foods experience more joint damage on a daily basis because sugar acts like an abrasive in the joints.[575, 576] At night, the small frays and tiny breaks in the collagen that formed during the day must be repaired. But inflammation interferes with healing. Instead of waking up feeling recovered, people on bad diets wake up with stiff joints.[577] Their scars and stretch marks will be more obvious, too, because inflammation disorganizes the collagen fibers so that, as tissue heals, it forms irregular lumpy mounds or deep pits, with more disfiguring results.[578]

SOUP UP YOUR COLLAGEN

One of the best ways to help collagen heal is, not surprisingly, to eat some. Eating collagen-rich organs (like tripe and tendon) or using bone broths in soups, stews, and sauces floods your bloodstream with glycosaminoglycans, which head directly to the parts of the body that need collagen most.[579] These extraordinary molecules attract enormous amounts of water, up to 1,000 times their own weight, which coats your joint tissues in tiny, electrically charged clouds, transforming ordinary water molecules into a protective layer of super-lubricating fluid.[580] Glycosaminoglycans will naturally adhere to collagen anywhere in your body, moistening dry skin, helping your tendons and ligaments stay supple, and generally making you look and feel younger.[581, 582]

Eating homemade bone stock in childhood has fantastic joint-strengthening and collagen-fortifying effects that can last a lifetime. The benefits are so dramatic that it's astounding to me that more people haven't noticed the connection. My patients who eat traditional cuisine with meaty stocks and rich bone broths on a regular basis tend to enjoy all the hallmarks of well-built bones and connective tissue—no matter their age. They have broad hands with wide knuckles and relatively large feet that are proportionately wide from toe to heel. Their skin is smoother, with tighter pores and smaller hair follicle openings, reflecting greater tensile strength. Because their bodies are so well built, these are the people who can enjoy their golden years to the fullest, or work past retirement if they so choose.

Even if you didn't get traditional soups as a child, regular infusions of stock convey bone-strengthening benefits throughout your life. An unusually holistic-minded bone surgeon at a prestigious university in Iraq recognized that "the use of bone broth dietary supplementation by the common folk for promoting the fracture-healing process is an old practice in our community" and designed a study to investigate whether the practice actually produced tangible benefits for healing fractures. He fed rabbits with fractures either normal chow (control group) or normal chow fortified with bone stock (study group) prepared in the traditional manner. He compared the density of newly built bone. At five weeks the density of the healing bone callous in the soup fortified study group was nearly twice that of the control group.[583]

If there is one beef I have with Nature's design for our bodies it's with our joint cartilage, specifically, its reaction to injury. While most cell types in the body react to injury by multiplying in order to fill in gaps left by their fallen comrades, the cells that build cartilage, called chondrocytes, have a tendency to undergo the process of self annihilation, called apoptosis, leaving fewer chondrocytes around to cultivate and support whatever collagen remains.

CELLULITE FAT LACKS ADEQUATE
COLLAGEN SUPPORT

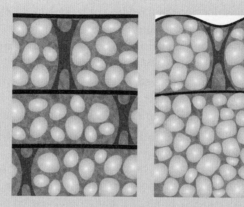

Left, normal. *Right,* cellulite. The fat under our skin is composed of individual adipose cells (light-colored blobs) surrounded and supported by three types of collagenous fibers, illustrated by 1) black horizonatally oriented lines (the topmost is skin); 2) X-shaped gray struts; and 3) lighter gray reticular matrix surrounding each fat cell. In those prone to cellulite, the skin has only two horizontal layers instead of the normal three, and all collagenous supports are substantially less robust. The less robust the supporting collagen, the more readily cellulitic dimpilng develops. This is why some people develop cellulite from only a few excess pounds while others can be quite overweight and still maintain smooth curves. Genes, age, and diet during childhood and adolesence all play major roles in determing the amount of connective tissue support you have. (Images based on MRI and ultrasound analyses.)

Over time, with repeated injuries, the collagen layer thins and weakens even to the point that the underlying bone is exposed—which is generally about the time joints becomes symptomatic with arthritis. Fortunately, there is something you can eat that will help curb your chondrocytes' out-of-control suicidal tendencies—and I'll bet you've already guessed it: bone broth. Research has shown that components in broth, including hyaluronans and collagen hydrolysate, are particularly efficient at preventing chondrocytes from undergoing apoptosis after injury.[584, 585]

Though I couldn't find a study showing a direct association between dietary bone stock and the reduction of cellulite, there are reasons to suggest that, in addition to healing bone and protecting cartilage, grandma's homemade soup might help smooth the appearance of lumpy collagen as well. A lot of people think cellulite comes simply from being too fat. But extra fat where you don't want it is only part of the problem. Lumpy, irregular cellulite forms in fat deposits that lack adequate connective tissue struts to support a smooth shape.[586] The connective tissue-creating cells I introduced earlier, called fibroblasts, are distributed throughout adipose (fat) tissues—including cellulite. Cellulite's lumpy appearance comes in part from the fact that cellulite contains less of the supportive collagen structure that helps to keep the layer of fat organized and smooth. When I see photos of celebrities with terrible cellulite on their thighs, I imagine how their nutritionists are probably telling them to avoid all animal products, which would include bone stock, and how frustrated they'll be as their cellulite hangs on. To get rid of cellulite, combine exercise with a diet full of healthy, natural fats (including animal fat) and collagen-rich stocks. This will send the message that you want your body to replace the saggy fat pockets with smooth, toned curves.

Now that you know why collagen health is important not just to skin, but to every organ in your body, let's learn how inflammation affects your collagen day to day, and over the years.

THE GOOD AND BAD SIDES OF INFLAMMATION

Inflammation, as the name suggests, creates a burning sensation—but only when it reaches our nerves. Skin is full of nerves, so inflammation in the skin causes irritating sensations, including burning, stinging, and itching. Inflammation in the joints may cause an aching feeling. In the head, a headache; in the gut, nausea or cramping; in the heart, a crushing chest pain; and in the lungs, it can make us wheeze and cough.

Like pain, which alerts us to the fact that something is wrong with us, inflammation does have a good side. It's supposed to signal the body's repair systems that a section of tissue needs special care. A bee sting is a classic example of an inflammatory event caused by toxins injected under the skin, which swells up as surrounding blood vessels leak in an attempt to dilute and neutralize the toxin. An ankle swells a little immediately after a sprain. But the real swelling begins hours later, when inflammation signals capillaries to begin leaking serum, stem cells, growth factors, and all the other materials needed to lay the groundwork for the creation of replacement tissue. One of the most dramatic examples of beneficial inflammation occurs during bacterial infection and abscess formation. Inflammation triggered by bacteria invading our tissues releases powerful enzymes that chew through collagen to help the body drain the abscess and expel the invaders. The resulting scar is the small price we pay for avoiding deadly sepsis.

In the setting of dietary imbalance, however, inflammation can go from the physiologic equivalent of a mild-mannered Dr. Bruce Banner into a destructive and uncontrollable Hulk. You may have just such a dietary imbalance and not have any symptoms, or only vague aches and a feeling of tiredness, but on a pro-inflammatory diet you are a true ticking time bomb. When inflammatory responses are triggered with little or no provocation, or are overly vigorous, swelling tissues and destructive enzymes may become life threatening. That's exactly what happened to Kyle when he turned strawberry-red.

RED RASHES—RED ALERT
SIGNALING AN IMBALANCED DIET

If you slap someone's cheek, it turns red. Ever wonder why? The injury triggers a healthy inflammatory response, which dilates the blood vessels of the skin. This allows more oxygen, white blood cells, and nutrients to give the injured tissue a little boost to regain normal function.

But what about red rashes that just appear for no apparent reason? I see patients with rashes every day in my clinic. And I take every one of them seriously because they're a sign that the body—and diet—are out of balance, maybe severely. In the most severe cases of imbalance, anaphylactic reactions like baby Kyle's are a real possibility. Even slight immune system imbalance leaves you vulnerable to all manner of recurring problems, feeling fine one minute and horrible the next.

All kinds of allergic reactions can occur whenever someone's immune system has been so overwhelmed by conflicting signals from excessive, ongoing inflammation that its chemical programming gets confused. The confused immune system interprets normal body proteins as foreign and launches an attack. The affected tissues then ooze chemicals that increase blood flow and cause serum to leak into their surroundings. On the skin, you may see a number of red, raised so-called *wheal and flare* reactions that look a little like mosquito bites. The affected blood vessels can be anywhere: sinuses, lungs, kidneys, joints, etc. Depending on the location and the severity of the immune response, a person's symptoms may be mildly annoying—a runny nose or watery eyes—or they may be life threatening. Immune system confusion will vary day by day depending on stress, degree of infection, sleep, and diet, making allergic reactions hard to predict. To get off the roller coaster, be confident that a good diet can straighten out even the most confused immune systems.

One of the most common rashes I see is eczema. People with eczema can develop itchy, blotchy red rashes all over their bodies. As with all allergic disorders, the symptoms of eczema can resolve but then flare up again and again throughout a person's entire life. People with eczema—just like people with food allergies—may also experience immune system imbalance elsewhere in the body, causing allergic rhinitis, sinusitis, and asthma. Food allergies, chronic runny noses, asthma—the underlying cause is the same: immune system imbalance caused by pro-inflammatory foods. And you already know what the cure is: eating the Human Diet and incorporating the Four Pillars into your daily routine.

When Kyle's pediatrician referred him for allergy testing, his mother learned that her ten-month-old had already developed allergies to proteins in milk, shellfish, green beans, and eggs—some of which he'd never even eaten. As Kyle grows and his airway enlarges and better tolerates small degrees of swelling, he may overcome the breathing crises. But if his mother keeps feeding him the standard food-pyramid-compliant diet, he will develop more inflammatory problems. One of the most common and most disfiguring is acne.

How Inflammation Causes Scarring Acne

Earlier in the book, I explained how oxidation damages fats, and how those damaged fats lead to inflammation, making it nearly impossible to lose weight. Oxidized fats in our skin lead to the pustular inflammation that teenagers, and many adults, dread.[587, 588]

Right now, you're covered in bacteria—billions of them. Don't bother running off to the shower; you'll never get rid of them all. These beneficial skin bacteria protect us from infection. They make their living off the shed husks of dead skin cells, which are so loaded with protein and fat that they offer a reliable food source for all kinds of microbes.

If bacteria were to penetrate the dead outermost layer of skin, patrolling white blood cells would go berserk. To them, the foreign proteins and oxidized fats adorning cell membranes of invasive bacteria are signs of trouble, and like beat cops spotting a couple of hoodlums carrying weapons into a playground, they sound the alarm.[589] Like a well-trained SWAT team, swarming white blood cells bust down doors and break through walls to get to their target, shooting free radicals and releasing collagen-chewing enzymes (called *collagenases*).[590]

If it was all a false alarm caused by diet-induced accidental inflammation and in reality no real infection—well, too bad. White blood cells aren't disposed to quibbling over such nuances, so you'll just have to deal with the scars. If

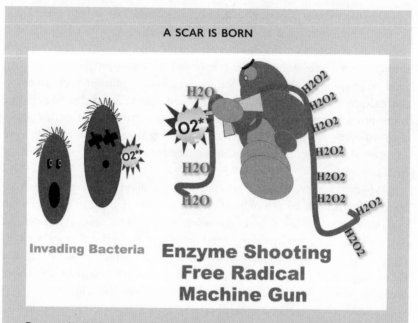

A SCAR IS BORN

Free radicals help kill bacteria but also damage collagen. Here we see an enzyme that generates free radicals to destroy bacteria. Without these enzymes, invasive bacteria would take over our bodies and kill us. Unfortunately, an enzyme's aim is not so accurate and many innocent body bystanders also get hurt—the cost of doing business.

you've ever had an abscess, you know that the first thing the doctor wants to do is drain it. That's all the body is trying to do by unleashing its collagenases.

Acne is a problem of oil oxidation. When we eat easily oxidizable, unnatural oils, they wind up everywhere—our arteries, our nervous system, and the skin on our face. White blood cells mistake oxidized oil for the fatty acids that coat the surface of invasive bacteria, and squads of white blood cells rush to the scene. And as you know, they show up swinging and strike at everything within reach. The acne lesion swells and reddens. Once the battle is over, the site is commemorated with a permanent pit. This is called *cystic-nodular acne*, an example of an inflammatory false alarm generated not by infection but by oxidized oils.[591, 592] So if you or your teen is fighting acne, step one is getting off of vegetable oil. And while you're at it, get off sugar, too. Sugar suppresses the immune system and feeds the bacteria living in acne pustules.[593, 594]

When I see a patient with acne, it suggests they've been eating pro-inflammatory foods full of sugar and vegetable oil. Pro-inflammatory foods send powerfully disruptive signals that will override signals for less urgent metabolic needs (like muscle development, as we saw in the last chapter). So I've found that people with bad acne are also prone to hormone imbalances, reproductive challenges, and a variety of other problems.

Today acne is the most common skin disease, with nearly 90 percent of adolescents affected.[595] But there's little evidence that acne occurred at anything near these rates in the distant past, and many dermatologists believe it is a modern disease.[596] Not only were the fats ancient people consumed healthier than what we eat today, they may have enjoyed protection from acne and other skin infections because of a secret ingredient in their makeup.

BEAUTY SECRETS OF THE ANCIENT EGYPTIANS

Archaeologists have found the earliest evidence of cosmetics being used in Egypt dating back to 4,000 years B.C. The Egyptians made their makeup using fat blended with special saps and either red ochre or ashes. Around the world today, indigenous people still go to great lengths to find the right ingredients to make their own makeup. For instance, the Himba, a nomadic tribe of goat herders in Northern Africa, mix goat butter with ochre and finely crushed herbs, and the paste gives their skin a beautifully smooth red-brown hue. In Hawaii, people used coconut butter that had been left in the sun for a few weeks to give themselves a shiny glow for (frequent) festival occasions. This common practice of applying carefully blended fats to our skin has several purposes.

For one, fat holds moisture in our skin, which helps it stay smooth and soft. Today, high-quality skin care products still contain cocoa butter, avocado, olive oil, and even egg yolk. As good as modern cosmetics may be, they lack the secret ingredient of their aboriginal counterparts: probiotics. The blends of goat butter, cocoa butter, and probably even the ash and fat the Egyptians used, were all loaded with beneficial bacteria, thanks to the fact that their raw materials and containers were colonized with microbes. Applying creams with beneficial bacteria has the same benefits to your skin that eating probiotic-rich foods like yogurt has to your intestinal tract: healthy numbers of beneficial critters outnumber any potentially invasive bacteria. This would have helped people in the past—who generally had little or no clean water to wash with—from getting infected after cutting their skin.[597]

Next time you're having lunch with one of your friends and she's pouring on the low-fat dressing, ask her if she'd use the same ingredients to condition her hair or moisturize her skin. Probably not. Quality beauty products are made with natural saturated fats. Vegetable oil is less suitable because it oxidizes too easily, gets sticky, and irritates our skin. The cosmetic manufacturers would probably love to use these cheap oils instead of more expensive natural fats, but they would never get away with it. Putting this stuff in makeup would lead to obvious allergic skin rashes and acne. Of course, food manufacturers *can* get away with putting vegetable oil in everything—while telling us that it's good for our hearts! Lucky for them, we can't see the inflammatory damage it does to our arteries. And because we don't have nerve endings in our arterial lumens, we can't even feel it. But we can think in the more naturalistic common-sense terms of our ancestors and say, *If I can't put it on my skin, I won't put it in my mouth.*

The Sun *Can* Damage Skin, But It Doesn't Have To

So far, we've seen that vegetable oils and sugar can create imbalances in the immune system and cause acne, and both diseases can damage our collagen. But one of the most well-known collagen-destroying factors is the sun.

Given the near-obsessive use of sunscreen in all but the dimmest of light, you'd think that UV radiation passed right through our bodies, like X-rays. In reality, UV has little penetrating power, and most UV (95 percent or more) is blocked by the rapidly regenerating epidermis. The collagen beneath the epidermis absorbs much of the rest.[598] Depending on your diet, that 5 percent may lead to inflamed, sunburned skin—or it may not. (Of course, if you get way too much sun, you'll get redness and inflammation even on the best diet.) Inflammation leads to the release of those collagen-chewing enzymes and can greatly exacerbate the damage done by UV light, leading to wrinkling down the road.[599] A diet full of nutrients will keep those enzymes on a short leash and keep your skin looking young.

So should we avoid the sun as much as possible? The more your diet is full of pro-inflammatory fats and sugar, the more my answer is yes. But if your diet is healthy, then your collagen won't be seriously injured unless your skin actually burns—which I would never recommend. The more vegetable oil in your diet, and the more PUFAs end up in your skin, the more readily you will get burned and the more extensive the invisible damage to the deeper layers of your skin. I recommend that my patients who follow a healthy diet enjoy sensible sunlight exposure. But what that means in terms of minutes in the sun will vary widely depending on your latitude, altitude, climate, the time of year, color of your skin, and your body's ability to tan.

Like plants, we use sunlight to grow. Plants use sunlight for photosynthesis. We use sunlight when our skin uses sunlight to make vitamin D, without which a child's growth will be severely stunted. We used to get much of our vitamin

D—the sunshine vitamin—directly from sunlight.[600] When UV smashes into the epidermis, it strikes cholesterol molecules, transforming ordinary cholesterol into a precursor of vitamin D, which gets fully activated in the liver and the kidney. We need D to metabolize calcium, so if a child doesn't get enough, the deficiency can weaken their bones and stunt their growth. As you know from

HOW SUN CAUSES WRINKLNG

On a pro-inflammatory diet, sun exposure (A) causes excess inflammation (B), which induces fibroblast cells to release enzymes that chew apart your collagen (C), leading to the imperfect repair (D) that distorts the smoothness of your collagen fibers and enables a wrinkle to form. The more cycles of collagen destruction your skin goes through, the more you wrinkle. Both inflammation and UV radiation damage your DNA, potentially leading to skin cancer.

Warning: To prevent aging, you have to block UVB *and* UVA, and no known sunscreen can yet block UVA. Fortunately melanin, which makes our skin dark, can. Sunblocks (opaque creams like zinc oxide) also block both UVA and UVB.

By the way, SPF reflects UVB blocking ability only. The FDA doesn't have any standards for UVA blocking creams, so labels claiming to block UVA are meaningless.

BATTLE OF THE DIETS

Compare how these two sixty-year-olds have aged. The man on the right has spent most of his life out in the sun eating a traditional Himba diet composed of 50–80 percent animal fat. His smooth, tight skin represents what everyone's skin could look like at this age had we all been raised on balanced diets. The kind-looking man on the left is Dr. Dean Ornish, a non-smoking American physician, and a well-intentioned proponent of a low-fat, industrialized interpretation of a Mediterranean diet. Unfortunately, his collagen is sagging and deteriorated due to lack of fat-soluble vitamins and unintentional consumption of pro-inflammatory fats (trans and MegaTrans; see Chapter 7).

Dr. Ornish is not overweight, yet we see fat deposits under his chin because of his pro-inflammatory diet. Inflammation also elevates insulin levels. Insulin is a powerful signal for storing both sugar and fat, and doing so in a hurry. The kind of fat receptors under our necks (and on our bellies) are called alpha receptors, which are the body's first responders to excess energy. So even on a low-fat diet, with alpha receptors turned on, your body is greedy for energy, and any sugar you eat is converted to fat and stored under your chin, on your belly, and around your internal organs.

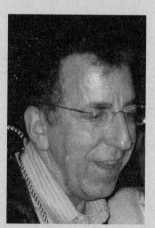 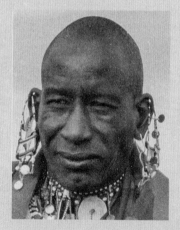

Low-fat *(left)* **versus high-fat diets** *(right).* **Who looks tougher?** Because sagging skin and bloated neck wattles belie a weakness within the connective tissues supporting our bones and joints as well as our skin, we can judge a person's potential strength by how well their skin holds up. Trans fat plus high carbs are largely responsible for the decline and fall of the American physique.

previous chapters, few of us get enough D these days. We used to eat a lot more liver than we do today, which happens to be the best dietary source of vitamin D. Even fortified milk rarely contains the amount of vitamin D it's supposed to, and only *cholecalciferol* supplements work like the real thing (*ergocalciferol* can even be toxic).[601, 602] No matter where we humans live around the globe, we've got to get our sunshine vitamin one way or another, whether directly from the sun or indirectly—as they do in Norway and Alaska—by consuming liver oils from fish and other animals that did get sunlight.

In the summer, a Caucasian sunbathing for twenty minutes at 35 degrees latitude on the outer banks of North Carolina or a beach in San Luis Obispo, California, at midday can make enough vitamin D to last at least a week.[603] After that amount of radiation, ideally, we'd shut off the supply of UV because too much destroys collagen and vital nutrients, *including* vitamin D. Fortunately, your skin has a way of regulating the dose of UV you get. A skin pigment called *melanin* accomplishes this for us. Our genetics so perfectly modulate the baseline amount of pigment in our skin that the skin tone of indigenous people can be used to predict their latitude of origin to within a few degrees.[604]

How does your skin manage its day-to-day regulation of melanin, say, when you go to the beach? By responding to an increase in the amount of radiation it gets. When UV light penetrates the thin outermost layer of dead cells, it enters special cells called *melanocytes*. Melanocytes, which live in the outermost layer of living skin (the epidermis), where they can best protect the layer of collagen beneath, contain a signaling chemical that acts like a tiny mechanical switch. When UV hits the chemical, it flips the switch to its "on" position. The chemical undergoes a shape change (because an electron is stripped away by the UV rays), which allows it to fit into an enzyme that turns on the melanocyte's melanin-production proteins, jump-starting your tanning systems. Within a matter of minutes to hours, depending on your genetics, your skin begins to darken. The faster your melanin appears, the more effectively your body protects you from the damaging UV rays.

Melanocytes, clothing, and opaque sun*blocks* effectively block both UVA and UVB. But while sun*screens* block UVB, which can damage epidermal cell DNA and increase your risk for skin cancer, they do nothing to stop the lower energy, more deeply penetrating UVA radiation.[605] UVA can penetrate to the deeper layers of the skin, where it can damage the collagen that keeps your skin looking smooth and healthy. While UVA does not have enough energy to directly damage DNA, it can—in much the same way as heat in a frying pan—interact with PUFAs to incite free radical cascades that will damage both DNA and collagen.[606] So while sunscreens do reduce burning and, importantly, the direct UVB-induced DNA damage, in a way they can also lull you into a false

TEST FOR PREMATURE WRINKLING

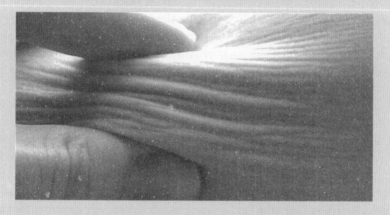

This is my forearm at age forty. My collagen was not formed properly, due to epigenetic damage on my father's side (he also aged prematurely), lack of cartilage/bone broth in childhood, and dietary toxins (my sugar habit, plus margarine). You can perform this test by starting with fingers two inches apart and pinching gently to bring your fingers one inch apart. Continuous wrinkling indicates inadequate elastin. If I don't watch my diet now, I'll age rapidly.

sense of security, letting you soak up far more UVA than you otherwise would. This may be one reason why sunscreens have never been shown to prevent skin cancer.[607] In my view, a complete strategy for preventing cancer-causing UV-induced DNA and wrinkle-promoting collagen damage includes more than just slopping on sunscreen and presuming you've done all you can. I also advise optimizing your diet to reduce PUFA oxidation and, if time permits, gradually coaxing your body into manufacturing more of the skin pigment melanin.

Many of us Irish folk have sluggish melanocytes that can't pump out the color fast enough, and so we tend to burn. Then, after a day or so, the redness starts to tan. How do we get tan *after* sun? Too much sun inflames the skin. The inflammation releases free radicals. And the free radicals trigger the melanocyte-signaling chemical, which gets the tanning engine running. This delay feature may be by design; in higher latitudes, a hyper-reactive tendency to tan wouldn't allow people to make enough vitamin D. Even on a good diet, that whopping dose of UVA on your first day of hanging out in the sun can damage

BRAINS LIKE IT SMOOTH

What happens inside our brains that makes us think young skin is more attractive? Like children, our brains can be easily frustrated. They can't stand confusion, even if it only exists at the subconscious level. When you look at someone, your eyes travel from feature to feature in jerky bursts of motion called *saccades*, darting between features as if magnetized by contrast. Young skin is smooth, with no distracting wrinkles. This enables us to focus on the person's expressions, facilitating safe and pleasant communication.

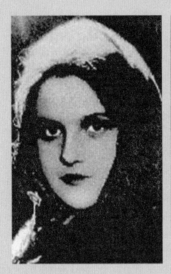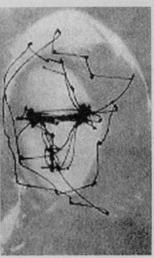

The picture on the right shows the trace of a person's gaze while examining the portrait on the left. These two pictures are taken from the work done by Russian psycho-physicist Dr. Alfred Yarbus in the 1950s. Yarbus demonstrated that human beings do not scan a scene randomly. Our eyes move deliberately between points of interest, which tend to be areas of contrast, particularly around the eyes and mouth. The quick darting from feature to feature strongly suggests that, rather than assessing features individually, we measure their relationships to one another and to the face as a whole. When those relationships conform closely to the Marquardt Mask (see Chapter 4) we want to keep looking!

your collagen down to the deep dermal layers and age your skin prematurely, but on a bad diet, the damage will be worse.

So get some summer sun, but pace yourself—especially if you're light-skinned. Ideally, before your Hawaiian vacation, get a base tan first. That melanin can protect your deeper tissues from UVA *and* UVB. I know you'll be tempted, but please, whenever and wherever you're getting sun, try to stay away from pro-inflammatory vegetable oils and sugar even if you're on vacation. Not only will you be protecting your skin, but that move will help steer you toward your vacation destination's best traditional cuisine.

DEFYING TIME AND GRAVITY

When we see a seventy-five-year-old who looks half her age, we might presume she's spent her whole life ducking into the shadows to avoid the sun. That, and maybe Botox. But when you hear that she loves the outdoors, hikes regularly, and spends three days a week out on the golf course, you think, *What gives? Why does her skin look so smooth?* The secret isn't avoiding the sun. It's avoiding inflammation.

If this woman, let's call her Mary, is so adept at avoiding inflammation, chances are good that the rest of her body is holding up just as well. She avoids inflammation by staying away from artificial fats and sugar—giving into none of those buffet-table temptations and steering clear of vegetable oil dressings and the sugary juices that could damage her nerves—so she's as sharp and feisty as ever. She remembers what happened sixty years ago and what happened sixty days ago. Mary and her husband have recently taken up ballroom dancing. Sometimes, when they get home after class, they waltz themselves straight into the bedroom to keep the music going. And they can, thanks to healthy arteries and the robust blood flow that comes with it.

Mary loves making stock, sauerkraut, her own fresh bread, and all the foods from the Four Pillars that her mother taught her to make and that keep inflammation away. When her friends come over for brunch, they compliment Mary on her amazingly smooth skin—especially lately, as they've been noticing more blotches on theirs. On imbalanced diets, something as minor as a pimple, a rap on the shin, or even friction around the neck from clothing and jewelry can produce enough inflammation to trigger the body's tanning machine by mistake, causing a dark spot. Their skin seems to have aged faster than Mary's. And it has: inflammation accelerates cell division, setting the aging process to fast forward, making skin thinner, weaker, and vulnerable to bruising. Mary's adherence to the Human Diet has slowed it all down.

Practically every nutrient studied plays a role in protecting collagen by acting as an antioxidant and/or growth factor. Vitamin A, vitamin C, glutathione, glucosamine, and omega-3 fatty acids have each been shown to cut collagen damage from UV radiation by up to 80 percent.[608, 609, 610, 611] Imagine the effects of getting enough of all of them combined, as Mary does. Cortisone has been studied too, and found to have similar anti-wrinkle effects. Cortisone is a hormone made from cholesterol by the adrenal glands, which, as with all organs, function best when fortified by a good diet, exercise, sleep, and avoidance of chronic stress. By eating poorly and suppressing adrenal function, we reduce our body's natural cortisone production and prematurely age all our collagenous tissues— most conspicuously, our skin. By eating real food, full of genuine vitamins (not synthetic counterfeits), Mary has kept her collagen in superb condition.

Mary does strength training, but toned muscles alone can't prevent "the sag" that we all dread, which develops as gravity relentlessly tugs our tissues downward. Mary has a built-in anti-gravity device, a latticework of sturdy collagen woven throughout her body fat. Having enough healthy collagen in the *subcutaneous* fat (just under your skin, where most body fat is stored) doesn't just prevent cellulite and keep your curves looking taut, as we saw earlier. It also prevents the development of the chin wattle, the droopy butt, the floppy underarm, and even those creases on the sides of the nose and mouth. Mary's mother didn't have these things, and neither does Mary. The reason is healthy subcutaneous fat.

THE ULTIMATE CONNECTIVE TISSUE
SUPPORT: ELASTIN

More than anything else, the ability of your collagen to stand up to gravity depends on a very special member of the collagen family called *elastin*. Think of elastin as a latticework of interconnected proteins that function like molecular springs. When we develop wrinkles, it's primarily because our elastin has sprung.[612] Skin, arteries, lungs, and ligaments have the most elastin, which gives these tissues their elastic consistency and the ability to rebound after stretching. Women like Mary have a healthy amount of elastin throughout their bodies, as does anyone who ages well or looks younger than they are. If any single molecule could be said to represent the fountain of youth, this would be it.

Mary's supple and resilient elastin molecules were built to last. With a half-life of seventy-five years, they're meant to last a lifetime. UC Davis anatomy professor Charles G. Plopper tells us that "the half-life of elastin matches the life-span of the species," [613] suggesting that elastin plays a central role in determining life expectancy. (Half-life means that half of something will be gone in the given time interval.)

Elastin's strength is also its drawback. Since it's supposed to be made to last, your body doesn't make much more after puberty. As far as we know, it's only possible to make elastin during periods of rapid growth. Elastin depends on a unique chemical bond, called the *desmosine cross-link*, that's extremely difficult to manufacture. It can be made only while your body is swimming in the hormones and growth factors that orchestrate its manufacture—during embryologic life, early childhood growth spurts, and adolescence. Although Mary's mother didn't know any of these physiologic details, she knew that the intricate and delicate growth processes going on inside Mary's little body were dependent upon the best nutritional environment she could provide. This applies especially to elastin, since elastin's complexity makes the process of manufacturing this vital tissue particularly easy to disrupt. Says Dr. Plopper, "It is now apparent that a range of intra-uterine and early postnatal factors, such as hypoxia, nutritional restriction, and FGR [not having enough room in the uterus] can affect elastin deposition."

Mary's upbringing was a lot different than Kyle's, the sickly baby we met at the opening of this chapter. Thanks to the fact that Mary's mother, and her mother's mother, did everything right—from planning conception to fortifying their bodies to breastfeeding and cooking from scratch—Mary's life has been blessed with superior health, good looks, and happy fortune. The same mixture of hormones and nutrients that ensured Mary's strong elastin also ensured balanced skeletal growth. Her wide jaw and strong cheekbones allowed for straight teeth and a beautiful smile. And because optimal facial development leaves enough room for the eyes to develop normally, Mary never needed glasses. Even now, much to her eye doctor's amazement, good quality collagen in the lenses of her eyes has delayed the onset of presbyopia (the age-related lens stiffness that necessitates reading glasses). Though she's always enjoyed the sun, Mary's anti-inflammatory diet has kept her free of cataracts, macular degeneration, and other degenerative diseases that make us feel old.

Even if your upbringing didn't provide you with an optimized complement of youth-promoting elastin, there's still a lot your diet can do to help you delay the aging process. In addition to avoiding harmful vegetable oils to reduce the tendency for inflammation to activate the elastin-destruction process, you can take another positive action. In 2014, Korean researchers studying the anti-aging effects of traditional bone stock discovered that a component of the stock, called bone hydrolysate, can help protect elastin from UV damage like that induced by overexposure to the sun.[614] Their work was done on a tissue culture Petri dish. Another group studying living mice exposed to UV light found that consuming the hydrolysate protected not just elastin but all forms of collagen as well as the fibroblasts cells that produce and sustain the collagen network supporting our skin.[615]

THE ANCESTOR'S TALE

Mary is the hero of this book. As is her mother, and her mother, and hers— all the way back to her most distant ancestors who followed dietary practices that ensured the benefits of beauty and health. Mary is the manifestation of that dream. And because she appreciates her ancestors' gifts, she has fulfilled her duty to protect them and has passed the genetic vessel unbroken to her son and daughter.

The vessel is her family's epigenetic code. And Mary's granddaughter now benefits from it. If she's careful, and willing to take seriously her charge as curator of her family's genetic heritage, then her ancestors' dream will live on in the healthy, beautiful body of Mary's great-granddaughter.

The sacred vessel of epigenetic integrity does not belong to us. We receive it, benefit from it, and then pass it on. During our lives on Earth we must also protect it. And by eating food from the Four Pillars and celebrating the living art of ancient, traditional cuisine, we can do exactly that, engineering our bodies, and those of our children, into the forms that best represent balanced, uninterrupted, natural growth.

The requisites of perfect health are not hidden. We know what keeps us well, and we know what makes us sick. When we allow real food to connect our bodies to nature, nature speaks through that sustenance directly to our DNA, to the living, intelligent engines that drive our physiologies. Health is beautiful. Food informs physiology. Source matters. Your family's physiologic destiny is largely under your control. These are the central tenets of *Deep Nutrition*. If you adhere to the principles outlined in this book, you'll soon feel healthier than you do today. You will support vital symmetry within your children's growing bodies and rig the genetic lottery to the benefit of those yet to be born. With every meal, you do the groundwork that will allow your legacy to sprout from the earth hundreds of years from now, in the form of a beautiful child. That child's beauty and health is your beauty and health, an unending renewal that promises to keep you forever young.

CHAPTER 13

Deep Nutrition

How to Get Started Eating the Human Diet

This section presents my clinic-tested approach to transitioning to a wholesome, new way of living.

After the first edition of *Deep Nutrition* came out and I started getting feedback directly from patients, I was pleasantly surprised by how readily so many folks adapted to this way of eating. It's a big change to go from pouring cereal out of a box and thawing foods in a microwave to planning healthy meals. But those who made the switch were happy to be eating their favorite foods again, and invariably came up with creative, easy ways to prepare them quickly, which I'll describe here.

I'm not going to try to convince you that adapting a *Deep Nutrition* lifestyle is something you can do overnight. Unless you're a chef, or majored in home economics, there are likely quite a few skills you may need to acquire. But there's no reason you must do it all at once. I waded into my new nutritional life by taking the simple step of cutting back on sugar while including more natural fats from foods I already ate, such as eggs, nuts, cream, and cheese. With more butter and delicious homemade dressings, vegetables tasted better, so I ate larger portions, making sure, when possible, that they were fresh instead of frozen. We went to farmers markets more often, and visited the local grocery stores on the days the fresh greens would be delivered.

The big hurdle was extracting the sweet tooth that had driven my appetites since I was two years old. I remember sitting in a booster chair, pouring a mountain of sugar on my bowl of Cheerios when my mother was looking the other way. Taking control of my sugar intake after a lifetime of fighting against cravings began with a decision to reduce the dose. I never believed I would ever stop craving sweets altogether. As I described in Chapter 9, cutting down gradually seemed less drastic and more doable than going cold turkey. And what kept me from relapsing was feeling better. I noticed a significant reduction in the inflammation in my sore knee the first day I skipped the sugar.

Many readers and patients have taken similar routes to better eating, switching out spreads for butter or just adding more natural fats they'd already been using while also cutting out some ritual around sweets, generally either soda or juice. The combination of cutting sweets while adding butter or cream (or some other natural fat) is extremely effective. The natural fats make us less interested in sugar, and the reduced sugar, in turn, enables us to enjoy our foods more, and it really helps with energy and mental focus. Such tangible results can snowball, giving us the energy to try something additional that often leads to another noticeable improvement: reinforcing the accumulating healthy new habits.

For those who don't have a sweet tooth to conquer, it's the reduction of fake, pro-inflammatory fats and excessive hormone-disrupting carbs that makes a big difference in their health. One of my most delightful patients in Napa was a foodie with a painful skin condition that had severely disrupted her daily life for more than thirty years. She switched out breakfast cereal for liver pate on toasted sourdough, her lunch sandwich for a bowl of homemade bone stock soup, and exchanged salad dressings made with vegetable oil for olive oil and vinegar. Just like me, she noticed a perceptible difference in her longstanding symptoms right away. That encouraged her to stay the course. And the longer she did, the more her symptoms continued to improve.

THE HUMAN DIET IN A NUTSHELL

An optimum diet allows you to extract the maximum available nutrition from the edible world. Most modern popular diets, such as the Paleo Diet, Atkins, or pescatarian, can readily be adapted to include all Four Pillars. Throughout this book, I've illustrated how and why following the Human Diet will optimize the function of every organ and tissue in your body—no matter your age.

Most of us are already familiar with the food groups codified by the U.S. government in the mid-twentieth century: fruits and vegetables, meats, dairy, and grains, beans, and legumes. While these can all be incorporated into the Human Diet, some traditional cultures—Hawaiians, for instance—do not include very much, if any, dairy. Other cultures did not have much access to fruits, vegetables, or grains; for example, native people living in what is now Canada and Alaska. This, of course, is another reason why we need to think in terms of strategy, not lists, and each of the Four Pillars represents a strategy we need to employ. Most people are not accustomed to thinking about food in terms of strategies. The following pages contain concrete examples.

THE HUMAN DIET AT A GLANCE

Pillar 1: Meat on the Bone
Some of my favorite meats on the bone:

- Roast turkey with stuffing and gravy
- Chicken soup with dumplings
- *Chile con carne*
- Barbequed spare ribs
- Mexican menudo soup
- *Pico de gallo* soup
- Thai *thom kha gai* soup
- Vietnamese *pho*
- Braised lamb shanks
- Southwestern green chile stew
- Grilled New York strip steak with demi-glace reduction sauce
- Burger (no bun) with mushroom in demi-glace reduction sauce. The original hamburger from Hamburg, Germany, was thin-sliced meat fried in a pan, and it did not have a bun. Only when ground beef in patty form was served in St. Louis, Missouri, at the 1904 World's Fair, where the vendor ran out of plates and convinced a neighboring bread vendor to sell him slices, did it acquire the bun.
- Wild rice cooked in chicken stock
- Greens braised in chicken stock
- Roasted butternut squash soup with chicken stock base
- Broccoli soup with chicken stock base
- French onion soup
- Beef Bourguignon

Pillar 2: Organ Meat
Some of my favorite organ meats:

- Sandy's miracle liver recipe (see recipes)
- Pakistani fried chicken liver
- Duck liver pate
- Chicken liver pate (i.e., Trader Joe's brand)
- Liverwurst (i.e., US Wellness Meats brand)

- Grilled beef heart strips
- Beef heart chili
- Beef sticks and organ meat (i.e., Pure Traditions brand)
- Filipino salmon head soup
- Roasted bone marrow
- Wild flying fish roe on buttered sprouted grain toast
- Mexican *menudo* with tripe
- Vietnamese *pho* with tripe
- Blood sausage
- Filipino *dinuguan* (savory blood stew made with pork shoulder and variety cuts)
- Sautéed sweetbreads with fava beans
- Beef tongue stew
- Pan fried lamb kidneys in butter
- Poached eggs. (If you can't do any of the above, eggs have many of the same benefits as organ meats. Keeping the yolk runny is the most nutritious way to eat eggs.)

Pillar 3: Fermented and Sprouted Foods
Some of my favorite fermented and sprouted foods:

(Note: Those marked "live cultures" contain beneficial probiotics. Those not marked no longer contain living microbes.)

- Yogurt (live cultures)
- Cottage cheese (live cultures)
- Sour cream (live cultures)
- Pepperoni
- Cheddar cheese
- Kombucha (live cultures)
- Sauerkraut (live cultures)
- Dill pickles (live cultures)
- Kimchi (live cultures)
- Tempeh
- Miso
- Fish sauce
- Soy sauce (only if naturally brewed, i.e., Kikkoman brand)

- Beer (unfiltered; glop at the bottom is made into Vegemite in Australia, a very salty but nutritious paste)
- Sourdough bread
- Sprouted grain bread (i.e., Ezekiel brand)
- *Chile con carne* with sprouted beans
- Sprouted almonds (i.e., Living Intentions or Go Raw brands)
- Old-fashioned oat porridge (oats fermented with whey overnight)
- Sprouted pumpkin seeds (i.e., Living Intentions or Go Raw brands)

Pillar 4: Fresh, Raw Food
Some of my favorite raw foods:

- Garlic
- Salad greens
- Bell peppers
- Any vegetable that you can eat without cooking (almost everything goes well in salad)
- Cilantro (and other fresh herbs)
- Poke
- Real milk and cream
- Ice cream
- Sushi
- Raw-milk cheeses
- Steak tartar
- Dried beef
- Prosciutto
- Pickled veggies (i.e., Mezzetta brand Giardiniera Italian mix)
- Dried seaweed (if possible, avoid brands with vegetable oil)
- Nuts
- Pickled herring in cream or wine sauce (the lowest sugar brand available)
- Seeds
- *Ceviche*
- Antipasto salad

The people who experience long-term success are able to accomplish these three things: cut down on carbs; swap out toxic fats for healthy ones; and add back missing nutrients. That's it. It's not all that complicated. We're stopping the toxins; unnatural fats are the most important toxic compounds to avoid. And we're reducing carbs to make space for more nutrient-dense Four Pillar foods.

This chapter will guide you through the process of easing into a new, healthy way of life. My goal is to help you understand how to integrate ancient principles of healthy eating into a modern diet. Here's how you can get started.

DAILY HABITS

- Drink a minimum of 64 ounces of water daily.
- Instead of soda, drink ice-cold sparkling water with a lemon wedge, herbal tea, or kombucha.
- For best results, do not snack.
- Take any supplements with meals.
- Consider sleep and movement as priorities.
- Plan your meals using the shopping and planning templates.

Water Intake

Drinking plenty of water is essential to helping your body adjust to the new nutrients. You can drink between meals to help deal with the urge to snack, or with meals to help your kidneys and digestive system adapt to any new foods you're eating. Or both. Every one of my patients who has developed kidney stones did not drink very much water. More than 16 glasses a day, however, is probably too much.

Beverages

If you've got a soda habit, you're not alone. Nearly half of all Americans drink soda on a daily basis.[616] Juice, often with added sugar but promoted as healthy, isn't much better. Both contain 16 to 20 teaspoons of sugar per 12-ounce serving. If you've already tried breaking the soda habit cold turkey and had no success, then I'd recommend trying these alternatives: ice-cold sparkling water with a lemon wedge, herbal tea, or 6 to 10 ounces of kombucha with the lowest amount of sugar you can find. I don't recommend diet soda unless you are using it as a bridge to kick the regular soda habit.

Snacks

The longer I've practiced, the more I've become convinced that there's just no such thing as a healthy snack. Snacking habits are a gateway to making poor food choices. Most ready-to-eat snack foods contain artificial flavoring agents that damage your natural appetite-regulation systems, disrupting your ability to enjoy simpler, high-quality foods that can form the backbone of a wholesome meal program. Even the so-called healthy snacks like food bars and trail mixes are typically loaded with toxic fats and/or excessive sugars. Planning and making snacks also takes valuable time away from planning and making meals. But the worst thing about snacking is what it does to your relationship with food. The habitual snackers I've worked with were thinking about food all the time. Only by breaking the snack habit did they gain freedom from these obsessive thoughts, opening up hours of time to immerse themselves in other activities, like family outings and exercise.

If you're hungry between meals, see the troubleshooting section below.

Supplements

Take these at meals or within an hour or two of eating in order to optimize absorption. The specific supplements you need will depend on your diet. See below for details.

Sleep and Movement

Real food is just one of your body's prerequisites for health. Your ability to use the building blocks from food for optimizing body composition depends on signals you generate during activity. Heavy lifting, for example, instructs your body to direct the raw materials for building muscle, bone, and joint material to the limbs you just exercised. And your body needs sleep to carry out this construction. So if you don't get very much activity, or if you lack adequate sleep, no matter how healthy your diet, your body will not be able to put the food you eat to optimal use building lean tissue. And that keeps you stuck in fat-building mode.

Planning Meals

Until you get used to shopping and cooking according to *Deep Nutrition* principles, it's useful to sit down for ten minutes or so once a week and plan out what you're going to buy and what you're going to cook. In addition to making a shopping list, it may also help to print out a blank weekly menu planner that you can fill in with seven days' worth of breakfasts, lunches, and dinners. Studies show that people who take a few minutes to plan things out are able to sustain new habits more successfully than those who don't.[617] You can find printable menu planners on my website at DrCate.com.

MACRONUTRIENT RATIOS

While I am generally not a fan of obsessively counting macronutrients, I've found that a good number of my patients eat far more carbohydrates than they realize and don't achieve the average minimum daily intake of protein, while those who follow a very low-carb diet often eat too much protein. This section will outline how much you need. Be aware that if you are an elite athlete, your needs may vary.

Carbs

If you only exercise moderately—jogging, tennis, biking, swimming—but don't make exercise a central part of your daily life, then you should consider 100 grams of daily carbohydrate intake to be your upper limit. Even so, most days you're better off keeping daily carbohydrate totals between 30 and 70 grams, because every gram of carbohydrates you consume but don't use to fuel intense activity (anaerobic exercise) must either get stored as fat or be burned as fuel. Burning sugar to fuel activity other than intense, anaerobic exercise gradually retools your cellular equipment to specialize in sugar burning, which impairs your natural ability to burn fat. Over years, your hormone and enzyme systems may adjust to facilitate this specialization in ways that lead to insulin resistance. Insulin resistance is a precursor to diabetes and makes it easier to accumulate body fat—even if you're a regular exerciser.

I've found that for most people the worst time of day to load up on carbs is at breakfast. Most of your carb intake should happen at dinner. (Carb timing is built into the meal templates you'll see later in this chapter.)

If you're an elite athlete who burns 600 or more calories a day doing intense exercises like sprinting or heavy lifting, those calories should come from an optimized balance of carb and fat. The optimal ratios depend upon a number of personal factors, including how much anaerobic activity you do, your muscle fiber types, and your metabolic health (a detailed discussion of which is beyond the scope of this book). Because protein cannot be burned for energy as easily as carbs or fat, I don't recommend eating more protein for the purposes of fueling intense exercise (as opposed to building muscle).

How to count carbs: I've provided a quick-reference guide to estimating the carb content in common foods; see the chart on page 431.

Protein

Protein is the "Goldilocks" macronutrient. Unlike carbohydrates, which have no minimum requirement, and unlike fat, which has no maximum (as long as you aren't generally overeating), when it comes to protein, you need to get enough and not too much. Inadequate protein reduces antioxidant enzyme capacity and stresses the nervous, immune, and skeletal systems—tissues that demand a good deal of protein every day—in ways that can lead to mood disorders, allergic problems and osteoporosis, just to name a few. The minimum average daily intake for a woman is 50 grams and for a man 70 grams. If you don't eat meat, eggs, or dairy with at least two meals per day, it's a good idea to tally your intake for a week to make sure you're getting enough.

On the other hand, if you don't eat many vegetables you may end up eating too much meat. The maximum your body can use is roughly 120 grams of protein for a woman and 150 grams of protein for a man (body builders and certain other elite athletes can use more). When we eat too much, our kidneys have to convert the unusable protein into either sugar or fat, which can increase the risk of a joint disease called gout.

How to count protein: If a vegetable is not on the list on page 433, it's got less than 5 grams per normal-sized serving. (For example, while spinach does provide protein, you have to eat 5 cups of it to get 5 grams of protein. Of course, if you're a big fan of spinach, there's nothing wrong with eating that much!)

Fat

I advise getting 60 to 85 percent of your daily caloric intake from fat. (Athletes' needs must be tailored to their training and body type, as this wouldn't necessarily be appropriate for, to use as an example, an elite athlete with lots of fast-twitch muscle fiber.) That probably sounds like a lot of fat. But realize we're not talking about percent by volume or weight. Fat is very calorie dense, so it doesn't take up much space on your plate. If you use 2 tablespoons of salad dressing on a giant salad with 4 to 6 cups of raw veggies (per the dinner salad on the template), that's about 180 calories of fat per 40 to 90 calories of veggies (depending on what veggies you add), which brings your percent of calories from roughly 65 to 80. Two tablespoons of butter on 2 cups of broccoli makes for 200 calories of fat per 70 calories of broccoli, roughly 75 percent fat calories. Most nuts and seeds as well as hard cheeses (like cheddar) are composed of roughly 75 percent fat, as are oily condiments like olives. Eggs, chicken wings, and 80 percent lean beef are all about 60 percent fat calorically. And butter, dips, and sauces often contain even more. So it's not like you have to go out of your way to get that ratio when you're eating a whole-food diet.

How to count fat: As long as you're eating nonrestrictive whole foods and are abiding by the guidelines for carbohydrates and protein, you don't need to extend a lot of mental energy tallying up this macronutrient, as you'll almost certainly be within the 60 to 85 percent range, or pretty close. If you're a vegan trying to avoid oils, I recommend you make a point of including plenty of avocados and nuts and other fatty vegetables to help ensure you're getting adequate natural fats.

On the next page you will see a quick and easy chart so you can see how the macronutrients of the *Deep Nutrition* approach compare with the standard American diet.

UNDERSTANDING YOUR CALORIC NEEDS

While I encourage you to use your appetite as your primary guide to how much to eat, realize that many people's appetites are overactive due to sugar cravings and blocked fat-burning ability. These issues will resolve with time, and you can

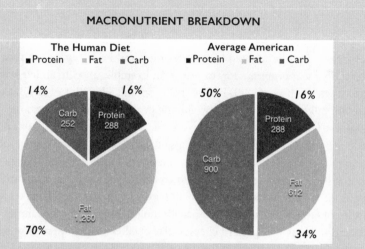

Macronutrients at a glance. Shown in terms of calories of each macronutrient as well as percentages of the total. The left chart represents a daily total of 1,800 calories on the Human Diet, which amounts to 75 grams of protein, 60 grams of carbohydrate, and 140 grams of fat. The chart on the right represents a typical 1,800-calorie American diet, composed of 75 grams of protein, 225 of carbohydrate, and 57 grams of fat. Both represent intakes of approximately 1,800 calories per day, the intake of an average American woman. Men report consuming approximately 500 additional total calories on average. The macronutrient breakdowns are similar in men and women.

recover your innate appetite regulation capacity. In the meantime, be aware that some of these foods (like cream, coconut, and nuts) are very calorie dense, making it easy to accidentally eat more than you need. So if you find yourself gaining weight, it's a good idea to check your portion sizes against the guidelines in the meal-planning templates. As you can see, there is a range of serving sizes for each meal, and so the sum total will end up being somewhere between 1,200 and 2,200 calories per day. You can estimate your calorie needs using any number of free, online calculators (I've provided my favorite at DrCate.com). If your size and activity level increase your caloric needs to greater than 2,200 per day, then adjust your portion sizes proportionately.

Online calorie counters can be useful, but you should use them only as a very rough guide. Because everyone's individual needs vary depending on genetics, age, activity, sleep, stress, and metabolic and hormonal health, even the best calculator can be off by 30 percent or more. This huge variability underscores one of the many reasons it's essential to eliminate habitual eating altogether and get in better alignment with your body's natural cravings and appetite. As you know, high sugar intake and vegetable oils derange appetite. But with these factors removed from your diet, your appetite once again becomes a far more trustworthy guide.

PLANNING YOUR MEALS AND SHOPPING

Whether you've decided to just focus on one simple change, like cutting out sweets, or you've decided to go all in, the planning templates on pages 340, 346, and 351 will give you some fast, healthy ideas. Let's go over how to get started one step at a time:

1. Select your "base" and "variations" from the meal plan templates.
2. Detox your kitchen.
3. Plan your first week of food, using the shopping planner.
4. Go shopping!
5. Follow the plan.

Let's take a closer look at each of these steps and how they work at each meal.

BREAKFAST

Select your "base" ingredient, and then choose "combinations and variations" from the meal plan templates.

The templates provide you a general outline of multiple options for different kinds of breakfasts, lunches, and dinners. I've found that most people need more help with breakfast and lunch than dinner because most of us are more pressed for time during the day but have carved out some time in the evening to make dinner. So the templates provide breakfast and lunch ideas you can make in minutes, with dinners requiring more time. The program included here is primarily geared toward beginner cooks, but it can also be a good guide for anyone looking to add variety into their routines.

The "base" is the main ingredient you're starting with, like eggs or yogurt, and combinations and variations are things you add to the base, like vegetables and herbs or nuts, so that you can convert the main ingredient into enough variety, day after day. Not getting bored is very important because any sense of

BREAKFAST		
Calories: 300–500		
Protein 0–15 grams / Carbs 0–10 grams / Fat 25–40 grams		
Base	**Instructions (per serving)**	**Combinations and Variations**
Fermented Dairy Parfait	■ Yogurt or cottage cheese: 6 ounces ■ Nuts and seeds totaling 1–2 ounces ■ Sweet/carb (optional): 1 tablespoon (max)	■ Vary nuts and seeds: cashews, pecans, walnuts, pistachios, pumpkin, sunflower, chia, flax ■ Vary sweet/carb: jelly, diced dried ginger, dried cranberries, no-vegetable-oil granola ■ Reduce topping by half and fold in 1/8 cup whipped cream
Breakfast Meat	■ Meats: 2–3 ounces ■ Veggies: 2–4 ounces ■ BREAKFAST STARCH (see below)	■ Vary meats: bacon, sausage, Canadian bacon, smoked salmon/lox ■ Vary veggies: sautéed onion, mushrooms, bell pepper, fresh tomato, kimchee
Eggs	■ Eggs: 2–3 chicken or 1–2 duck/goose ■ Cooking fat: 1/2–1 table-spoon ■ Cheese and/or meat fat totaling 1–2 ounces ■ Veggies: 2–4 ounces ■ BREAKFAST STARCH (see below)	■ Vary egg-cooking technique: poached, steamed, scrambled, frittata ■ Cheeses: cheddar, goat, parmesan, meunster ■ Vary meats: (see above) ■ Vary veggies: (see above) ■ Substitute toast for cheese or meat (to keep calories in range)

Base	Instructions (per serving)	Combinations and Variations
Wake-Me-Up Shake	▪ Coffee or tea, brewed: 1–2 cups ▪ Whole milk: 1–2 cups Cream: 2–4 tablespoons	▪ Vary coffee/tea flavors ▪ Try cold-brewed coffee (grind 1/8 cup, soak in 8 ounces water overnight, pour through filter in the morning)
Low-Carb Custard/ Pudding	▪ Custard or pudding: 1½–2 cups	▪ Vary textural and flavor ingredients: peanut butter, pumpkin, herbs ▪ Google "low carb custard recipes" or "savory custards"
Breakfast Smoothie (2–3 cups)	▪ Ice cubes: 6–12 ▪ Milk or yogurt (4–8 ounces) ▪ Veggies: fresh, 3–4 cups ▪ Fat source from cream (2 tablespoons) or coconut oil (1 tablespoon) or avocado (1/2) or nuts (10) ▪ Fruit: ½–1 piece	▪ Vary milks: cow/goat/soy/almond (must be unsweetened) ▪ Vary ice: freeze juice or milk ▪ Vary flavoring extracts (vanilla, almond, orange) or herbs/spices (tarragon, allspice, nutmeg, cinnamon) ▪ Vary veggies: spinach, kale, celery, tomato juice
Crepes	▪ Crepes: 1–2 ▪ Filling: sautéed veggies (1/2–1 cup total) or fresh berries (1/8 cup total), soft cheese or whipped cream (1–2 ounces total) ▪ Finely chopped nuts (sprinkle half on top)	▪ Vary flours: wheat, spelt ▪ Vary veggies: spinach, radish, beet tops, onion ▪ Vary fruit: blueberries, strawberries, preserves (1 tablespoon) ▪ Vary dairy/cheese: goat, chevre, farmer's crème fraiche, yogurt
Leftovers	▪ Any leftover meals 3–6 ounces	▪ The sky's the limit!
Breakfast Starch (choose one)	▪ Toast: 1 slice ▪ Fermented or sprouted porridge: 1/2 cup ▪ Muffin, small (2–3 ounce size) ▪ Fruit (berries or melon): 1/2 cup	To keep calories in range, when including a starchy side with your breakfast, you must reduce the meat, cheese, or cooking fat (i.e. eggs poached or hard-boiled so no cooking fat is required, and no cheese).

tedium will tempt you to slide back into old habits.

The reason base foods are broken out this way is that I'd like you to start seeing them as the main ingredient staples that you'll be using in a variety of dishes throughout the week. Many keep more than just one week, or will freeze well, so you can buy plenty and not worry about them going bad. I suggest you pick at least two base foods for each mealtime (breakfast/lunch/dinner) to rotate through the week, and use the different combinations and variations to keep them interesting. For example, if you're thinking that for next week you want to alternate eggs and porridge for breakfast, you'll want to make sure you buy plenty of eggs and have properly prepped grains for porridge, in addition to the ingredients with which you will create the variations.

Look over the template to find a base you like. Let's say you don't have time to cook. The top three options don't require cooking at all.

Let's go over each of the breakfast choices in detail.

Base: Fermented Dairy. Your choice of cottage cheese, OR Greek or regular yogurt (4 to 6 ounces, more if you like).

> VARIATION: Top the fermented dairy with your favorite combination of nuts and seeds, which I call a Parfait Blend and describe in more detail in the breakfast template. Use your favorite nuts, seeds, or other items to vary the blend, keeping the total of nuts and seeds to 2 ounces if you are watching your weight. If not, feel free to add more nuts or even a couple teaspoons of your favorite jam or jelly.

> **Dr. Cate's Notes:** One of my favorite combinations is cottage cheese topped with a handful of pistachio nuts, adding a few drops of vanilla extract, a dusting of cinnamon, and a sprinkle of orange zest or dried orange peel. (I eat this for lunch or dessert.)

Base: Coffee/Tea Milk Shake. 6 to 8 ounces of coffee/tea.

> VARIATIONS: Add a ton of milk and cream. The cream provides a fat source to help your body stay in fat-burning mode, and the milk provides just a little protein and carb for satiety and nutrition.

> **Dr. Cate's Notes:** I like my coffee cold, so I soak about 1/8 cup of grinds in 10 ounces of water overnight and pour through a paper filter in the morning, producing just under a cup of coffee. This is actually what I've had every day for breakfast for years and it is rich enough to hold me all the way to dinner, which, on days I don't have time for lunch, comes in handy. I would not recommend making your diet so repetitive unless you can get the best possible quality milk and cream, which I try to do. The dairy is raw and comes from 100 percent pasture-raised cows.

Base: Breakfast Smoothie (see template). Most smoothies benefit by starting with ice instead of water. Avoid smoothies that have more than one piece of fruit per serving; the fruit should be used as a sweetener, not the main ingredient, so that you can enjoy a larger "dose" of vegetables.

> VARIATIONS: To make sure the smoothie fills you up, I recommend adding additional fat sources as described. There are other good fats you could use in addition to those listed, i.e., macadamia nut oil, so this is a very rough guide.

Base: Breakfast Meat. The fastest option here is to use 2 to 3 ounces of smoked salmon, or other breakfast meats include sausage (turkey, pork, etc.), bacon, Canadian bacon, or leftovers. Breakfast meats tend to be lower in protein and higher in fat, which makes them more satisfying and more likely to hold off your hunger till lunch (or longer).

> VARIATIONS: Combine the smoked salmon with tomato slices, capers, and a dollop or two of cottage cheese. If you're not watching your weight, spread your favorite brand of cream cheese, ideally something organic or grass-fed if you can find it, on some sprouted grain or sourdough toast and plop the fish on top. It's a higher protein version of lox and bagel (lox would work too, but it tends to be so salty you can't eat very much, and most people end up eating too much bread with it).

> **Dr. Cate's Notes:** Most breakfast meats go really well with a small portion of breakfast porridge (see list of breakfast carbs in template). But if you have a habit of snacking between breakfast and lunch, be aware that the high-carb content of the porridge may make you hungry before lunch, so this may not be the best option for you.

Base: Eggs. Entire cookbooks have been written on great things you can cook with eggs. Enjoy them any way you like: hard-boiled, poached, scrambled, as an omelet, etc. Remember, the yolks are healthier the less you cook them.

> VARIATIONS: A classic breakfast combination is eggs with sautéed onions and green peppers. Kimchee goes surprisingly well with sunny-side-up eggs. And if you're not worried about your waistline, go ahead and enjoy them with a slice of sprouted grain or sourdough toast.

Base: Low Carb Custard/Pudding. This is a great make-ahead option for the week or for entertaining. Choose a low-sugar or sugar-free savory custard recipe.

PORTIONING AND CALORIES

The amounts indicated in the templates provide a guide to portioning that will help keep you in the 300- to 500-calorie range. Let's walk you through a few examples.

To keep calories between 300 and 500 for the Breakfast Parfait, use 6 ounces of yogurt, mixed with 1 to 2 ounces of your choice of nuts or fruit or both, keeping in mind that if you add fruit, then you need to cut back on nuts to keep the calories in range. Nuts are very rich foods, each ounce having between 150 and 200 calories.

The coffee/tea option. To keep calories closer to 300, use only 2 to 3 tablespoons of cream with 1–½ cups of whole milk. If you're okay going up to 500 calories, then use more cream, 4 to 5 tablespoons.

Let's do one more: the smoothie. Choose your base, either yogurt, cow, goat, almond, or soy milk. Add 6 ounces to the ice cubes. Choose two fats: for example, either cream and coconut oil or avocado and nut, or double up on any one. In the amounts indicated you'll get about 100 calories from each (one walnut half equals one nut, by the way), so if you're okay with a 400- to 500-calorie smoothie, you can choose 3 of these different sources of fats. Then toss in your non-starchy veggies. These are so low-calorie (for example, 4 cups of spinach has 27 calories), you don't generally have to bother counting. If you're in this for weight loss, caution on using fruit because it may make you hungry before it's time for lunch.

One of my favorites is "hot pumpkin," listed on my website, made with ricotta, egg, and ground flax.

> VARIATIONS: Add peanut butter instead of ground flax to the hot pumpkin recipe. Or add different spices. Savory custards can also be made with cheese combinations—semi-hard with hard—for example, a Gruyère, Comté, or Emmenthal with parmesan, which pair well with thyme.

Base: Crepes. If you have a hankering for pancakes, try making crepes instead. Just a little flour really holds the eggs, and if you fully melt the butter to sizzling, you can end up with an unbelievably scrumptious treat. Luke has made delicious crepes with as little as 1 teaspoon of flour per crepe. Non-wheat flours are less glutinous and require a little more volume.

> VARIATIONS: For fillings, we've used all kinds of sautéed vegetables or fruit. Instead of syrup, top with vanilla whipped cream, slightly sweetened, or, for savory crepes, use crème fraiche.

LUNCH

As with the breakfast template, start by looking over the options to find a "base" you like. If you don't have time to cook, the top five options don't require cooking at all.

Just as with breakfast, check the shopping guide for tips on finding the healthiest versions of all these ingredients. So under deli meat, for example, you'll see that I advise nitrate-free, and under bone stock I advise you to read the label to make sure it's not just reconstituted bullion (which won't offer you the benefits of real bone stock).

Let's go over each of the lunch choices in detail.

Base: Picnic Lunch. Whether you pack your lunch for work or school or eat at home, there's no reason your approach can't be a fun-filled finger-food adventure through your fridge and cupboards. Just grab an ounce or two of two to four of your favorite ready-to-eat nuts, cheeses, and/or kale chips.

> VARIATIONS: One of my favorite combinations is 1 ounce cheddar cheese, ½ ounce sprouted almonds, a half ounce of sprouted pumpkin seeds, and an ounce of kale chips. But I also enjoy Swiss cheese and provolone, cashews, macadamia nuts, and sprouted sunflower seeds. If you keep two to three kinds of hard cheeses, various nuts and seeds, and kale chips in your house, a picnic lunch is always an option for you.

> **Dr. Cate's Notes:** You can keep a few of your favorite stock items at work, if the fridge there is big enough, or toss them into a storage container on your way out the door in the morning. For a beverage? Bring a kombucha.

Base: Fermented Dairy.

> VARIATIONS: When choosing this option for lunch your carb count can be as high as 30 grams, which means you can enjoy more fruit or even a healthy (no-vegetable-oil) granola.

> **Dr. Cate's Notes:** There's no reason you can't have any breakfast idea for lunch or lunch idea for breakfast. These are all arbitrary tastes; traditional people had no such arbitrary distinctions outside of the aristocracy. The only thing to keep in mind is that if you have hunger or energy problems, keep your breakfast carb counts to under 10 grams.

LUNCH
Calories: 300–600
Protein 15–30 grams / Carbs 0–30 grams / Fat 20–40 grams

Base	Instructions (per serving)	Combinations and Variations
Picnic-Lunch	■ Nuts, seeds: 1–2 ounces ■ Cheese: 1–2 ounces ■ Veggies: 1/4–1 cup AND/OR ■ Veggie preserves: 1–2 ounces	■ Vary nuts and seeds: as with breakfast (see FERMENTED DAIRY PARFAIT) or spread nut butters on celery or ½ apple ■ Vary cheese: cheddar, manchego, Swiss, Al-penal, provolone ■ Vary veggies/preserves: fresh carrots, snap peas, dill pickle, sauerkraut, kimchee
Fermented Dairy Parfait	■ See instructions for breakfast	■ See instructions for breakfast, keeping in mind that total carbs at lunch can go up to 30 grams.
Seafood, fresh	■ Fresh fish: 3–6 ounces with optional ■ SPREAD/DIP (see below)	■ Vary fish: pickled herring, poke, sashimi, sushi (without the rice), shrimp (available precooked)
Deli Meat	■ Precooked/cured meat: 3–4 ounces wrapped in ■ Deli-sliced cheese: 1–2 slices ■ SPREAD/DIP: 1 tablespoon (optional, see below)	■ Vary meats: smoked turkey, roast chicken, sliced ham, roast beef ■ Vary cheese: cheddar or Swiss (for ham), provolone or Havarti (for roast turkey or beef) ■ Vary preparation: add mustard or SPREAD/DIP, wrap with lettuce/kale, micro-wave to melt cheese
Drop-In Soup	■ Bone stock: 1–2 cups ■ Precooked/cured meat: 3–4 ounces OR ■ Eggs: 2–3 dropped into *hot* broth	■ Vary veggies: try kale chips, other precooked (i.e. frozen peas) or dehydrat-ed vegetables ■ Vary crouton substitute: pumpkin seeds, crumbled pork rinds ■ Vary cheese: substitute half the meat or eggs for your favorite cheese
Seafood, canned	■ Tuna, salmon, sardines, mackerel, oysters, herring: 2–4 ounces ■ Cottage cheese: 2–3 ounces OR ■ Mayo: 2 tablespoons ■ Optional veggies/veggie preserves: ½–1 cup	■ Smoked sardines taste okay on sauer-kraut ■ Tuna salad: add chopped carrots, celery, cilantro, capers ■ Salmon or mackerel salad: see above ■ Smoked oysters straight from the can go well with mustard

Smoothie	▪ Follow instructions for Breakfast Smoothie ▪ Add your favorite protein powder, which must contain less than 7 grams of carbs per 20-gram protein portion	▪ See Breakfast Smoothie (above) ▪ Use different flavored protein powders as desired (protein powder not recommended more than 2 meals per week)
Meat over Salad	▪ Cooked meat: 3–4 ounces placed over: ▪ Vegetables: 3–4 cups ▪ Dressing: 2 tablespoons	▪ Instead of dressing use ½ an avocado and ½ an orange, sliced ▪ Add cheese/bacon/nuts and reduce dressing
Leftovers	Any leftover meal, 3-6 ounces	The sky's the limit!
Spread/Dip	▪ Cream cheese whipped with soy sauce in equal parts plus horseradish and/or sesame seeds ▪ Mayo + ketchup + relish combined in equal parts	▪ Mustard, mayo, mustard and mayo combined in equal parts ▪ Sour cream and any style plain yogurt combined in equal parts plus herbs ▪ Cream cheese whipped with milk in equal parts plus herbs

Base: Fresh Fish: Sushi (skip some or all of the rice), sashimi, poke, pickled herring, precooked shrimp.

VARIATIONS: Shrimp with salt and lemon, cocktail sauce, or Spread/ Dip (see recipe).

Dr. Cate's Notes: Poke is a raw fish salad made of chunks of ahi tuna or other fish mixed with salt and other seasonings. You can find good deals in Costco, especially on weekends. Herring in wine or sour cream sauce is basically Northern European sushi. It's extremely healthy, especially if you can find a brand that has less sugar than protein per serving. One of my favorite ways to enjoy herring in wine sauce is topped with additional sweet onion slices and drizzled with olive oil.

Canned or Marinated Fish. Salmon, mackerel, sardines, herring, tuna, clams, crabmeat, and oysters are all available preserved in cans, usually in water, oil, or sauces.

VARIATIONS: Smoked sardines taste pretty okay on a bed of sauerkraut (they taste better after a hard workout), and all the fish tastes passably good combined with cottage cheese. The smoked oysters taste quite good with mustard and, as long as you don't mind the oily mess on your fingers, a small slice of Swiss cheese. Open a can of tuna and add 2–3 tablespoons of mayo or, if you want to really ritz it up, then slice up half a stick each of carrot and celery, or add some capers.

> **Dr. Cate's Notes:** While not the ideal way to eat seafood, canned seafood is nevertheless going to provide excellent high-quality protein. Preserving in olive oil or mustard sauce that does not contain any vegetable oil helps to preserve the omega-3 fat. These make excellent travel foods and are also far better alternatives for after workouts than protein powders. One benefit of canned food is that you can eat the bones, which are extraordinary sources of bone-building minerals, so if the bone-in, skin-on versions don't weird you out, they are the healthier option. The skin will also convey some glycosaminoglycans (the same collagen supporting compounds you get from bone stock), and the fat under the skin is a rich source of omega-3.

Deli Meat. Nitrate-free deli meat is best. Use one third to half the package per meal and combine it with 1–2 slices of deli cheese. Each pack will stay good for about one week.

> VARIATIONS: Smoked ham, smoked turkey, roasted turkey, and roast beef pair well with sliced cheddar, provolone, or Swiss. You can melt them together in a toaster oven or microwave and turn it into a real high-class dish by adding a layer of Spread/Dip or wrapping around a dill pickle. If you aren't severely restricting carbs, you can melt the cheese on a 6-inch tortilla round (15 grams of carbohydrates), toss on 3–4 slices of smoked chicken or ham, and slather a bit of mustard and top with sauerkraut for a deconstructed corn dog—one of my personal favorites for Superbowl Sunday.

Drop-in Soup. This is extremely filling and easy. If you've made your own stock, it tends to taste better, but you can buy boxed pre-made chicken and beef stock. Heat 1–2 cups in the microwave or, when working with raw ingredients like eggs, on the stovetop.

> VARIATIONS: 1–2 eggs with ½–1 cup peas and 1–2 ounces mozzarel-

la cheese. Or if you're not in the mood for that much work, heat up in a bowl in the microwave for 1–2 minutes. Meanwhile, slice up 2–4 ounces of your favorite deli meats, grass-fed hotdogs, or other random scraps. Surprising tasty combinations are waiting to be discovered!

> **Dr. Cate's Notes:** One of my fastest favorites is to add 1 ounce of sprouted pumpkin seeds and 1 ounce of sliced Swiss cheese. This sounds really weird but it tastes great.

Smoothie. Using the same principles as for the breakfast smoothie, make yourself a smoothie for lunch. If your diet is generally low in protein, this is a good time to use a protein powder (I do not generally recommend protein powders at breakfast). While I definitely prefer real foods to protein powders for a number of reasons having to do with damage done during processing and the effects of essentially predigested protein in the body, some folks swear by their protein powders. Choose one without artificial flavors or sweeteners.

VARIATIONS: For protein, if you're not worried about salmonella—because you have a great source of healthy eggs and you follow a careful protocol—you can whip up a wonderful smoothie using 1.5–2 cups milk, a tiny splash of vanilla extract, a small banana, and an egg yolk (the whites contain anti-nutrients, so I'm not a big fan of eating raw egg whites). For variations on this or other smoothies try hazelnut or chocolate extract, orange zest, cinnamon, or other spices.

Leftovers. Done. That was easy. You can even have leftovers for breakfast; it's always a great time for leftovers.

Meat over salad. First, the meat. You can use the deli meats for this purpose, or you can buy ready-to-eat meats from the grocery store, or you can use meat you cooked yourself (see dinner template). Ready-to-eat meats from the deli section of the grocery store include smoked trout, salmon, and whitefish, or anything appealing from the deli section.

Now, the salad. Use 1–2 cups of greens and, if available, additional vegetables like sliced carrots, celery, and onions. For dressing you can splash on your favorite oil and vinegar combination or just use half an avocado and, if you're not over your carb budget, half an orange. Don't forget salt, or even soy sauce. Both can really help blend the flavors together.

VARIATIONS: Endless options using different kinds of salad greens, dressings, and toppings.

DINNER

This template relies on cooking more than the breakfast and lunch templates do. So the first thing to consider is whether or not you are able to implement all of these cooking techniques. Do you have the right pan to stir-fry? Do you have a good pot for slow cooking? Do you have a toaster oven? Are you comfortable with grilling?

The next consideration in terms of planning is not just what kind of meat but also the cut, because the cut must be amenable to the cooking method(s) that you're comfortable with. A rib-eye steak tastes better if it's been grilled or cooked in a toaster oven than if it has been slow cooked or stir fried, for example. Fish doesn't stir-fry well, but shrimp does. If you're comfortable with all these cooking methods, then your choices are much more varied. If you're not, then limit what you buy to ingredients that you feel confident about preparing in the time you have set aside to cook.

If this seems obvious, then that's good news. Planning is the hardest part, particularly for my patients who are dealing with being overweight. In fact, research suggests that obesity may be caused in part by difficulties with executive functioning[618, 619] (the medical term for planning), making it easier for advertisers and food manufacturers to manipulate you at mealtimes.

Let's go over each of the dinner choices in detail.

Stir Fried Meat, Fish, and/or Veggies. Chop everything to half-inch pieces. Ideally using a hot wok, first brown the meat in oil, remove, add more oil, then add veggies, add back meat, and then add sauces to taste. Veggies that taste good with just about any stir-fry variation (below) include onions, carrots, celery, green and colored peppers, water chestnuts, bamboo shoots, and spring peas.

> VARIATIONS: Some tasty combinations: beef and broccoli; shrimp, ginger, and coconut; and chicken, peanuts, and red bell peppers. Try also experimenting with combinations of soy, fish, or oyster sauces and Thai green and red chili pastes.

> **Dr. Cate's Notes:** When stir-frying, for best flavor, brown the meat slightly first, remove from wok, then cook the vegetables (thickest first), and then add the meat for a few more seconds to finish cooking. Choose skin-on chicken and brown the skin during the first step by cooking skin side down for a few moments.

	DINNER	
	Calories: 600–1,100	
	Protein 30–50 grams / Carbs 30–70 grams / Fat 40–50 grams	
Base	**Instructions (per serving)**	**Combinations and Variations**
Stir Fry	■ Protein: 4–8 ounces ■ Veggies: 2–4 cups ■ Nuts: 1–2 ounces ■ Oil: 2 tablespoons ■ Sauce, to taste	■ Meat (chicken, beef, turkey) sliced thin or shrimp ■ Veggies, sliced thin: onions, celery, broccoli, carrots, bok choy, snow peas, bell peppers ■ Oil: peanut, sesame, olive ■ Sauce: soy, fish, oyster, hoisin
Baked/ Roasted	■ Protein: 4–8 ounces ■ Veggies: 2–4 cups ■ Oil, to coat	■ Meat (poultry, steak, roast, fish) ■ Thick cut or starchy veggies (green beans, sliced squashes, onions, bell peppers, mushrooms) ■ Vary spices/herbs, premixed rubs
Stewed/Slow Cooked	■ Stew meat or braising meat: 4–8 ounces ■ Veggies for braising: 2–4 cups ■ Stock (chicken/beef) or canned tomatoes: 1–2 cups	■ Ask at the butcher counter for help choosing stew meats ■ Veggies for braising are typically tough: carrots, parsnips, kale, collards, asparagus, string beans, onions ■ Herbs for braising include bay leaves, rosemary, thyme, sage
Ground Meat	■ Ground meat: 4–8 ounces ■ Spices/herbs (see Resources) ■ SALAD or STEAMED VEGGIES	■ Meat (beef, bison, turkey, loose sausage) ■ Formed into patties, meatballs, meatloaf or cooked loose in pan with tomato and veggies for Italian style meat sauces, stroganoff, or sloppy joe
Egg-Based	■ Eggs: 2–4 with 2 ounces of optional other meats ■ Optional cheese: 1 ounce ■ Optional DINNER STARCH ■ SALAD, salsa, or STEAMED VEGGIES	■ If using other meats (sausage, ham, ground beef), use only 2 eggs ■ Cook all ingredients into frittata, crustless quiche, or omelet ■ Top a corn tortilla with a fried egg, sausage, salsa, and cheese
Casserole	■ Protein: 4–8 ounces ■ Veggies: 2–4 cups ■ Optional SPICE BLEND ■ Stock: 1–2 cups ■ Cheese, for topping	■ Brown ground meat/sausage and/or veggies first on stovetop for added flavor ■ Place casserole with stock to bake ■ Google "low-carb casserole" for more ideas

Base	Instructions (per serving)	Combinations and Variations
Meat over Salad	▪ Protein: 4–8 ounces ▪ Large DINNER SALAD	▪ Cooked poultry, salmon, trout, beef ▪ Place over salad, slice first if needed ▪ Dress with three of these: DRESSING (2 tablespoons); avocado (1/2); crumbled soft cheese (1½ ounces); mixed nuts (1 ounce); crumbled bacon (1/2 ounce); vegetable condiment like olives, capers (1 ounce)
Salad	▪ 4x4 rule ▪ DRESSING, 2 tablespoons	▪ 4 cups veggies (2–3 cups lettuce, 1–2 cups other mixed veggies) ▪ 4 colors of veggies (salad greens, carrots, red peppers, celery)
Dressing	▪ Oil to vinegar 3:1 ▪ Oil to vinegar to soy sauce 4:1:1	▪ Olive + balsamic + optional minced garlic ▪ Peanut + sesame + vinegar + soy sauce + optional minced ginger
Steamed Veggies	▪ Veggies: 2–4 cups ▪ Butter/sauce: 1–2 tablespoons	▪ Garlic butter: melt butter on stovetop, add crushed garlic, stir till aromatic ▪ Cheese sauce ▪ Other sauces: aioli, hollandaise, etc.
Dinner Starch	▪ 1–2 of the following:	▪ 6-inch corn masa tortilla (no vegetable oil) ▪ 1 slice sourdough or sprouted grain bread ▪ 1/2 cup beans (sprouted, if possible) ▪ 1/4 cup ancient grain/wild rice

Dinner Salad. 4–6 ounces of tender, easy-to-slice meat (or if a tougher meat then pre-slice the meat) tossed across the top of a large salad.

> VARIATIONS: Think Cobb or Caesar or chef salad. Or think in themes like Mediterranean (chicken or lamb with Greek olives, feta, sundried tomatoes, and pine nuts) or Asian (chicken or pork with bamboo shoots, palm hearts, garbanzos, and a soy-sauce dressing).

> SALAD TIPS: Use at least four different kinds of vegetables in all your salads as often as possible. For savory crunch, instead of croutons use nuts or even pork rinds. Try a variety of condiments like sun-dried tomatoes, capers, olives, and pepperoncini over mixed baby greens. We often use celery, carrots, sunflower seeds, and olives. Another popu-

lar combination is palm hearts, garbanzos, red bell peppers and thinly sliced shallots over butter lettuce drizzled with an Asian dressing. Always eat from a really big bowl so you can more easily poke around and try different flavor combinations without knocking things off your plate. We eat our salads from the large metal bowls many people use as serving bowls.

SALAD DRESSING: One of the easiest ways to add variety to your salads is by using different oils. I advise keeping two or three vinegars on hand (for example, balsamic, apple cider, and a flavored vinegar like fig) and several oils (we use olive, peanut, and sesame). So instead of needing to make a salad dressing you can simply splash these over your bowl using roughly three times as much oil as vinegar. For an Asian-flavored dressing, combine peanut, sesame, about half the normal amount of vinegar, and a splash of soy sauce roughly equal to the amount of vinegar used. If you want to get even fancier, add finely diced ginger to the Asian dressing or, if sticking with olive oil and vinegar, add finely diced garlic. And don't forget to sprinkle your salad with salt to taste.

Baked or Roasted Meat, Fish, and/or Veggies. The idea is to do the veggies and the protein at the same time. When cooking for just one or two people you may be able to fit everything into a toaster oven. Whenever possible, use fat and/or skin of the meat for additional flavor and moisture. So for example instead of boneless skinless chicken breast, use thighs and wings.

The veggies may need to go in twenty minutes or so ahead of the meat depending on how thick they are and what kind of meat you have. Try dusting a spice mix or rub over the oil-coated veggies before or midway through the roasting process (depending on temperature, the spices may burn).

VARIATIONS: Keeping a variety of spice mixes or rubs on hand can generate a lot more dishes using the same protein: BBQ ribs one night, Cajun ribs the next, Mexican chicken thighs one night, Indian chicken the next.

Stewed or Slow-Cooked Meat, Fish, and/or Veggies. If you have a slow cooker, you can fix it and forget it. If you have a Dutch oven, the advantage is that you can brown it right in the same pot before turning down the heat. Either way, these techniques are more ideal for the tougher cuts of beef, lamb, and free-range chicken. Vegetables that can tolerate all-day cooking tend to be higher in carb, like carrots and other root vegetables. So if you want to keep the carbs down, toss in more tender vegetables for the last thirty to sixty minutes of cooking.

VARIATIONS: One of my favorite resources for low-carb easy slow-cooker recipes is Dana Carpender.

> **Dr. Cate's Notes:** Sprouted beans make a great addition to many low-carb slow-cooked stews and crock pot recipes. The low-carb books are a great place to start because they generally won't be super starchy or overly sweet and then you can add small to moderate amounts of your own healthy carbs like sprouted beans, or wild rice, or root vegetables.

Steamed Eggs, Fish, and Veggies. Steam gently cooks food and, when properly done, is one of the healthiest methods of cooking. Brussels sprouts, asparagus, kale, broccoli, string beans, and cauliflower are some of our favorite veggies to steam.

VARIATIONS: The key to enjoying steamed veggies and fish is the sauce, and garlic butter with salt is our go-to fast solution for veggies. Béchamel sauce and hollandaise go great with a variety of fish and veggies, and cheese sauces work will with many veggies.

> **Dr. Cate's Notes:** Steaming is the easiest way to bring out the best in your veggies. The only tricky part is timing it right. Once you can poke a fork through, they're done. But the real secret to making them delicious is liberal use of garlic butter. We use about 4 tablespoons of butter and two cloves of garlic for the two of us over two to slow down, drink water, and give three cups of steamed vegetables each. Since fat is very calorie dense, it's important to slow down, drink water, and give yourself time to feel full.

Ground Meat. Buffalo and grass-fed beef are cost-effective ways to get high-quality red meats, but any ground meat (chicken, turkey, pork) can make for a quick and tasty meal.

VARIATIONS: Everything from stovetop goulash and burgers to meatballs to meatloaf can be made more varied using ready-made spice mixes. And you can sneak vegetables into the goulash and meatloaf really easily. One of my favorites is just combining a load of butter-fried mushrooms with an equal volume of ground beef. Pork sausage also blends well with ground beef.

> **Dr. Cate's Notes:** One of our favorite ways to use ground beef is homemade grass-fed ground beef pasta sauce, without the pasta, fortified with added beef stock. Luke makes his sauce using grass-fed ground beef and pork sausage, onions, green peppers, diced canned tomatoes, mushrooms, zucchini if in season, garlic, and Italian herbs.

Eggs. Eggs go well with almost any meat, vegetable, or cheese. You can combine all three into a single one-dish meal with endless possibilities.

VARIATIONS: Aside from the basic omelet and scrambled, there are quiches, frittatas, and soufflés. These can include a good deal of vegetables as well, making for a potential one-pot meal.

> **Dr. Cate's Notes:** One of our favorite so-easy, fast meals is a huge, colorful salad and three fried eggs (per serving) with runny yolks over a 6-inch corn-masa tortilla with 2 ounces of cheddar melted over the top.

Casserole. You can make any casserole using recipes you already have by reducing (by half or more) or eliminating whatever starch (pasta, potatoes, etc.) it calls for and increasing the protein or vegetable content. For example, if you like mac and cheese, turn it into a tetrazzini by cutting the noodles you add in half and adding tuna and finely diced vegetables like red peppers, celery, and onions.

VARIATIONS: Some classic casseroles are tettrazinis and lasagnas. Layering makes the presentation and seems to help the flavors meld nicely. To make them more nutritious, as with the example above, just cut back on the noodles and pump up the veggies and other ingredients.

> **Dr. Cate's Notes:** To make casseroles more flavorful you can brown the protein and/or sauté the vegetables on the stove top first (if you have extra time). The key to success with any casserole is making sure the vegetables are sliced thin enough to cook through so they're done at the same time as the meat. You can mix everything together with tomato sauce, stock, or a very soft cheese, like ri-

cotta. If you want to step it up, use a sauce like Béchamel (the creamy sauce used to make mac and cheese), or any cream-based sauce or aioli.

DETOX YOUR KITCHEN

If you haven't already done so, now's the time to go through everything in your kitchen and to throw away anything that contains vegetable oil as one of the top six ingredients. Go ahead. It will feel good. Get rid of all that junk that's been making you unhealthy. (One exception may need to be mayo, at least until you get the knack of making it yourself. Or buy the one national brand that does not use toxic oils, Primal Kitchen, which you can order online.)

Once you've made space in your kitchen, you're ready to go shopping.

PLANNING YOUR WEEK: STOCKING STAPLES AND CHOOSING FRESH FOODS

I've provided a list of staples that you can review to select which ones you think you'll eat. Once you establish your new routines and learn which ones

WHAT ABOUT DESSERT?

It's a slippery slope for some people, and if you have to get a sweet tooth under control it's best to try with no dessert at all for at least the first six months. Once your sweet tooth is tamed, you can better control the portion sizes, and a small taste of dark chocolate or a few ounces of a dessert wine can be a nice way to finish off the night. If you still feel hungry, instead of more food, try drinking a big glass of water and then find some excuse to bend over—put a few dishes away, sweep the floor, or take off your shoes. Bending forward can activate the stretch receptors, jolting a sluggish stomach to action and convincing it to send an overdue "I'm full!" message to your brain.

you use most consistently, then just as with everyday household supplies like soap and paper towels, you'll want to check on your stocks of these before each shopping trip.

As opposed to staples, which keep for extended periods so you can keep all your favorites on hand, you can only use so many fresh foods each week. This is why it's a good idea, at least initially, to write out your meals for the week before you go shopping. (Eventually you will get expert enough to adjust your plans based on what's fresh and available at your local grocer or butcher, but this may not be possible at the beginning.) I strongly recommend that you plan to shop one to two days a week, and not necessarily all at the same store. Shopping less often may mean you don't get enough fresh foods, and shopping more often may indicate you're not planning ahead effectively and can waste valuable time.

Now let's tally how much you'll need to buy to stock up for a week. While this may seem like a pretty basic exercise, if you've never done it before, it's helpful to have someone walk you through it the first time.

Planning Your Breakfast for the Week

Choose one or two "base" choices to use for the week that you plan to vary. Let's say you like the fermented dairy and the egg options, and will do yogurt for the weekdays and eggs on weekends. Since both of these are perishable, they're not staples, and you'll want to match how much you buy with how much you think you'll eat. To figure out what you need to buy, first figure out how many people are on board with the plan, then do the math using the serving sizes as a rough guide. In this case, each serving calls for roughly 6 ounces of dairy and 2–3 eggs. So if you've got a family of four more or less adult eaters, then start out with 6 x 5 x 4 = 120 ounces of yogurt, which means buying 4 quart-sized tubs of yogurt, and 3 x 2 x 4 = 24 eggs, which means buying 2 dozen eggs. If it's just you, then a dozen eggs and a single quart will be plenty and you'll have enough for the same thing a few days next week.

Now decide what variations you'd like to try.

Let's review the Yogurt Parfait first. Nuts and seeds can be bought in bulk whereas you can get smaller amounts than what typically comes in packages, but that's only useful if you're on a tight budget and the bulk is kept very fresh. Most people buy 6 to 16 ounces of each and keep five or six varieties on hand. (We use pistachios, brazil nuts, almonds, walnuts, cashews, sesame seeds, and pumpkin seeds most often.) If you want to add some fresh fruit on the Yogurt Parfait, be sure not to get too much because you're only using a small quantity per serving. Dried fruits, on the other hand, keep much longer but are very potent sugar delivery vehicles.

Next, the weekend eggs. In this example we'll imagine everyone eats the same meal, and you're starting with a simple omelet with cheddar and sautéed mushrooms and green bell pepper. A pound or two of cheddar (the common, economical amounts) will be way more than you need for this breakfast, but cheese keeps about a month and, as long as plenty of people like it, you'll find other uses. An 8-ounce pack of mushrooms will likely leave you with extra as well, but that's okay if everyone likes them raw because you can just throw the extra on a salad. One or two bell peppers should be enough but if you get extra you can toss them on the salads, too. Don't forget to consider the cooking fat. We use butter and bacon grease most often for our eggs.

So far your shopping list looks like this:

- Yogurt, plain whole milk: 4 quarts
- Eggs: 2 dozen
- Cheddar cheese: 2 pounds
- Almonds: 8 ounces
- Walnuts: 8 ounces
- Pistachios: 1 pound sack (from Costco)
- Sprouted pumpkin seeds: 12 ounces (available online)
- Brazil nuts: 6 ounces, from the bulk section at the market
- Butter: 1 pound (Kerrygold brand or other grass-fed variety)
- Dried goji berries: 2 ounces (from the bulk section)

Planning Your Lunch for the Week

Just as with breakfast, figure out how many people are on the plan and do the math based on serving sizes. We'll stick with the family of four for the rest of this exercise.

Let's say you want to do the deli slices three days this week, for a total of 12 servings, each 3–4 ounces: that's 36–48 ounces. If you buy six 8-ounce packs, you're set. (The packages last only about a week, so you have to use them up.) Now the cheese. Most pre-sliced cheeses weigh an ounce, and packs have 8 slices. Buying three packs gets you 24 slices, which is enough for each person to have two slices per serving. If a zero-carb lunch seems lacking and you want to pack some fruit or carrot sticks or a dill pickle or crackers for your kids to enjoy as well, then toss those in too. Just make sure the crackers are vegetable-oil-free.

Now let's say you want to do the Drop-in Soup for the other four lunches this week, amounting to 16 servings. Make sure to have 2–4 ounces of meat per serving, so your total for this week will need to be 1 to 2 pounds (any extra deli meat can be used here, too). Hotdogs or chicken tenders, available precooked and frozen, also work really well and come in packages of

1-pound packs. So does precooked sausage.

Along with the meat, your soup is going to contain an ounce or so of Swiss or cheddar cheese, a handful of kale chips, and your adventurous family will try the soup with about an ounce of sprouted pumpkin seeds instead of croutons. So you'll need a half pound of each cheese, 4 or 5 sacks of kale chips, and a pound of pumpkin seeds.

You can heat the soup in the microwave if one is available, but if not, or you want to have it already hot, heat up the broth and meat together at home and pour into a thermos. Be sure to include a bowl to pour it all into so they can add the toppings (seeds, chips, and little rectangles of sliced cheese) last, keeping the crunchy things crunchy and preventing the cheese from getting too glommy.

For stock, use either homemade or a good quality bone-stock like Pacific Organic (see preferred brands on page 437), which comes in 32-ounce packages. Each serving will use 8 ounces, so you'll want 4 boxes for the week. Since homemade stock keeps for months in the freezer and the unopened boxes keep for months, you should always have some on hand so that, in the future, if you like this option then all you have to think about adding to your list for the week are the foods you want to "drop in."

For lunches, add the following items to your shopping list:

- Boxed chicken stock: at least four 32-ounce boxes
- Hotdogs: preferably 100 percent grass-fed, 1 pound
- Chicken tenders: preferably organic—see recommended brands in the Resources section at the back of this book.
- Swiss cheese: 1 pound
- Kale chips: five 2.2-ounce packages
- Deli-sliced roast beef: two 8-ounce packages
- Deli-sliced smoked chicken: two 8-ounce packages
- Deli-sliced provolone: three 8-ounce packages
- Water crackers (or artisanal crackers without vegetable oil): one package
- Carrots: 5-pound bag
- Dill pickles: one 32-ounce bottle (fermented)

Planning Your Dinners for the Week

Meat (by which I mean any animal product, including fish and seafoods, poultry, pork, beef, lamb, etc.) is often your most expensive food investment, particularly when it's well-sourced. Which makes being able to buy what's on sale especially important. Fortunately, with many of the dinner templates, you can use multiple different protein options so you're free to improvise in the

Sample Meal Plan				
	Breakfast	Lunch	Dinner	Dessert
Monday	Yogurt Parfait with slivered almonds, cacao nibs, coconut flakes, and dried goji berries	Drop-in-Soup (see recipe) with smoked turkey breast, kale chips, and sprouted pumpkin seeds	Stir-fried skin-on chicken breast with onions, carrots, celery, green pepper, peanuts, peanut and sesame oils, soy sauce, oyster sauce, and fish sauce	1 ounce dark chocolate with espresso beans and 1 ounce sprouted salted almonds
Tuesday	Coffee with milk and cream	Cottage cheese parfait with pistachios, macadamia nuts, and finely diced dried ginger	Fried eggs over cheddar melted on a 6-inch corn tortilla topped with fresh salsa; salad of spring greens, green olives, sunflower seeds, carrots, and celery	2 ounces Chardonnay with 4–6 ounces GT Dave Synergy brand kombucha, original flavor
Wednesday	Pan-fried breakfast sausage with sautéed mushrooms	Smoked turkey breast rolled together with provolone cheese, fermented dill pickle	Grass-fed beef hamburger with minced, roasted (in the toaster oven) onion, mustard, and ketchup added to the beef before cooking, topped with provolone cheese and sliced tomatoes; frozen green peas stir-fried in butter	1 ounce dark chocolate with almonds and sea salt, and 1 ounce salted, roasted Macadamia nuts
Thursday	Two hard-boiled eggs, sliced, with salt and pepper, with kimchee	Drop-in Soup with chicken stock, sprouted pumpkin seeds, scissor-cut smoked turkey breast, and 2 organic ricotta-spinach ravioli (store bought)	Homemade grass-fed ground beef pasta sauce (without the pasta!), with added beef stock; salad with fresh baby greens, thin-sliced purple onion, thin-sliced red bell pepper, Kalamata olives, carrots, celery, and feta cheese with Italian dressing (see recipe)	2 ounces Chardonnay with 4 ounces GT Dave Synergy brand kombucha, Trilogy flavor, and 3 Brazil nuts

	Breakfast	Lunch	Dinner	Dessert
Friday	2 eggs steamed in ramekins with finely diced sun-dried tomato and feta cheese	Duck liver pate (store bought) on vegetable-oil-free rye and raisin crackers with mustard and a thin slice of Swiss cheese	Chicken vegetable soup; salad with butter lettuce, sliced green cabbage, avocado, pistachio nuts, olive oil and balsamic dressing and sprinkled with fresh ground parmesan cheese	Cottage cheese, with cherry jelly, vanilla extract, pistachio nuts
Saturday	Herbed tea with milk and cream	Sardines and (fermented) sauerkraut	Sprouted split pea, vegetable, tongue, and bacon soup; salad of shredded carrots, raisins, lemon juice, dried orange zest, salt	Hot pumpkin low-carb "cereal"
Sunday	Steel-cut oatmeal (1/4 cup dry) soaked overnight in water with a spoonful of yogurt, warmed in the morning stirring in milk (or yogurt), topped with nuts, ground flax seed, spices, and butter	Grass-fed beef hotdogs with finely diced purple onions squeezed dry (in a paper towel) with Kalamata olive hummus (make your own or use a store-bought brand made with olive oil)	Salmon with mustard caper dill sauce; steamed green beans with kalamata olives, capers, lemon juice, and salt	Vanilla custard (low sugar) sprinkled with lemon zest and spices (we use Penzy's brand "cake" spice mix)

store as long as you know, walking into the store, how much you need to buy for the week.

It's all about the amounts. When it comes to meats, you'll want between 4 and 8 ounces per person for each dinner. So if there are four of you, then for a week's worth of dinners you'll need 7 to 14 total pounds of meats for the entire week.

The same math applies for the vegetables. Usually Luke and I have really big salads four days per week and the other days we make steamed veggies. On days when the main dish includes a lot of veggies, we have smaller side dishes of salad or veggies, or none.

Let's say you plan on having an egg-sausage scramble with salsa over corn tortilla plus salads for two days (3 eggs x 4 people x 2 days = 2 dozen), roast turkey thighs with roast veggies for one day, stir-fry chicken with lots of veggies for two days, and stewed meat sauce with steamed veggies for two days.

Add these dinner-recipe items to your shopping list:

- Cashews (for stir fry): 6 ounces
- Soy sauce (for stir fry): 1 large bottle
- Peanut oil (for stir fry): 1 large bottle
- Sesame oil, toasted (for stir fry): 1 bottle
- Corn tortillas: two 1-pound packages
- Oyster sauce (for stir fry): 1 bottle
- Herbs and spices for roasting: to taste
- Salad greens: two 1-pound tubs
- Carrots (for salads and roasting): already included in lunch list
- Celery (for stir fry, meat sauce, and salads): 1 bunch
- Onions (for stir fry, meat sauce, salsa, and salads): 1 large bag (these keep well)
- Green onions (for salsa): 1 bunch
- Cilantro (for salsa): 1 bunch
- Garlic (for salsa, meat sauce, and stir fry): 1 sack of multiple bulbs (these keep well)
- Cheddar cheese (for sausage scramble): already included in breakfast list
- Canned tomatoes (for salsa and meat sauce): eight 12-ounce cans (these keep well)
- String beans (for roasting): 2 pounds
- Broccoli (for steaming): 2 pounds
- Green bell peppers: (for stir fry): 4
- Red bell peppers (for stir fry and salad): 2
- Frozen peas (for steaming): 2 pounds
- Winter squash (for roasting): 1 pound
- Butter (for basting turkey and for steamed veggies): already included in breakfast list
- Olive oil (for salad dressing and meat sauce): 1 large bottle
- Balsamic vinegar (for salad dressing): 1 large bottle
- Mushrooms (for meat sauce and salads): 2 pounds
- Eggs: 2 dozen (additional)
- Pork sausage: 1 pound
- Ground beef: 4 pounds
- Turkey thighs (one feeds about two people): 2 thighs
- Chickens, whole: 2

GO SHOPPING!

This part will take some practice. And time, to get acquainted with new stores, butchers, farmers markets, or other purveyors of real food that may be available in your area and, importantly, convenient enough not to require you to turn your life upside-down. Buying better quality animal products, in particular, may take some legwork to identify what stores carry, for example, grass-fed dairy. Still, I'm rooting for you and I know you'll get the hang of it.

The shopping guide provides tips on buying the healthiest versions of all these ingredients. (See also the list of recommended brands on page 437.) So under yogurt, for example, you'll see the recommended brands, and under nuts and seeds you'll see my tips on avoiding toxic oils.

You will probably end up needing to shop at stores you've never been to before. That can be stressful, but it might help to think of it as a new adventure. The first time you do this, you'll probably be buying a bunch of staple items. You may also need to read lots of labels. So you want to give yourself plenty of time.

Some of your shopping may be online, especially if you live in a rural area.

You can use online services to order sprouted nuts and seeds, quality oil and vinegar in bulk, lots of seafood, kale chips, herbs and spices, a starter culture, and even fermented veggies.

If you only shop once a week, you may want to freeze the meat you'll use toward the end of the week, or simply plan on using the most perishable meats earlier in the week.

SHOPPING RULES FOR FINDING QUALITY FOOD

1. **Natural:** If something couldn't have existed 200 years ago, skip it.
2. **Variable:** If all units (chickens, eggs, tomatoes, etc.) are identical in size and shape, that's a bad sign.
3. **Flavorful:** Intense flavor indicates nutrient density, but not when it comes from ingredients like sugar, MSG, or hydrolyzed protein.
4. **Seasonal:** Avoid foods that are frozen or canned.
5. **Buy local:** Packages should identify the source of the item.

FOLLOW YOUR PLAN

If I've done my job right, now the rest is easy. *Bon appetit!*

SUPPLEMENTATION

You may wonder why you have to take supplements if you're following a balanced, traditional eating plan. There are two reasons: (1) because most of us don't exercise all that much, we don't get to eat as much food as our more active ancestors, offering us fewer opportunities to get a full complement of vitamins and minerals from our diets; and (2) because soils in many areas have been depleted of minerals. Keep in mind that plants need soil minerals in order to make vitamins. So that means today's food is a relatively poorer source of not just those missing minerals but all the nutrients the plant would make were it supplied with more optimal nutrition.

On the other hand, I don't recommend supplementing with nutrients other than vitamins and minerals (for example, lecithin, creatine, or any of the other thousands of products out there) without a specific reason and careful analysis of your current diet.

What I recommend for everyone:

- Vitamin D 2-4000 IU. I recommend 4,000 international units daily unless you get a lot of sun, in which case 2,000 IU is enough.
- Magnesium oxide, 250 milligrams.
- Zinc gluconate, 15 milligrams. By the way, zinc deficiencies have been shown to negatively impact appetite, so if you're dealing with picky eaters, supplementing may help.
- A standard multivitamin with 100 percent of the RDA of vitamins (Mason One-A-Day is the only brand currently nationally available that meets this criteria).

Magnesium and zinc come in many formulations, and folks will tell you that you need a different formulation that's more bioavailable than what I've listed here. However, I've selected these for the greatest bioavailability per volume ratio. For example, the evidence suggests there's maybe a 10 percent difference between the most bioavailable form of magnesium and the least, but the most bioavailable forms are up to five times larger. Massive size makes them difficult to swallow and some are even too large to fit into a single capsule, so you have to take several throughout the day.

In my accounting, that's not worth the trouble.

What I recommend for people who don't eat red meat or liver:

■ Desiccated liver pills

What I recommend for people who don't do dairy or bone-in fish or frequent bone stock:

■ Calcium citrate, 250-milligram tablets, twice per day, divided at different meals. I don't recommend coral calcium, as it's not a sustainable source.

If you can't get grass-fed dairy fat (from cheese, butter, or cream, for example) then I also recommend:

■ Vitamin K2, 1.5 milligrams per day. If you can't find one that small, then do the math and figure out how often to take it for an equivalent daily dose. (It's fat soluble, and your body can store fat-soluble vitamins more effciently than water soluble vitamins.)

■ Omega-3. My preferred method of omega-3 supplementation is with flax seeds that you grind fresh before using. You can stir 1–2 tablespoons into hot water and drink like a tea, or plop on top of your yogurt, or anywhere else they taste good. Getting ½ to 1 tablespoon per day with this method will provide 4,000–8,000 milligrams of omega-3 each week, which is plenty. I don't recommend supplementing with encapsulated fish or liver oils unless they're of exceptional freshness and quality.

What I recommend for vegetarians:

■ Iron, 325 milligrams every other day

For vegans, non-dairy consumers, and for vegetarians, add

■ Iodine, from dulse seaweed, one ounce per week

WEEKLY SHOPPING PLANNER
(Only buy items you know someone will eat, don't buy stuff nobody likes.)

PERISHABLE VEGGIES: EAT WITHIN 7 DAYS
(Choose 4 to 6 of the following, most perishable on top.)

Salad tub: 8–16 ounce tub (16 ounces will make 4–6 servings)

Romaine, red leaf, or butter lettuce: 2–3 heads, each head makes two very large salads

Fresh herbs: 1–2 of the following: basil, chives, cilantro, green onion, parsley, tarragon

Tops: Beet greens, radish greens: 1 bunch makes 2 servings

Spinach tub: 8–16 ounces (cooked, 16 ounces will make 2 servings: as salad will make 4-6 servings)

Avocado

Tomato

Bell peppers: 1–2 green / yellow / red

Asparagus: 1 bunch makes 2–3 servings

Green beens: 1 pound makes 2–3 servings

Swiss chard or Kale: 1 bunch; each bunch makes 2 good size servings

Broccoli: 1 bunch, makes 2–3 servings

Mushrooms: 1–2 pints for sautéeing and/or meat sauces

Radish: 1 bunch for 4 salads

Zucchini, Spaghetti and Summer Squashes

PERISHABLE MEATS:
BUY A TOTAL OF 3–4 POUNDS/WEEK PER PERSON
(Choose 2 to 3 of the following.)
(double poundage for cuts that include bone)

Chicken: i.e. breast, fingers (unbreaded) wings, thighs, drumsticks, whole, livers, ground meat

Pork: i.e. loin, chops, ribs, sausage, bacon, ground meat

Beef: i.e. steaks, ground, chuck, ribs, oxtail, liver

Turkey: i.e. breast, thighs, drumsticks, groun sausage, whole with giblets

Lamb: i.e. chops, ribs, ground liver, kidneys

Buffalo: i.e. ground

Fish: i.e. salmon, cod, tilapia, ahi, mahi mahi, herring

Shellfish: i.e. shrimp, oysters, scallops, lobster, crab

Eggs: 1/2 dozen per person

Storage and timing of fresh meats
Freeze half of what you buy. If you shop on Saturday, thaw out second half on Tuesday (day 3 of 7-day cycle)
Fish Preserves
Pickled herring, smoked trout, or salmon, lox

DAIRY STAPLES
Most perishable on top

Milk: 1–2 pints per person for coffee/tea, smoothies
Buttermilk: small amount only, for dressing
Dairy fats: cream, cream cheese, sour cream
Cottage cheese: 2–4 percent dairy fat, 1–2 tubs per person
Yogurt: 1 quart whole milk plain, Greek, or regular style
Hard cheese: 2–3 pounds of your favorites at any given time: cheddar, colby, farmers, gruyere, manchego, Monterey jack, mozzarella, muenster, provolone, Swiss. Note: parmesan and romano will keep for months.

VEGGIE STAPLES AND PRESERVES

Store 4–6 weeks	Store for months
Beets	Artichoke hearts
Cabbage (green/red)	Capers
Carrots	Frozen green beans
Celery	Frozen lima beans
Garlic	Frozen spinach
Ginger root	Giardiniera (Mezzetta brand)
Jicama	Horseradish
Kimchee (fermented)	Kale chips
Onions	Olives (green, black, Greek)
Pickles (fermented)	Mixed bean salad (jarred)
Shallots	Pepperoncini
Sauerkraut (fermented)	Roasted red peppers
Turmeric root	Salsa (green, red)
Turnips	Sun-dried tomatoes

EXTENDED SHELF-LIFE STAPLES
**(Always have these on hand. Don't buy stuff you don't eat;
do buy more of the stuff you eat more often.)**

FATS / OILS

Butter (or ghee, okay to freeze)	Peanut oil
Coconut oil and cream	Toasted sesame oil
Olive oil	Avocado oil

PROTEIN STAPLES

Canned salmon (bone-in is best)	Canned tuna (in water or olive oil)
Chicken and beef stock (i.e., Kirkland Organic, Pacific Organic)	Sardines (in olive oil; bone-in is best; avoid those containing vegetable oils)
Oysters (in olive oil)	Canned chicken
Tofu (fermented is best)	Canned tuna
Anchovies	Canned mackerel
Kippered herring	Beef jerky

NUTS / SEEDS / BEANS

Nuts (6 to 16 ounces of at least three of your favorites): almonds, Brazil nuts, cashews, macadamia nuts, pecans, walnuts. Store in fridge for better flavor. Sprouted nuts or raw nuts are better than roasted. Avoid those in vegetable oils. Nuts roasted in peanut oil or coconut oil are okay.

Seeds (2 to 16 ounces of each): sunflower, pumpkin, sesame, chia, poppy.
Sprouted or raw are better than roasted. Avoid those roasted in vegetable oils. Sprouted sunflower and pumpkin seed brands include Go Raw, available at Costco or health food stores, and Living Intentions, available at health food stores.

Canned or dried beans, i.e., pinto, black, kidney, garbanzo, your favorites; dried are recommended over canned as they can be sprouted.

VINEGARS / SAUCES / CONDIMENTS

Balsamic or flavored vinegar (i.e., cherry, red wine, infusions)

White vinegar (i.e., apple cider, rice vinegar)

Soy sauce, naturally brewed (i.e., Kikkoman or Yamase)

Tabasco and/or hot chili sauces

Worchestershire sauce

Ketchup (Trader Joe's has lowest sugar content)

Mustard (yellow and/or brown and/or Dijon)

Mayo (toxic oil–free brand: Primal Kitchen, available online)

DRIED HERBS AND SPICES

Allspice, basil, cinnamon, chile flakes, coriander, cumin, dried orange peel, nutmeg, powder, oregano, paprika, parsley, pepper, rosemary, salt (see Himalayan), thyme
Handy spice blends: barbeque, buttermilk-ranch dressing, cajun, chile powders, curries, Italian, Mexican/taco

STARCHY STAPLE FOODS

Sprouted grain bread (i.e., Ezekiel brand) or dense rye (keep breads in freezer/fridge)
Corn masa tortillas (6-inch, store in freezer/fridge)
Potatoes (white or sweet)
Crackers (i.e., water crackers or flax crackers; avoid those with hydrogenated oil or vegetable oils)

EXOTICS

Seaweeds: dulse, wakame
Pastes: miso, shrimp paste, Thai chili pastes (red, green)
Sauces: fish, hoisen, oyster

PANTRY STAPLES

Canned tomatoes (diced and tomato paste)
Jams and preserves (choose brands and flavors with less than 9 grams of sugar per tablespoon)
Extracts, all natural (i.e., vanilla, chocolate, almond)
Honey (raw is best, if available)
Agave nectar
White granulated and brown sugars
Flours (white wheat flour stores longer than whole wheat flour, which can be refrigerated to extend shelf life)

BEVERAGES / TREATS / DESSERTS

Coffee and teas, dried herbs for brewing (i.e, peppermint, chamomile, lemon balm)
Wine and spirits (i.e., red and white wines, tequila, vodka, bourbon, brandy, whiskey)
Kombucha (GT Dave Synergy brand is low in sugar)
Chocolate (70 percent cocoa or more; avoid vegetable oils; cocoa butter is preferred)
Dried fruits, candied nuts, herbed coconut flakes (unsweetened)
Cacao nibs

EATING WELL WHILE TRAVELING AND DINING OUT

Tips for Dining Out

No matter if you're at a five-star restaurant or McDonald's, the management will pinch pennies by serving you vegetable oils instead of natural fats. If you're not vigilant, you can end up eating a lot of toxic oils that can—especially if you've been avoiding them for a while—give you heartburn and make you feel noticeably worse the next day. This occurs partly because your body is no longer geared up to defend itself against them and partly because you'll be feeling so much better that the oil's toxic effects will be that much more noticeable.

The two biggest sources of toxic fats in a restaurant will be the fried foods and the salad dressings. Avoiding fried foods (especially deep fried) and asking your server for olive oil and vinegar as a dressing will cut your exposure to these toxic fats by more than half.

If you are at a sit-down (as opposed to fast food) restaurant, there's a good chance that you can work with the server to help you get better quality fats. Be sure to tell your server that you are okay with butter, cream, and olive oil, but that you need her help to identify which items can be made using those ingredients. Encourage her to take her time and ask the chef for help. This exercise in taking control of your nutrition can sometimes make you feel like you're being a pain in the neck. Just remember to be patient with your wait staff. Whether they appreciate it or not, you are educating the server and the chef, and some day they may elect to look into why vegetable oils are unhealthy and improve their own health.

Tips for Travel

Whenever possible, I bring frozen milk and cream in my check-in luggage. I also scope out hotels that are located near Whole Foods stores or other grocery stores.

Here are a few of my favorite travel meals and survival strategies:

- An 8-ounce tub of salad greens with ½ an orange, ½ an avocado, and 6 to 8 ounces smoked fish
- Sourdough bread with fresh tomato and Brie or Manchego cheese
- If I'm at a nice hotel with a chef who makes his or her own bone stock (most of the high-end hotel chefs do), I'll order the soup.
- If I'm at a function where the food is not that good, I'll choose eggs or fish or whatever dish looks least oily, along with salad greens topped with the meat and some fruit or other fresh veggies (no dressing). I skip the

dessert and any fried foods and don't load up on the free bread—bypass it altogether if they don't serve it with real butter. When served a sandwich, I skip the bread and, when possible, eat the filling with a knife and fork so that hardly anyone notices what's going on. If you exercise a lot and the bread is of high quality, you can go with one slice or even eat the sandwich as served.

- Emergency travel foods I'll pack include mostly canned fish, like tuna in olive oil, canned sardines with a pack of mustard (from one of the fast food vendors in the airport), canned smoked oysters, kale chips, nuts, cheese, chocolate, peeled carrots, and dill pickles.
- Airports at any midsize or larger city usually offer one or more of the following: sushi, hard-boiled eggs, Cobb salad (skip their dressing). Anything oil-free and low-carb will do.

KIDS AND SPORTS

These days, it seems like sporting events and other activities are an excuse to refuel kids with junk food. If your kids are on board enough that they're not going to insist on partaking, and you want to give them something as a snack, you have options. Here are snacks from the PRO Nutrition Program we designed for the L.A. Lakers:

- A charcuterie tray with cheese slices, pepperoni, other cured meats, and light hors d'oeuvres
- Kale chips (many brands and flavors are available)
- Nuts, either dry-roasted or roasted in peanut or coconut oil
- Sprouted nuts and seeds
- Olives
- Dill pickles

BABY FORMULA

A baby's complexion often reveals telltale bumps or rashes, indicating they're on commercial formula, the first two ingredients of which are vegetable oils and sugars. The vegetable oils will concentrate in a baby's fat, so that a baby's chubby cheeks are going to be loaded with it. The sugar has detrimental effects on the immune system that can lead to auto-immune skin rashes. What's more, the formula is produced using aluminum equipment, and many formula products exceed the aluminum limit set by the European Food Safety Authority (1 milligram/kilogram/bodyweight per week).[620] This limit has been imposed based on research that shows that above this threshold the aluminum can cause neurologic damage. Cow's milk formulas fared slightly better than soy, at 0.9 versus 1.1 mg/kilogram/bodyweight per week of use. Compare these to breast milk, which conveys an average of less than 0.07 mg/killogram/body weight per week.[621] But even if you can't breastfeed, you don't have to use a commercial infant formula. You have another choice—homemade.

While a complete set of instructions is beyond the scope of this chapter, I want to provide you with at least some resources for making a natural product that will be leaps and bounds more capable of promoting your baby's optimal growth than commercial formula.

Two of my favorites are:

■ www.wellnessmama.com/53999/organic-baby-formula-options/
■ www. thehealthyhomeeconomist.com/video-homemade-milk-based-baby-formula/

TODDLERS: TRANSITIONING FROM MILK TO MEALS

When your baby is ready to transition to real food, cereal is quite possibly the last thing I would recommend. Unfortunately, that's exactly what I was trained to tell mothers, and what many influential pediatricians still advise.[622] Other countries are more forward thinking, however, and in 2012 Canada changed its recommendations to include egg yolks and pureed meats among baby's first foods.[623] My sister weaned her first baby on Brie cheese, butter, and chicken liver pate, along with soft-boiled egg yolks and pureed cow's tongue soup—cow's tongue was cheaper than other cuts of meat. As soon as her daughter was ready for solids, that's when she added more plants, in the form of, among other things, sauerkraut and dulse seaweed. Fruits were one of the last foods she introduced, and now, at age four, the child still has not had instant cereals.

For more specifics on what to offer kids when, you can refer to the websites above. You can also use information from any of the hundreds of parenting websites now available. However when referring to a mainstream website, you'll need to focus more on the texture and consistency rather than the recommendations for ingredients. For example, instead of starting rice- or noodle-based soups, start with a more nutritious beef and bean stew. Or instead of finger foods like yogurt melts or Cheerios, go for sausage balls or chunks of cheese.

CHILDREN: CHANGING HABITS

As restrictive eating habits are growing more common and food allergies are on the rise, fewer families are able to sit down to a meal where everyone eats the same foods. This can drive parents crazy. Unfortunately, there's no instant fix. The best advice I've heard comes from a wise grandmother who never kept cookies or other sweet junk foods around for her (thirteen) grandchildren, and amazed many parents of the kids for whom she babysat because after a few weeks with her they'd go home and ask for foods like dill pickles, tomato slices with salt, and celery sticks with peanut butter.

Here are some tips:
- Lead by example.
- When introducing new foods, offer small pieces and ask kids to just try a taste.
- Don't make them finish anything if they don't want to.
- Be gently consistent. It can take several dozen tries for a kid to start liking a new food.
- Don't use food or drink as a reward for good behavior, especially not sweets.

TROUBLESHOOTING

I'm hungry between meals. What do I do?
If you've noticed that you get hungry like clockwork at certain times each day, this is actually good news. As long as you don't have symptoms of hypoglycemia (headaches, shaking, irritability, concentration problems, etc.), it's likely just habit hunger. Habit hunger is trained into the memory of your circadian clock much in the same way a dog will bark at the mailman and, like a pet, can be retrained. But just as with retraining an animal, the most important thing is to be consistent. If you intermittently reward yourself with snacks, then you are intermittently reinforcing a bad habit, and that can make it take even longer to break.

If your hunger is accompanied by hypoglycemic symptoms, then your problem may be metabolic.

The fastest fix for this is reducing your breakfast carbohydrate and/or protein intake. A high-carb breakfast sets you up for a day of metabolic problems. When your breakfast contains too much carbs or protein and not enough fat, your body needs to release a lot of insulin to store the extra nutrients, and this can make your blood sugar drop, creating an energy crisis that puts your body in panic mode, releasing the adrenaline that helps your damaged metabolism access energy stores that should be more readily available. Energy crises are particularly common between breakfast and lunch in folks who are used to eating low-fat or high-protein and so are not quite adapted to burning fat. The solution is to select a breakfast with higher fat counts, and pull back a bit on the carb and/or protein.

I don't feel right on this diet. What do I do?

When cutting carbs, your body must make a lot of adjustments. The most common issues causing symptoms are fluid or deficiency of sodium (from salt), calcium, potassium, or magnesium. Very often a person is either not drinking enough water or not getting enough salt, or both. To address mineral deficiency, if you've not evaluated your need for supplements, you should do that now.

I'm getting bored with my routine. What do I do?

This may seem too obvious, but the number-one reason for getting bored is not having enough variety, which comes from not buying enough variety. So the simple solution is to expand your shopping list. If you're not sure what to do with what you have on hand right now, it's time to hit the internet for recipes or check out the Resources section at the end of this book.

The number-two reason for getting bored is that you're actually not that hungry. If you were truly hungry, then the nourishing foods you have in your fridge would seem more appealing. If nothing in front of you is turning you on, rather than heading out to McDonald's, you might consider just skipping this meal and waiting for the next.

I'm not losing weight. What do I do?

More than anything, success with the plan depends on not being hungry. If you're hungry, see above.

If you're not hungry but not losing weight, you can probably guess what I'm going to say next: eat less! The easiest thing to do is skip a meal once in a while.

I miss my breakfast carbs. Do I really need to be so strict?

Of course not! If you're not dealing with excessive hunger or energy swings, or struggling with your weight, as long as you keep your daily carbohydrate totals in the range of 30 to 70 grams, with 100 grams of carbohydrates per day being your absolute upper limit (unless you're an athlete; see prior comment above), you can certainly enjoy some carbs at breakfast. I don't generally recommend making carbs the center of the meal, however, because they're generally relatively devoid of nutrition. Try a slice of sourdough or sprouted grain toast with eggs, or oatmeal (or other whole grains) that's been enhanced by soaking in whey overnight or sprouting and then fortified with plenty of other ingredients, like plenty of nuts and seeds in the oatmeal example and fruit instead of sugar or honey. Traditional breakfast porridges, cereals, and muffins are generally enhanced not with sweetness (because traditionally sugar was a rare treat and fruits were not available for much of the year), but with sprouting and/or fermentation. Both procedures reduce anti-nutrients, enhance the complexity of flavor and nutrition, and go well with savory tasting herbs.

If you're avoiding grains and you want your breakfast carb, then try some winter squashes instead. You can also use nut flours to make breakfast pastries. But because nut flours go rancid rapidly, I'm not a huge fan of them unless you grind the nuts into flour yourself.

Because carbs can sneak up on you if you're not accustomed to a lower-carb lifestyle, be sure to acquaint yourself with the highest-carb foods on your own list of favorites (see Dr. Cate's simple Carb-Counting Tool, in the Resources section).

Adding organ meats to my diet sounds difficult and disgusting. How do I get started?

I have to admit I sometimes find the intense flavors a little unappetizing. Two simple tricks Luke and I use are to cook with soy sauce or strong spices. Sandy's Miracle Liver recipe, page 380, for example, uses soy sauce to make cow's liver taste surprisingly good, and the same recipe can work on chicken livers. Liver pate or liverwurst (available in many grocery store delis) tastes better when combined with mustard and/or fermented horseradish spread on (vegetable-oil–free) crackers and, if you're feeling fancy, garnished with olives or cheese. You can also use your favorite blend of Indian spices to liberally coat chicken livers, and stir-fry them in peanut oil.

Roasted bone marrow is so buttery and delicious you don't have to cover it up. It tastes great spread on toast or with a beef-based demi-glace reduction sauce. The same goes for sweetmeat, which is super mild and tastes good simply pan fried or grilled. Finding a place to buy it will probably be the hardest part.

Don't forget that you can outsource the organ-meat cooking to a pro. Either look up a local nose-to-tail eatery or (this will probably be easier on your wallet) find a nearby Vietnamese or Filipino restaurant, as these two cuisines seem to have endured Americanization better than the rest.

A last resort that will enable you to enjoy some of the nutrition in organ meat without ever looking at an organ is to eat a lot of eggs because the yolks have a somewhat similar nutritional profile to liver.

Is there a way to add bone broth to my diet that doesn't mean I'm eating soup all the time?

One of our favorite dishes is steak with demi-glace-reduction. You can thicken the demi-glace further with a roux, turning it into a silky gravy, and pour over any simply cooked cut of meat. Demi-glace also tastes fantastic with caramelized onions and/or sautéd mushrooms. You can also add stock in place of water for rice or risotto.

Sandra Padilla, head chef at the L.A. Lakers facility, slips stock into grits, whips it into mashed potatoes, and uses it to braise collards and other vegetables. Aside from using stock for classic Mexican soups and old-fashioned chicken soup, she also adds it to every kind of vegetable soup—from butternut squash to asparagus to broccoli. Kobe Bryant is now so enamored with Sandra's incredible soups that he gets them delivered to his doorstep!

I want to get healthier, but this feels overwhelming. Where should I start?

The best place to start is with breakfast. Once you're comfortable with a new breakfast, then you're ready to move on to incorporating healthier lunchtime meals. Likewise, when you've mastered breakfast and lunch, you're ready to complete the transition to a *Deep Nutrition* lifestyle by adding dinner. There are, of course, other methods to going gradually, but this is what my patients have shown me seems to work the best.

SELECTED RECIPES

8 NORTH BROADWAY HEIRLOOM GAZPACHO

Nothing beats the infusion of freshness like a cool cup of gazpacho on a hot summer day. On a recent trip, we stopped for lunch at a wonderful restaurant in Nyack, New York, called 8 North Broadway, or 8NB. I enjoyed what is, without question, the best gazpacho I'd ever had. Chef Constantine Kalandronis was kind enough to give me the recipe.

- 4 Persian cucumbers, grated and strained through cheesecloth or a clean kitchen towel to remove excess liquid
- 12 red beefsteak tomatoes
- 4 large ripe heirloom tomatoes
- 4 cloves garlic
- 1 cup pepper vinegar
- 2 jalapeño peppers, seeded
- 1 red onion, sliced
- 1 can organic tomatoes
- 1 cup basil leaves
- 1 cup chopped mint leaves
- 1 cup chopped parsley leaves
- 1 cup chopped cilantro
- 2 tablespoons freshly ground horseradish
- Juice of one lemon
- Juice of one lime
- Salt to taste
- Extra virgin olive oil, as needed
- Garnish of choice

Place all ingredients in a bowl and let flavors marry overnight. After twenty-four hours, blend to a chunky puree and serve with more organic olive oil and garnish.

8 NORTH BROADWAY TZATZIKI

This simple Greek condiment is a refreshing accompaniment to raw veggies or grilled meat, especially spicy grilled meat like lamb souvlaki.

- 2 English cucumbers
- 2 cloves garlic, grated
- 1/4 cup extra virgin olive oil
- Juice of 1 lemon
- 4 tablespoons distilled white vinegar
- 4 tablespoons minced red onion
- 4 cups local sheep, goat, or cow yogurt, strained in sieve
- Chopped parsley, mint, and dill to taste
- Salt to taste

Squeeze out excess water from grated cucumber through a clean kitchen towel. Add all ingredients except yogurt and herbs in a bowl. Allow to macerate and mix for about 2–3 minutes so flavors can develop. Add yogurt, herbs, and adjust salt to taste. Straining yogurt for an hour will yield a better, thicker tzatziki. Use a fine mesh sieve or cheesecloth. Fage and Skotidakis tend to be thicker yogurts and need less straining.

LIVER AND ONIONS

The secret to this simple recipe is to avoid overcooking the liver and to sauté the onions slowly, so that they can develop a complex, caramelized flavor. Beef liver is typically sold already "cleaned," but if it still has silver skin around it, carefully remove it from the liver first.

- Fresh liver
- 1/2 cup butter
- 2 tablespoons olive oil or avocado oil
- 2 cloves garlic, whole
- 1 large yellow onion, sliced
- 1 cup beef stock
- 1/4 cup red wine
- 1 teaspoon balsamic vinegar
- 1/8 cup flat leaf parsley, chopped
- 1/2 cup mixture of equal parts flour, sea salt, and fresh-ground pepper

Boil 4 cups of water. Cut liver strips into ¼-inch slices and place in a metal colander. Pour the boiling water over the liver, making sure all the liver surface is exposed to the water (this removes some of the blood and bitterness and prevents clumping when you drench the liver in the flour mixture). Pat the liver completely dry with a paper towel.

In a medium-sized sauté pan, add the butter, 1 tablespoon of the olive oil, and garlic cloves. Add the onion to caramelize it, stirring often to prevent burning. Once onion is golden brown, smelling slightly sweet, add the beef stock, the red wine, and the balsamic vinegar. Simmer sauce until reduced. Be careful not to over-reduce, as the sauce will thicken a little once removed from the heat. A minute or so before removing from heat, add the chopped parsley.

Heat up another sauté pan and add the second tablespoon of olive oil. Place the flour mixture in a large bowl and quickly drench each strip, coating lightly. Sauté the liver strips over medium heat until they brown, then flip and continue to cook for another minute or so.

Serve liver with caramelized onion sauce.

SANDY'S MIRACLE LIVER

We include this second, super-fast and easy organ meat recipe to show you that it doesn't take a culinary arts degree to get such tidbits to taste good. Sandy is a nurse I worked with for years in the Kaleheo Clinic on Kauai, and this Filipino adobo-style (marinated in soy sauce) dish is her own creation. Her children love it and so do we!

- 1 pound cow's liver, cleaned
- 4 to 6 cloves garlic, diced
- Black pepper to taste
- 1/8 cup soy sauce (naturally brewed, not hydrolyzed)
- 2 to 4 tablespoons olive or peanut oil
- Pepper

Slice the liver into one-inch cubes. Pour oil into a large, flat-bottomed frying pan, coating the bottom. Turn heat to medium, toss in the garlic, and heat until it starts to sizzle. Sauté garlic for a few seconds, stirring. Add liver and cook briefly on each side until evenly brown and blood starts oozing out, about 2 to 3 minutes. It should smell savory and good by this point.

Working quickly, grind about 1/4 to 1/2 teaspoon of black pepper over the meat, then add the soy sauce into the pan, being careful not to pour it over the liver (to avoid washing off the pepper) and cover pan. Turn off heat, leave on hot stovetop for five to ten minutes until the blood turns pale brown. Serve with juice over rice, or over noodles with a sprinkle of parmesan cheese. Oddly enough, this liver will also taste good the next day!

HOMEMADE CHICKEN STOCK

The most common cooking question I get is, How do I make bone stock? Here is an easy chicken stock recipe from my friend Larry Ells, executive chef at the Grand Hyatt Kauai in beautiful Poipu. We've added white wine to his recipe for flavor and because the acid extracts more bone minerals to be released into the broth.

Use this stock for making mashed potatoes, gravies and sauces, or quick soups for the family, with the addition of fresh vegetables and meats.

This recipe yields about 3 gallons of very good stock. The shelf life if refrigerated is three days. If frozen, three months.

- 5 pounds chicken bones, either fresh, or freshly frozen (If you can find a butcher who sells them, include up to 50 percent chicken feet, thoroughly washed and toenails clipped off, for extra collagen.)
- 2 medium carrots, washed and cut into slices or cubes
- 3 stalks celery, washed and cut into slices or cubes
- 1 leek, well washed and cut (optional but very tasty)
- 1 large onion, peeled and diced
- 4 to 6 ounces white wine
- 2 bay leaves
- Pinch of kosher salt
- 6 to 8 black peppercorns
- 1 small bunch Italian parsley, fresh and rinsed, whole

Cover the chicken bones and feet with cold water. Bring to a simmer and drain, and then rinse well. Return the bones and feet to the pot. Again cover with cold water and add all other ingredients. Bring pot back to a low simmer, and simmer uncovered for about 4 hours. As the stock cooks, some gray foam will collect on top. Skim the foam with a spoon and discard.

When the stock is done, allow to cool for about 10 minutes and then very carefully strain stock into a metal or glass container and cool, loosely covered, at room temperature for about 30 minutes. Then chill thoroughly. Use immediately or store in 3/4-full plastic containers and freeze. (The stock will expand on freezing.)

(continued)

BROWN BEEF STOCK

This is difficult but worth the trouble. You're dealing with large, heavy items here: big pans, lots of water, giant bones. It can be a little intimidating. But when you're done, you'll have around a gallon of stock, which will last for at least a month.

- 1 tablespoon olive oil
- 4 ounces tomato paste
- Beef bones (with joint material) and tendons (enough to fill stock pot half way)
- 1 cup red wine
- 3 cups mirepoix (onions, carrots, and celery), diced large
- 1 tablespoon sea salt
- Sachet d'Espices (parsley, thyme, bay leaf, cracked peppercorns, and, optionally, garlic)

Preheat oven to 400 degrees. Combine olive oil with the tomato paste and use to lightly coat the bones and tendons. Roast bones and tendons until they turn a fairly deep brown, stirring and turning occasionally to prevent burning. Trust your instincts here. When it looks and smells appetizing, that's brown enough. Any further, and you risk introducing bitterness into the finished stock.

Transfer bones into a large stock pot and cover with cold water and a 1/2 cup of the red wine. Bring to a simmer slowly—never to a full boil!

(continued)

Lightly coat mirepoix and roast in a roasting pan at 400 degrees, stirring occasionally, until a deep golden brown. Remove mirepoix from roasting pan and set aside to be added to the stock after it has simmered for 5 to 8 hours. Deglaze the pan using the remaining red wine (or water). Add deglazed liquid to the stock.

Simmer the stock for 5 to 8 hours, skimming scum off the top often. Stir bones occasionally so that different parts of the bones are sitting on the bottom of the pot. At this time, add the mirepoix.

Simmer for an additional 4 hours. During the final half hour, add the spices. You may add the spices directly or place inside a large tea infusion ball and then drop the ball into the stock.

Remove stock pot from heat and carefully remove the large bones. Using a chinois strainer and/or cheesecloth, strain stock into another large pot. Salt just enough to be able to better taste the stock, as any reduction in the stock will intensify the salty flavor.

Stock can be used now or cooled in an ice bath in the sink (stir ice water one direction while stirring the stock in the other), then refrigerate.

After the stock has cooled, you may remove the crust of fat that will have formed at the top. If the bones you used had plenty of joint material on them, then the finished stock should have firmed up noticeably, and even congealed into a wiggly, jelly-like consistency. The stock liquifies again once heated.

SAUERKRAUT

To make sauerkraut, you need a large, food-safe crock. We've got a couple two-gallon Ohio Stoneware crocks, and they're bigger than we need. Since it's just the two of us, we could easily have gotten by with the single gallon. As two-gallon crocks are quite heavy, and can be unwieldy when cleaning, I recommend going with a one-gallon size. Once you discover how ridiculously easy it is to make big batches of sauerkraut, you will always have a batch fermenting in the coolest spot in your house.

- 3 to 5 large cabbages, green or purple or both, sliced
- 1/4 cup sea salt
- Starter culture (pickle or sauerkraut juice)

The best method of slicing cabbage for sauerkraut is with a mandolin slicer. But mandolins are notoriously dangerous. Luke severed a tendon on the middle finger of his right hand using one. Celebrated Michelin-starred chef Eric Ripert says he won't use them, they're so dangerous. So feel free to use a sharp chef's knife to do the job. Just remember, the thinner the cabbage slices the better. Slice the cabbage in one direction. Don't crosscut. You want long, thin strands.

Combine the sliced cabbage in a big mixing bowl with the salt and starter culture (juice from a previous batch of sauerkraut or from a real, fermented pickle, like Bubbies brand). The exact amount of salt needed can be a little tricky, because different salt varieties vary in intensity. Master of All Things Fermented, Sandor Katz, recommends roughly 1-1/2 to 2 teaspoons per pound of cabbage, but advises that you also rely on your taste to determine the perfect salinity. My personal rule is this: make the cabbage just a little saltier than you think it should be. By the time the kraut is mouth-puckeringly sour, the high acidity and the high salinity will balance each other out.

(continued)

Pack the salted cabbage into the crock, handfuls at a time. Use your fist to punch the cabbage down flat. Then add a couple handfuls more, and punch it down again. Place a plate that's nearly the size of the interior of the crock (but not precisely the size, as it can get stuck; I learned this the hard way!) on top of the cabbage and then weigh it down with a sealed jar of water. Then cover the crock with a breathable towel and secure it around the edges with a large, thick rubber band.

Place the crock in the coolest part of your house (not anywhere that might freeze) and wait. Check the progress every week. If you see mold, carefully remove it with a spoon or moistened paper towel. Once the kraut tastes plenty sour, pack it into a jar and store in the fridge.

TEN-MINUTE ITALIAN DRESSING

If your heart and your kidneys are in good health, you don't have to worry about salt. I mention this because many people worry about sodium, often under-seasoning their homemade salad dressings, which makes other family members reach for store-bought stuff, which is loaded with vegetable oil and pumped up with sugar and "natural flavorings."

I make this dressing in a small Mason jar with a tight lid. This way, I can emulsify the finished dressing with twenty seconds of vigorous shaking.

- 2/3 cup extra virgin olive oil
- 1/3 cup balsamic vinegar
- 5 drops roasted sesame seed oil
- 1 teaspoon prepared mustard
- 1/8 teaspoon raw honey (optional)
- 1/8 teaspoon dried Italian spices (Penzey's spices are good)
- 1/2 teaspoon fresh-ground pepper
- 1 teaspoon sea salt, Himalayan salt, or other quality salt

Place all ingredients in a jar with a tight-fitting lid and shake for twenty seconds. Add more salt and balsamic vinegar to taste. Store in the fridge. Remove 10 minutes before using again to allow it to liquify. Shake vigorously before each use.

BUTTERMILK DRESSING

Why don't people eat more salad? The answer is usually because they're not thrilled with the dressings they are offered. Here's a great, rich, tangy, zippy dressing whose buttermilk base provides probiotics and calcium.

- 2/3 cup buttermilk
- 1/3 cup olive-oil-based mayonnaise (homemade, or Primal Kitchen brand)
- 1 teaspoon lemon or lime juice
- 1 teaspoon mixture of dried onion powder, garlic, parsley, thyme, and basil
- 1/4 teaspoon fresh-ground white or black pepper
- 2 teaspoons sea salt
- Fresh chopped chives (optional)

Place all ingredients in a jar with a tight-fitting lid and shake for twenty seconds. Season to taste.

CHAPTER 14

Frequently Asked Questions

As I mentioned in the Author's Note, this now-expanded volume of *Deep Nutrition* owes itself to the hundreds and hundreds of intelligent questions from readers, patients, conference attendees, and folks who follow me through social media. I've done my best to build as much of that insight into the body of the book as possible, but there are always great questions that fall outside the purview of the chapters.

The questions I like best are the ones that catch me a little off guard, those for which I have a decent answer but that expose a weak spot in my own knowledge of a given topic, an area deserving of further investigation. But most of the following questions and answers below are of the practical variety, specific tips and instructions to make it easier for you to apply the concepts in the book in a real-world context. If you're just embarking on a *Deep Nutrition* lifestyle, you'd be right to think that living this way at least in the beginning is going to make you feel a bit different, perhaps even slightly alienated from friends and family who still march by the everything-in-moderation mantra—which is another way of saying that nutrition doesn't really matter. The fact that you're reading this means you think it does. Questions and insight from the growing community of people who place food right at the center of their healthy lifestyle strategy keep the nutrition conversation interesting, informed, and practical. *So please keep 'em comin'!*

What kind of animal bones should I use to make broth?
The kind of animal doesn't matter. Get organic if you can. Free-range or grass-fed is the very best. The stuff that helps your joints the most comes from the cartilage-rich joint material. Marrow bones, used in a minority of beef stock recipes, don't contain joint material and do contain a lot of fat that typically will just get skimmed off the top, so we prefer not to use them.

What can I do with bone broth?

Broth is put to so much good use that the famous French chef August Escoffier said, "Without broth, nothing can be done." You can use it almost anywhere you'd add water: for braising vegetables like collard greens, green beans, carrots, parsnips, sweet potatoes, turnips, onions, and beets; for vegetable purees and soups made with asparagus, squashes, leeks, cabbage, onions, broccoli, collards, or anything else. Broth serves as the tastiest base for all the most familiar kinds of soup, including the familiar chicken soup, *chile con carne,* minestrone, and cream of broccoli. A much-reduced beef stock is called demi-glace. Add demi-glace to butter-sautéed mushrooms or caramelized onions for a wonderful addition to grilled steak. With stock on hand, you can boldly foray into less familiar soups from other great culinary cultures. *Thom Kha Guy,* the spicy coconut Thai soup, is one of my personal favorites, as are green chile, *pico de gallo,* and Mexico's national soup, *menudo.*

How often should I drink broth, and how much?

You can certainly have broth every day if you like, with a meal or even as a meal (see below). Just keep in mind that the more concentrated the broth, the less you need to eat in order to enjoy its benefits. Store-bought broths tend to be fairly weak and don't even gelatinize in the fridge, so it's perfectly okay to have a couple of cups of this every day. A reduced demi-glace sauce is intense both in taste and in nutrition, so just a couple tablespoons makes for a healthy dose.

Can I just drink it?

Yes, of course! This is a common practice around the world. For example, Koreans will make stocks using a base of leeks, daikon (a mild-flavored white radish), onion, and garlic to sip like a tea, infusing it with extra flavors depending on the bones used. Ginger and ginseng are added to the chicken stock, and seaweed and mushroom are used for beef. Heat it up in a pot or in a cup in the microwave and enjoy it like tea.

Can I heat broth in the microwave?

Absolutely, because it's a liquid. The primary problem I have with microwave cooking is that the microwave cooks unevenly and you can get overdone sections. But for heating up broth (or other liquids), no problem.

Does freezing negatively impact the nutritional value of bone broth?

Freezing does reduce the content of some nutrients, like for vitamin C, for example. But we don't drink bone broth for its vitamin C as much as for the sturdier glycosaminoglycans, hyaluronans, and collagen hydrolysates. These are still present in bone stock after freezing and thawing.

Can I get Mad Cow disease from bone broth?

Theoretically, yes. Though it's not more likely to cause Mad Cow than muscle meat, because the agents (called prions) that cause Mad Cow disease live in the nervous tissue, not in the bones. If the bones come from 100 percent pasture-raised cows, it's even less likely because these cows won't ever be eating other cows—which is how some of these prion diseases are transmitted.

I heard bone broth might contain a lot of lead. Is that true?

An article in the journal *Medical Hypothesis* entitled "The Risk of Lead Contamination in Bone Broth Diets"[624] made headlines when it came out in 2013, triggering a flurry of emails to my inbox. The article shows that bone stock made according to a standard recipe and not concentrated further contained just over ten times the concentration of lead as the tap water control (9.5 micrograms of lead per kilogram of liquid stock versus 0.89 per killogram of water). So yes, bone stock contains a good deal more lead than tap water. But keep in mind, many foods contain lead. So for the lead level report to be more meaningful, I think we need to compare broth to something other than water. Lead levels are not reported for most foods, but I was able to find the following data (all units in microgram kilogram or kilograms): kale,[625] 200.3; hake fish,[626] 7; performance protein drinks,[627] 15, urban-raised chicken eggs,[628] 30-80; infant cereal formula,[629] less than 20 (threshold of detection) -180; canned sardines,[630] 60-270; mussels,[631] 150. So it appears that bone broth's lead level of 9.5 is relatively low.

Can I use a pressure cooker to make broth?

We found that pressure cookers aren't large enough to be practical for making beef stock, but they can shave an hour or two off the minimum time required to make chicken stock (two to four hours). It does change the flavor a bit, in our experience—still pleasant but less bright and more industrial tasting. It's also a cloudier, less gelatinous end product. So it's slightly more convenient but slightly less tasty and probably also slightly less nutritious. For these reasons, we generally use a seven-gallon stock pot for making stock, and the pressure cooker for other dishes (primarily bean-based).

Why isn't gelatin as good as bone stock?

Gelatin is made from bones and not from cartilage, so while it does contain one of the components of broth, called *collagen hydrolysate*, it provides none of the hyaluronans, glycosaminoglycans, or other complex components of broth.

What can vegetarians do to get bone stock?

If you eat fish, you can make fish stock. If not, there's no exact substitute. However, seaweed and bacteria can produce a molecule in the glycosaminoglycan family, which is one of the families of compounds in broth. (See the next question.)

Is there a vegan substitute for bone stock?

Compounds in bone stock were originally invented by the most primitive multicellular life forms billions of years ago, called stromatolytes, dome-shaped structures about a foot in diameter, which to this day continue to grow in Australia's shallow coastal waters. They are composed of colonies of single-celled microbes called *cyanobacteria*. The bacteria are held together with a rudimentary form of connective tissue, composed, in part, of one of the families of special connective tissue compounds found in our own collagen, the glycosaminoglycans. The concentration of glycosaminoglycan molecules varies from 0.5 to 1 percent, depending on the seaweed species.[632] Of all the different seaweeds, kelp is thought to contain some of the highest concentrations of glycosaminoglycans.

Preliminary cell-culture research investigating the potential for using plant-derived glycosaminoglycans to improve joint health indicates possible anti-inflammatory benefits.[633]

One caveat to the idea that we can get significant benefit to our collagen from eating seaweed or algae comes from the often overlooked molecular detail that many of these plant-derived glycosaminoglycans contain bonds and sugar molecules that are unique to plants, and so they may not convey the same benefits as glycosaminoglycans derived from simmering joint material. So, while this avenue of nutritional substitution is still promising, the reality is that the health effects remain largely unexplored.

I had a recent angiogram and they found a 50 percent blockage in one of the major coronary arteries. Can your diet help to clean the plaque from my arteries?

You might be surprised to learn that cardiologists disagree on whether or not arterial plaque can be reduced significantly with diet. Even research specifically funded to prove benefits of powerful cholesterol-lowering drugs shows almost no plaque reduction unless the drugs knock your LDL cholesterol down below 70. Unfortunately, there's been no research to date investigating whether or not a low-sugar, natural-fat traditional diet can reduce arterial plaque, so we have to rely on those markers known to be associated with the formation of arterial plaque, namely high triglycerides, small LDL particles, and low HDL cholesterol, and hope that, as plaque-markers diminish, so too does the amount of plaque in your arteries. Over the past decade and a half, I have seen hundreds of my patients improve all these lipid markers following the Human Diet. What's more, in all my years of practice, I have yet to see anyone who strictly limits sugars and categorically avoids vegetable oils go on to suffer a heart attack, which is pretty extraordinary given that each year one in 300 Americans over age eighteen has a heart attack. On the other hand, every patient I've encountered who has had abnormal blood sugar or regularly consumes vegetable oil (or both) very often has eaten something fried in vegetable oil on the day of the attack.

I heard that milk from A2 cows is better than A1, what's that all about?

If you don't have an allergy to milk, there's no qualitative difference between milks from these two cows, as far as your body is concerned, because they're nearly identical.

A2 versus A1 refers to one of the gene-encoding milk proteins, called casein. Caseins represent about 30 percent of the total protein present in milk. The difference in casein produced by the A2 gene versus A1 is a single amino acid change in the nearly 200 amino acid protein sequence. Where A2 has the amino acid proline, A1 has the amino acid histidine instead, and the rest of the amino acids are all entirely identical.[634] Some argue that the substitution of this single proline for a histidine is enough to make A1 milk pro-inflammatory. Given that goat and cow caseins differ by far more than one amino acid, as do sheep and human casein, the change in and of itself is unlikely to be an issue. These proteins, like most dietary proteins, are digested into peptides and then into individual amino acids. After digestive enzymes have broken them all down, the body has no way of identifying which of the many histidines is the extra, among all the multitudes of amino acids swirling about in the gut fluids.

If you do, however, have a milk allergy, there's a small chance that your immune system has developed antibodies to one kind of milk but not the other. In fact, I found at least one study indicating that if you have a milk allergy, switching from A1 to A2 might help.[635]

The A1 type variant arose in European herds from the original A2 type some 5,000–10,000 years ago. Some breeds produce mostly A1, like Holsteins, some mostly A2, like Guernseys, Jerseys, Brown Swiss, Normandes, and breeds native to Africa and India.

Is raw milk safe?

An average of 28 people are sickened by raw milk annually,[636] out of 9.4 million raw milk drinkers[637] compared to an annual average of 2.3 people sickened annually by pasteurized milk, out of something like 150 million pasteurized milk drinkers (a very rough estimate).[638] If these epidemiological statistics are to be taken at face value, you might conclude pasteurized milk is by far the safer choice. But there's reason to conclude that the raw-milk/sickness stats may not represent the reality.

And here's why: knowing how doctors take histories, when faced with a sick child and we hear that they've consumed raw milk, we're likely to blame the raw milk. Period. This is based on bias that is so strong that even when parents report their children ate other suspect foods, the doctors won't change their report.[639] One woman told me her three-year-old was hospitalized after drinking raw milk, and while no one else who'd consumed the milk got sick, the doctor nevertheless reported that the infection came from the milk. But after the child recovered, it was discovered he and another toddler had gnawed on chicken bones dug out of the trashcan—a much more likely source. These sorts of errors appear to happen all the time.

If you want to significantly reduce your risk of food-borne illness there is a step you can take that would be more effective, in my opinion, than avoiding raw milk: that step is cooking for yourself.

I'd like to take a moment to put the risks of eating anything in perspective, whether cooked or raw, if it's put on your plate by a stranger. According to the CDC, more than half (52 percent) of all food-borne illnesses between 1998–2004 came from eating out, in restaurants, hotels, and delicatessens. Add to that an additional 4 percent from schools, 22 percent from "other" (hospital and other institutions, take-out, catering, and civic and church buffets), and you've got 78 percent of the roughly 77 million annual food-borne illnesses coming from outside the home.[640] Given that most people eat at home most of the time, it's safe to estimate that eating out increases your risk of getting sick by anywhere from five to ten times.

Another way to reduce your risk of food-borne illness is to avoid the foods that the CDC has identified as the top ten culprits:[641]

1. Leafy greens: 13,568 reported cases of illness

2. Eggs: 11,163 reported cases of illness

3. Tuna: 2,341 reported cases of illness

4. Oysters: 3,409 reported cases of illness

5. Potatoes: 3,659 reported cases of illness

6. Cheese: 2,761 reported cases of illness

7. Ice cream: 2,594 reported cases of illness

8. Tomatoes: 3,292 reported cases of illness

9. Sprouts: 2,022 reported cases of illness

10. Berries: 3,397 reported cases of illness

In spite of the apparent risks I'll not be cutting these categorically from my diet for the simple reason that I like all kinds of real foods.

Bottom line: I personally drink raw milk daily and I've never had a problem. But if you're worried about it, don't drink it.

I usually don't drink milk but I'd like to try raw milk. How do I get started?

If you don't usually drink dairy, then the microbes in your gut aren't necessarily going to help protect you from the minuscule but real chance of pathogenic infection. So I recommend you first reintroduce the micro-organisms in your gut to the nutrients in milk by eating two to four ounces of plain yogurt (you can add a little low-sugar jelly for flavor) daily for two to four weeks before you add raw milk. After this reacclimatization, you can begin with two to four ounces of raw milk and work your way up gradually to however much you want, never doubling the intake more than once in a week. Do not drink raw milk if you cannot get it from a trusted source.

Do I have to drink raw milk to get the benefits of dairy?

You don't have to drink milk to get the benefits of dairy.

Fermenting milk into cheese makes it even more nutritious. Fermentation can reduce the sugar count to near zero because the microbes eat it up, while producing a variety of nutrients, including amino acids, and essential fats along with several vitamins like K2 and B12. Even if the cheese is not raw, because prolonged fermentation increases the complexity of the nutrition and in some ways rehabilitates the nutritional damage done by pasteurization, as long as it's grass-fed it's still going to be an extremely healthy food. Other extremely healthy forms of dairy include kefir, cottage cheese, and yogurt (not the pre-flavored kind).

How do I find grass-fed dairy?

Common commercially available grass-fed brands of milk, yogurt, cottage cheese, and other delicious dairy products are Kolona Supernatural, Organic Valley, and Wallaby. Regardless of the brand you buy, always read the label carefully to make sure it's grass-fed or pasture-raised—because brands can change their values or be bought out by larger commercial entities with less interest in your good health. For local farm sources, see www.eatwild.com and www.realmilk.com.

Does raw milk provide beneficial bacteria?

Raw milk does contains beneficial bacteria, but not many.

Farmers go to great lengths to avoid introducing bacteria to the milk, wiping down udders with iodine, flushing collection lines, sanitizing tanks, and constantly keeping everything properly chilled. Colony counts of harmful bacteria can be kept to near zero using these methods. And since sanitizers kill beneficial bacterial along with the bad ones, we can presume their numbers are drastically reduced as well.

A better source of beneficial bacteria will be live-cultured products, like yogurt, kefir, cottage cheese, sour cream, and buttermilk.

There is some evidence that commercially prepared yogurts contain bacteria that don't readily survive stomach acid, and that wild-fermentation products might contain beneficial bacteria colonies that are hardier and more likely to survive the trip through your acid stomach. This may be the case. But whether wild-cultured or not, the more good bacteria you eat, the more will make it through.

I heard milk leaches calcium from my bones because it's acid-forming. Is that true?

No. It's not true.

If you haven't heard this claim before, the argument is that since acidic food products like milk acidify the body, and since the acidified body takes calcium from the bones in attempt to neutralize the pH, milk, though rich in calcium, ironically takes more than it gives. This simply does not happen. The notion that foods we eat can significantly alter the body's acid base balance, as measured by pH, stands in direct conflict with what we know about chemistry, metabolism, and kidney physiology.

One of the main functions of the kidney is to ensure that your body never wanders outside a very narrow pH bandwidth of 7.4–7.44. Outside of a few extreme circumstances like septic infection, poisoning or kidney failure, your kidney is able to keep you in the pH "Goldilocks" zone day in, day out, and unless you're on a starvation diet, it doesn't need to rob any materials from your tissues in order to do this.

Second, milk is not a strong acid; the pH is 6.5–6.7, barely below that of distilled water, which is 7.0 (pH values below 7 are acidic; above 7 are alkaline). Orange juice has a pH of 3.3–4.1, bananas 4.5–5.2, vinegar 2–3.

As long as your kidney is healthy, be assured that you could have a whole jar of pickles and not significantly alter your body's pH.

I heard dairy makes you insulin-resistant. Is that true?

A 2005 article in the *European Journal of Clinical Nutrition* may have sparked this rumor.[642] The article compared eight-year-old boys consuming either 9.6 ounces of lean meat or two liters (seven cups) of skim milk over a one-week period as their major protein source, and compared their insulin and blood-sugar levels at the end of the week. The boys who got the milk showed roughly double the levels of fasting insulin in their blood as compared to the boys who got the lean meat.

The article used this evidence to conclude that the boys had developed insulin resistance. I'm not sure that's an accurate conclusion, since their blood-sugar levels were nearly identical to what they were at the beginning of the study, and insulin elevation without blood sugar elevation is not the same as insulin resistance, nor is it known to be a problem. Insulin resistance is bad. But a temporary rise in insulin levels in kids without attendant elevation in blood sugar level has not been associated with any detrimental consequences. It is likely that as soon as their milk consumption returned to a normal level (seven cups is a lot of milk), their insulin levels would, too.

Might there in fact be a benefit to a temporary increase in insulin levels in children of the kind brought on by drinking milk in this study? Possibly.

The same study group that published the above article used their data to write a second article concluding that drinking milk supported better bone health than meat consumption.[643] A third article showed that two-year-old children who drink less milk have lower insulin and fewer blood markers of bone growth, suggesting that children who drank more milk would likely develop stronger bones and possibly even grow taller.[644]

What is lactose and why are so many people lactose intolerant?
Lactose is the primary sugar in milk. It's composed of glucose and galactose bonded together. In order for the glucose and galactose to get into the body, the bond needs to be broken by an enzyme called lactase. When we are born, our intestinal lining possesses plenty of lactase activity. But when we stop drinking milk our intestines may stop producing lactase, so not all adults retain the ability to break down this sugar. Without the lactase enzyme, undigested lactose sugar can pass downward to the colon, which normally does not see sugar of any kind. The presence of sugar in the colon can draw too much water into the colon and cause bloating, or promote the growth of unwanted bacteria, causing symptoms. So lactose intolerance is not due to a milk allergy, it's more like a kind of atrophy; if you don't exercise the enzyme for digesting lactose often enough, you can lose the ability altogether.

Another way you can lose your intestinal lactose-digesting enzyme capacity is through intestinal infection, which can denude the fragile cells lining the intestine down to the basement membrane. When the cells grow back, they may not immediately regain the capacity to generate all the enzymes they were producing previously. But a little patience and practice may reboot your intestinal enzymes, and by slowly re-introducing dairy, you may regain the ability to digest lactose once again.

I'm lactose intolerant. Can I still include dairy products in my diet?

Absolutely. All you need to do is avoid lactose, not the rest of the components in dairy. Butter and ghee (clarified butter) have almost no lactose, so many people who are lactose intolerant can enjoy them. Cream is also naturally low in lactose, so some people who are only mildly lactose intolerant can enjoy cream and products made using cream. Store-bought ice cream, however, is quite often made with milk solids that do contain lactose, so check the ingredients carefully.

The bacteria that turn milk into cheese digest most or all of the lactose in the process of fermentation, converting it into protein and other nutrients, which is why cheese is one of my favorite fast foods. Thanks to the bacterial action during fermentation, most people with lactose intolerance can eat long-fermenting hard cheeses like parmesan, cheddar, and Swiss. People with milder lactose intolerance can enjoy softer cheeses like Gruyere and cottage cheese. Mozzarella is not fermented, so those with lactose intolerance typically cannot eat pizza.

My friend's children had eczema that got better when they switched to raw milk. Why is that?

Eczema is an inflammatory skin condition characterized by patches of itchy, flaky dry skin, typically on the cheeks, the insides of the elbows, or behind the knees. Long, hot showers or dry air can exacerbate symptoms. Like many other auto-immune disorders, including celiac disease, the underlying cause is inflammation in the gut, which causes the immune system to mistake a protein from food for an invading pathogen, launching an attack. When the protein under attack happens to resemble proteins in the skin, white blood cells can attack the skin, causing a number of auto-immune skin symptoms including eczema, psoriasis, and other forms of dermatitis.

The underlying mechanisms of any food-triggered auto-immune problems are all very similar. And the best long-term strategy to avoid developing all kinds of auto-immune disorders is to avoid heavily processed foods, particularly those high in protein (such as dairy, eggs, and soy), because processing denatures proteins in ways that can make your immune system more likely to launch an attack. Add pro-inflammatory vegetable oil and sugar to the mix and an attack becomes even more likely.

The best strategy to alleviate eczema is to remove the "suspect" food from the diet along with excess sugars and vegetable oil until an improved diet allows the gut inflammation to recede and the immune system overactivity to calm down. (Some people can slowly reintroduce the offending food and have no further problems with it.)

If you believe milk might be causing eczema, you should know that the offender protein present in typical store-bought milk may be completely absent in raw milk. Pasteurization and homogenization necessarily denature some of the milk proteins, making them appear very different to your body than their unprocessed counterparts. So different, in fact, that your body is more likely to mistake these novel proteins for an enemy, attacking them (and similar-looking proteins in your body) on a large scale, and then keeping a record of their appearance (in the form of antibodies) so that, should the protein ever show itself again, the body will remember to wage war once more.

So although removing the provocateur protein from the diet is a smart move, it's important to recognize that eczema, or any autoimmune symptom, is a sign that your entire dietary program may be in need of revision.

What is gluten?

Almost nobody asks this question. But they should, because most people don't know what it is—even when they're avoiding it. Without knowing what gluten is, it's easier to be seduced into buying something thinking it's a healthier choice simply because it's "gluten free."

Gluten is the protein in wheat that makes it gluey and enables it to hold starch together. It's the reason air produced by yeast gets trapped in holes that makes bread rise. Gluten is not a carb. But because wheat and other grains that contain gluten also contain a lot of starch, by avoiding gluten you avoid a lot of starchy carb-rich foods.

Is gluten bad for me?

I don't buy the idea that gluten is bad for everyone. In fact, purified wheat gluten has been crafted into a staple of Chinese, Japanese, and other Asian cuisines for many hundreds, if not thousands, of years. In my estimation the origin of most people's troubles with gluten is the inclusion of gluten in junk food, and not any inherent problem with the gluten itself.

Gluten is simply a protein that the wheat plant produces for its own uses—to enable the seed to germinate. Because it's a protein, our bodies can develop antibodies to it, and that can lead to symptoms, very much the same way that milk proteins can lead to symptoms in people allergic to milk.

It just so happens that, as discovered centuries ago, when wheat is ground to flour and kneaded with water, the wheat proteins (gluten is composed of glutenin and gliadin) align themselves in such a way as to make a uniquely flexible dough. This dough can then be used to make a huge variety of food products because of its unique ability to trap air. Gluten is now added to a huge variety of processed foods in order to craft them into just the right shape with just the right amount of crunch or fluffiness to be irresistible. So we find gluten-rich foods hard to resist and easy to overeat. And that's another problem.

Gluten is added to so many junk foods rich in vegetable oil and low in nutrients and antioxidants that the body often encounters gluten proteins accompanied by oxidative stress and inflammation. Lots of inflammation. When the immune system sees a certain degree of inflammation, it has to presume there's an infection because throughout the majority of our human history the only things that triggered massive inflammation were immediately life-threatening circumstances—infections, poisons, penetrating trauma (which opens the door to infection)—where harmful proteins or bacteria containing proteins needed to be neutralized. This is why inflammation triggers production of the protective, bacteria-fighting proteins we call antibodies.

The impact of inflammation in the gut on overall immune function is enormous. The immune cells patrolling the gut see more antigens in a day than the immune cells patrolling our bloodstream see during our entire lifespan. The health of your body depends on the ability of your gut immune system to ignore most of those antigens.[645] If it can't, that's going to lead to problems.

So now, back to our person eating too many starchy treats (crackers, pizza, waffles, for instance) and let's say this time they eat so many of these foods that they over-distend their intestines and/or over-expose themselves to pro-inflammatory oils, and develop a stomach ache. Now the immune system is on high alert, furiously making antibodies that will bind to proteins relatively indiscriminately. It is supposed to be making antibodies that bind to proteins on the surface of pathogenic bacteria or to poisonous, accidentally ingested compounds. But in the context of inflammation, the body takes an attitude of "make antibodies first, ask questions later." It will make antibodies for as many proteins as it encounters. And if, as in this particular hypothetical scenario, gluten proteins happen to be the primary protein around, then gluten antibodies are likely to get manufactured.

If the body doesn't recognize its mistake and delete the antibody against gluten (this procedure is called *developing immune tolerance*), then the antibody sticks around. So now, the next time this person eats foods containing gluten, the antibody reaction is likely to trigger the immune-patrol system into taking offensive action—even though there's nothing around but little ol' gluten. Regardless of its pointless, quixotic nature—the immune system is figuratively tilting at windmills here—the immune reaction can cause a variety of symptoms.

But as I suggested a moment ago, it's not just gluten proteins. A similar process can lead to any food allergy: peanuts, tree nuts, eggs, shellfish, milk proteins, soy, and so on. Food allergies are dramatically increasing in the U.S.

GLUTEN, ZONULIN, AND THE MYTH OF HARM TO HEALTHY PEOPLE

Scientists have sorted out many key details linking gluten to celiac disease over the past decade. Perhaps no one has done more to improve our understanding of this connection than a scientist at Harvard's teaching hospital, Dr. Alessio Fasano.

Beginning with a quest to immunize people against cholera in the 1980s, Dr. Fasano accidentally created a vaccine that caused terrible diarrhea—a tragic outcome after years of hard work. Instead of moving on to a different area of research, the doctor decided to dig deeper, and launched an investigation to discover what had backfired. He soon identified a protein made by our bodies called zonulin, which loosens connections between intestinal cells (called tight junctions), allowing fluid to pour into the gut. Cholera bacteria produce a toxin that mimics this effect to generate such massive diarrhea that, without adequate IV rehydration, those infected can die in a matter of days.

Fasano realized that his discovery of zonulin had implications beyond infectious disease. After all, he figured, the body wouldn't leave zonulin-receptors laying around in our digestive cells if all they could do was hurt us. The leakiness stimulated by zonulin very well might have a purpose, he hypothesized.

Soon, Dr. Fasano's team discovered that zonulin plays a key role in defending against parasitic infections. White blood cells walking the beat of the intestinal immune ststem do much of their work in special surveillance centers called Peyer's patches, which function a little like the TSA checks at an airport, randomly singling out travelers for a thorough pat-down and then, after clearance, releasing them to continue on their way. Without zonulin, white blood cells can't squeeze through the spaces between cells in the intestinal wall in order to get into their Peyer's patch work stations, and security in the intestine is compromised—particularly when it comes to parasites. Zonulin, it seems, serves as a kind of workplace key card, allowing white blood cells access to their surveillance centers in the intestinal wall.

Hoping to put his new discovery to clinical use, in the late 1990s, Dr. Fasano's team focused on diseases mediated by an overzealous repsonse to zonulin, crowding the security stations (Peyer's patches) with too many white blood cells, thus throwing the immune system into a state of confusion. His main interest was celiac disease. He wanted to understand how, exactly, gluten exposure could, in some people, translate to celiac disease. So he went to work again. Several years later, he published his findings.[646] It turns out that a minority of the population has a genetic tendency to develop an immune-system malfunction that makes their bodies respond to gluten as if it were a parasite rather than a benign protein, launching an unnecessary and ultimately painful attack on the innocent gluten protein.[647]

Zonulin is a very important link between gluten exposure and celiac disease. However, it's only a link; it's not the whole story. Dr. Fasano never said that gluten causes zonulin-mediated celiac disease in this subgroup of people genetically predisposed to celiac, only that it's a key step in the process. The real problem underlying celiac is not gluten or zonulin; it's an immune system malfunction. In folks with celiac, their immune systems erroneously trigger an exaggerated and sustained zonulin release and, in turn, the exaggerated and sustained zonulin-stimulated increase in gut permeability (i.e., gut leakiness).

One of the reasons people reading Dr. Fasano's articles might jump to the conclusion that gluten is harmul to those without celiac is that Fasano's research shows that gluten does, in fact, induce a limited zonulin release in non-celiac patients. However, there is a very important dose-response difference in the reaction to the zonulin so released. In celiac patients, the reaction is extreme. In non-celiac sufferers, the reaction is muted: "Biopsies from non-celiac patients demonstrated a limited, transient zonulin release paralleled by an increase in intestinal permeability that never reached the level of permeability seen in celiac disease tissues."[648]

This relatively modest permeability modulation may be completely normal and may indeed be essential to normal gut/immune function. To get back to our analagy of white blood cells as TSA employees working at security check points in the intestinal tracts, gluten's ability to stimulate a small amount of zonulin may be necessary to ensure that, in response to proteins coming through the sytem, at least a few TSA workers have key cards in hand and show up for duty at the inspection stations.

It's likely that it is only the over-the-top zonulin release and subsequent extreme immune-system discombobulating reaction to zonulin that promotes the excessive permeability that leads to celiac symptoms.

Another reason Dr. Fasano's work might mislead folks to believing gluten always overstimulates the immune system comes from the choice of protein Dr. Fasano used as his control. As a scientist, Dr. Fasano needed to see if zonulin release was perhaps just a general reaction to the presence of proteins in the stomach. So he compared the amount of zonulin release induced by gluten to the amount of zonulin release induced by the milk protein called casein. He found that gluten triggered a small amount of zonulin release even in normal, non-celiac patients, while casein triggered none at all.[649, 650]

But here's the problem. Casein is not your average food-derived protein. In fact, casein's unique properties may be precisely why Dr. Fasano chose to use it as a control. Casein comes from milk, the only thing we eat that is manufactured for the express purpose of nourishment. Because of this, the body quite possibly treats casein proteins the way TSA treats approved pre-check passengers, with a nod and a wave as they walk right on through. So casein may be one of the rare foods that does not cause zonulin release. To date, I have been unable to find any foods other than gluten and casein that have been tested for their ability to trigger zonulin release.

Unfortunately, these nuances are not always properly understood, which is why, in my opinion, many people—from respected scientists to your local yoga instructor—recommend that gluten is so inherently harmful that everyone should avoid it like a protein plague, lest they risk developing a serious auto-immune disease. I agree entirely that a small percentage of people have bona fide celiac or gluten intolerance. But I believe that these anti-gluten-gladiators leading the angry mob to the bakery are telling the gluten/auto-immunity story backward. The immunity impairment comes first, setting the stage for gluten and any number of other intolerances. If you don't have immune system problems, you don't get celiac disease. End of story.

population particularly among kids, but none of these proteins are inherently bad for you.[651]

I feel better since I stopped eating gluten. Does that mean I have gluten intolerance?

First, if you feel better, that's good. Next, let's discuss why you might be feeling better.

Many times when I ask patients what they did to go gluten free, they say they stopped eating take-out pizza, and often stopped eating fast food of all kinds—so no fries or sodas—in addition to cutting out hamburger buns. At the same time, they also cut down candy and quit the weekend twelve-pack. *Hmmm.* So there's more to their diet change than simply cutting out gluten. That's cutting out a lot of carbs, which most of us overeat, a lot of vegetable oil, and the alcohol binges that can overwhelm the liver's antioxidant capacity. So while at the surface, it can look as though you've just run a successful test to see how you do off of gluten, you've actually made a far more comprehensive dietary change—and a really good one!

For this reason, there's really nothing wrong with avoiding gluten, even if you don't need to. But try not to take it so far that you end up restricting your diet unnecessarily. I had a friend who stopped going out for sushi because he wanted to avoid the few micrograms of gluten in naturally brewed soy sauce (something that's been an important part of Eastern dietary culture for a couple thousand years or so).

The best way to determine if you have gluten intolerance is not through a blood test. It's through working with an allergist M.D. or D.O. who specializes in food-related allergies or who has completed a three-year residency training in allergy and immunology after completing medical school. It's worth the time it takes to find a doctor you trust and with whom you can work closely. But be patient, as it often takes a number of visits to nail down the individual food item causing the problem—or to rule out the possibility of a food allergy altogether.

If liver is the detoxification organ, doesn't that mean it contains toxins that make it unhealthy to eat?

There is no organ in the body devoted exclusively to storing toxins. The liver does play a big role in eliminating useless molecules of all sorts from the body, and once they're eliminated, they're gone. The same goes for the kidney, which plays another key role in eliminating useless molecules. Unfortunately, all organs, even muscle, can accumulate toxins over an animal's lifetime. So this makes it particularly important to pay attention to the source of your food.

What makes that very challenging is the fact that even if the farmer you buy your eggs from treats his chickens like feathered royalty, providing top-quality forage and access to the sun, etc., if the soil he happens to have built his farm on was used for industrial purposes or fell within the shadow of an industrial plant at any point in the past, that soil may contain high levels of a wide variety of industrial toxins that wind up in the chicken. This is a sad legacy of our industry-centered economy.

Outside of harassing your poor local food producers to provide soil-testing results, what can you do? According to a number of articles, the more urban an area, the more likely the soil is to be contaminated.[652, 653] If you live in an urban area and don't want to drive yourself insane worrying over this, then be assured that if your farmer is providing organic feed and doing his best, the toxic burden in the final food product is still likely to be less than anything produced by the larger food conglomerates.

How often should we eat organ meat?
Between once and three times a week, depending on portion size.

I'll never get my kids/spouse/myself to eat organ meats. What can I do instead?
There's no substitute for the nutrient intensity packed into foods like liver, heart, kidneys, and bone marrow from grass-fed animals. But if you don't think you'll be able to include them in your diet anytime soon, then it's important to optimize the nutritional value of the other foods you do eat by following the nutrition-intensifying principles outlined in the previous chapter.

I had a blood test for food intolerance but I'm not sure I trust the results. How accurate are they?
Blood tests are not accurate enough to be used on their own. Unfortunately, they are marketed directly to consumers, so anyone, with or without adequate training in the physiology of the immune system or the limitations and inaccuracies inherent in the tests, can now order them.

Based on this kind of practice, a couple of my professional athlete clients who had been told they were dairy intolerant even though they'd never experienced any symptoms went years with dietary calcium intakes well below normal. When I began working with them, I'd learned that one had been diagnosed with osteoporosis and another had recently suffered a low-impact fracture that was complicated by a protracted healing course such that he was unable to play for a large part of the season. Both players were able to add dairy back without any allergic symptoms, but years of inadequate nutrition had already taken a toll.

The gold standard for evaluating food intolerances is not a blood test, but rather a very strict elimination diet, where you eat nothing but lamb, carrots, pears, and rice (because these foods are rarely a cause of reactions) for an extended period, and then add back new food items one at a time. This is best accomplished by working with a dietician or other expert trained and experienced in the use of elimination diets.

I heard peanut oil was not Paleo. Why do you recommend it?
Technically, no oil is Paleo, because extracting oils requires equipment not particularly suited for the mobility typically associated with a hunter-gatherer lifestyle. But this book moves beyond the strictest definitions of Paleo to include

some of the culinary advancements that bring us things like butter and bone stock and fermented wheat products and, yes, healthy oils. But even if you are willing to incorporate peanut oil into your personal Paleo playbook, you might still be concerned after hearing that peanut oil "contains too many PUFAs" and that it "contains aflatoxin." Let me address these concerns here:

First, a little background. Peanut oil has a long history of use beginning with cultivation in South America several thousand years ago and spreading throughout the rest of the world after Marco Polo's visit in 1500 A.D. New World peanuts eventually replaced indigenous versions of the peanut plant in Africa and Asia (where it's called groundnut, because it grows on the ground as opposed to in trees). Presumably, the replacement occurred because New World peanut plants grew faster or the nuts tasted better. It's also not entirely clear whether people used the seeds to make oil, but it wouldn't have been terribly difficult, as peanuts are quite oily, and so peanut oil is easily extracted with the same simple equipment used to extract oil from other traditional oilseeds.

The peanut's natural oiliness is one of the main reasons peanut oil has the potential to be healthy; it means that a lot of oil can be extracted easily without doing much molecular damage—at least during the first pressing. This is why I recommend you buy cold-pressed unrefined peanut oil if you can, which will ensure the oil molecules are still relatively intact.

When it comes to cooking oil, keeping molecules in their original configuration is always the goal. You can't see distorted molecules, but you can detect their presence, because oils with distorted PUFAs—which have been refined, bleached, and deodorized—generally lack flavor.

Which brings me back to the first of the two above objections to using peanut oil: the relatively high PUFA content.

Peanut oil is only good as long as it tastes good. This is true for all oils. But peanut oil is right on the edge of having too many PUFAs. Peanut oil has 5 to 10 percent more highly oxidizable omega-6 (a PUFA) than olive oil, but it also has 3 to 10 percent more naturally oxidation-resistant saturated fat. This fatty acid profile means that only the highest quality peanut oil (first pressed, unrefined) will be good to eat. If you don't detect any peanut taste, and it's before the expiration date, then the problem may be that it is a lower grade of oil. So take it back.

The second objection to peanut oil pertains to the potential for toxic contamination with *aflatoxin.*

Aflatoxin is produced by a mold in the Aspergillus family. We often hear about it potentially contaminating peanut butter (although there have been no reported outbreaks in the United States), but the mold can grow on just about anything—corn, rice, cotton, cosmetics—and so the problem is not at all unique to peanuts. The best way to avoid aflatoxin is by avoiding foods where the off-flavors that mold growth would normally produce can be hidden behind strong-tasting additives, like sugar, MSG, and other artificial flavorings generally found in processed foods.

Considering that peanuts cause such serious allergy problems for so many people, why is peanut oil okay for the rest of us?

The fact that some people have serious allergic reactions to a food does not in any way indicate that the food is harmful to the rest of us. I wouldn't want to suggest that everyone avoid dairy, tree nuts, soy, eggs, and seafood just because some people need to!

If my child is autistic, how much improvement can I expect from better nutrition?

As I described in Chapter 9, autistic children are not just different from typically developing children, they're different from one another. So the results of dietary improvement are going to vary greatly. It's a shame there's been so little research into the benefits of an improved diet, particularly the good-for-everything improvement of switching out vegetable oil and reducing carbs, but hopefully that will change. In the meantime, there are a couple reasons to believe that better diet could lead to significant changes in mood, socialization, and learning.

Reducing pro-oxidative, inflammatory compounds (found in vegetable oils and processed foods) will help them in the way they will help anyone else: they aid in mental acuity, reduce symptoms of allergic disorders, and improve digestive health. Additionally, research has shown that many autistic kids' brains are dealing with an ongoing immunologic attack[654, 655, 656] that I believe may be brought under control if the inflammation can be subdued through diet. Another reason to be hopeful is the concept of the plasticity of the brain, which speaks to the fact that our brains continue to develop new connections throughout our lives. So it's common sense to suppose that all the brain benefits of reduced inflammation discussed in Chapter 9 will apply also to the autistic child.

That said, autistic children are notoriously finicky about food, and any dietary change will likely be met with resistance. Because it's such a common issue, there are now dieticians who specialize in autism, and if you can find one, he or she may help guide you through the process.

I have non-celiac gluten sensitivity. If I change my diet and my health improves, could I have moderate levels of properly prepared gluten again?

As with other immune-based diseases, I do believe it's possible to put your gluten-sensitivity into remission. So you may be able to enjoy foods containing minimally processed forms of gluten, like those you'd get from wheat berries or sourdough bread. I would not advise adding back gluten-containing foods without working closely with a practitioner who understands your issues.

I have heard that the bacteria involved in the production of sourdough breaks down gluten. Is that possible?
Bacterial action can break down some gluten, but I would not count on it to break down all the components you might have reactions to. If you still want to try, start with just a few bites.

We have just cleared our kitchen of vegetable oil and are weaning our kids off sugar, which seems more difficult. Do you have any tips?
The best thing for weaning kids off sugar (aside from patience and time) is helping them love new foods. The best way to build healthy new food habits is to introduce new items when they're really hungry. So add new foods strategically, like after they've been playing outside all afternoon. And just offer a taste! Forcing them to finish something is a sure-fire way to turn them off to that food for a long time. If all goes well, they'll gradually begin to ask for those new foods.

I've read your sugar chapter and I'm convinced I should reduce my sugar. But can I have just one soda at work to get me through the afternoon?
You can have your can. But I'd much rather you do what billions of other Earthlings do for an afternoon pickup: have a cup of lightly brewed tea. I advise this because studies done in the United States in 2014 and in Korea in 2016 showed, respectively, that a single soda per day can increase the calcium deposits in your arteries by 70 percent[657] and your chance of having a heart attack by 30 percent.[658]

I've cut my carbs but now I'm constipated. Help!
This often occurs in folks who are not also drinking enough water or including enough fiber-rich vegetables (particularly fermented veggies) and nuts, so try that first. Something else that has helped many of my patients is flaxseed: 2 tablespoons ground (you can buy pre-ground flax meal or grind the seeds in a coffee grinder) stirred into a cup of hot water. You can use cold water, but hot water helps prevent clumping.

Does your restriction on sugar mean no dessert?
No, but do seek out those desserts that are less sugary, and, of course, portion size is important. Desserts in the United States probably have ten times the

sugar of desserts in Europe. And anyway, dessert is not something you should eat every day.

Tofu is a traditional food. Can I eat that?
Traditional tofu is fermented. Most of the stuff in the stores, however, is not. If you can find fermented tofu, go for it. If you can't, regular tofu is still okay.

I'm currently breastfeeding. I find that if I cut carbs too much, or lengthen time between meals, my milk supply decreases. Do you have any advice on ways to increase milk production?
Breastmilk contains sugar, roughly 7 grams per 100 milliliters (but it varies widely). So if you're producing a liter of milk for your baby each day, that's 70 grams of sugar your body needs for milk production alone. While your liver can make the sugar you need out of protein if your diet is high enough in protein, that seems like a waste of good protein to me. You might as well get the carbs you need from your favorite carb-rich foods, be it whole grains, root vegetables, beans and peas, or fruits. Just try your best to mix it up; variety is always important!

By the way, stress and sleep deprivation can increase your body's demand for sugar—and what new mom isn't sleep deprived? So listen to your body and use common sense in choosing how you increase your carbs.

After doing the low-carb Atkins Diet for four months I lost nearly fifty pounds and felt great at first. Then the fatigue started, the dry skin, and worst, all of my hair is falling out like crazy. (My doctor says my tests are all normal.) I really don't want to go back to eating bread and sugar but I've read that it helped other people. What do you advise?
Atkins is not necessarily a balanced diet (several of the Four Pillars are missing from the Atkins Diet), so I'd start by identifying what you are missing and add that to your diet. Meanwhile, depending on what kind of exercise you do, it may be beneficial for your metabolism to get a break from severe carb restriction for one or two days per week by eating fruits, sprouted grains, or beans—whatever suits you best.

I have been wary of maintaining a low level of carb intake during pregnancy. What do you think about that?
I understand your concern. But given that 18 percent of pregnant women are now diagnosed as having gestational diabetes, it's safe to say that these fears are rooted less in medical science and are more the product of the fact that our diets have slid so far over to the high-carb end of the scale that our idea of "normal" is skewed. By the way, the first-line treatment for

gestational diabetes is now a carb-controlled diet.

I have been following your diet for about ten days now in addition to exercising. I have lost about five pounds. I am happy but I also feel tired, foggy, and lethargic during certain times of the day. Is this diet for me?

If you're diabetic or prediabetic and on meds to lower your blood sugar, you may endanger your health by cutting carbs without the ability to check blood glucoses. Make sure to discuss this sort of diet change with your healthcare professional.

If you are not on blood sugar meds, then it may simply be that you are adapting to a new, fat-burning metabolism, and I would say you should expect your energy to improve in short order. You may need more carbs because of the kind of exercise you do. Or—and this is very common—you may not be getting enough salt, calcium, magnesium, or zinc (see Chapter 13 for how to supplement). Fatigue persisting beyond four days is a red flag and you need to discuss your case in detail with a good low-carb doc in your area before continuing (see Resources).

Do I count carbs from all the veggies I eat?

Carbs from every source count. But undigestible fiber doesn't. However, the label won't tell you what portion of the fiber is digestible, so the recommendation is to cut the fiber content in half and subtract that figure from the total carb count.

What about liquor, wine, and beer? These break down into sugars, so how do they fit into the equation?

It's a common misconception that alcohol breaks down into sugar. In reality, alcohol is metabolized into acetic acid and that is a precursor for triglyceride fats. Different alcoholic beverages have different amounts of carbohydrate, and mixed drinks that taste sweet typically have loads of sugar. Beer is quite high in carbs, whereas dry wines and hard liquors that don't taste sweet (such as vodka and tequila) are quite low.

How much alcohol can I have?

A better question might be, How much alcohol is too much? Studies show that four drinks or more per day is clearly associated with bad health outcomes. Women who drink any alcohol appear to have an increased risk of breast cancer compared to women who do not drink, so if you have a bad family history you may want to consider not drinking. When I lived in Napa, I came to appreciate how wine is integrated with a healthy social life, but still recommended my patients keep it to two drinks per day. One of my favorite desserts is about 1–2 ounces of white wine mixed with kombucha.

What do you recommend for intestinal upset, like indigestion and bloating?

The solution to intestinal upset depends on the cause! But one thing that may help is to eat something acidic before the meals that bother you—like a (fermented) pickle or half a teaspoon of vinegar. If that doesn't help, see your doctor.

I've lost about 40 percent of my hair as I've gotten older, which wasn't great to start, but had been in much better shape. Is there anything I can do?

I've heard from people who are enjoying a cup or so of homemade bone broth at least five days per week that it helps hair, skin, and nails. Trimming any excess carbs and eliminating pro-inflammatory oils is key to enabling your body to respond to the collagen-stimulating effects of broth. You may also want to eat liver, rich in biotin and other vitamins that support healthy hair growth. Desiccated liver pills are an alternative for those who cannot do liver.

Also, if you haven't already done so, be sure to get checked out by your doctor, because auto-immune disease and thyroid can cause hair loss—just to name two of the more common conditions that should be ruled out.

I have reduced my intake of breads and grain substantially, but then I realized that so many other foods have carbs in them such as rice, potatoes, fruits, etc. I don't understand how I will be able to maintain all of these restrictions without severely restricting my diet to mostly fat, vegetables, and meat.

Rest assured that if you cut out a good portion of the empty-calorie carbs, you have opened the door to expanding the nutritional variety of your diet, not shrinking it. The reason it can feel restrictive at first is that you might imagine 80 percent of the products in the middle aisles of your go-to grocery store now have been cordoned off. So in the beginning, moving to a lower-carb diet can feel limiting, especially if you are trying to avoid vegetable oils at the same time.

Expect a six-month period for transitioning to new habits. During this time you may need to learn new cooking skills (steaming vegetables, making salad dressing, working with new ingredients); you may also need to find new grocery stores, new restaurants, even new people to hang out with.

I have found that many of my patients on the standard high-carb diet are eating a lot more convenience (junk) foods than they realize. It's not because they're lazy. It's because no one ever told them that you do have to learn at least a few basic cooking skills to eat anything other than a high-carb diet.

This is much more easily said than done, I realize, which is why this question touches on an essential solution to the puzzle of achieving long-term success with healthy eating. One mental trick that may help you make the adjustment is rather than thinking of it as cutting down or focusing on how much you're missing, try to think of it as opening up space in your daily routines for greater variety.

One great way to accelerate this transition process is by joining a social media group to meet other people trying to go low-carb and to learn about the best farmers markets, gardening clubs, grocery stores, butchers, and restaurants in your area.

Do dehydrated foods count as raw? Would making a bunch of organic jerky be a good way to get in raw meat?
No. The drying alters the molecules in ways that make them less bio-active. Still, jerky is a great grab-and-go food.

What is your opinion of the popular topic in holistic nutrition circles regarding the acid/alkaline balance and the notion that most people need to consume more alkalinizing/catabolic foods and less acid-forming, anabolic ones?
The acid/alkaline balance theory originated in a time before physiologists had a solid understanding of renal function, and this theory is incompatible with our current understanding of human physiology. (See question on milk leaching calcium from bones, page 396.)

Is soy sauce is okay or not? Would you recommend any brand?
Fermented soy sauces are fine! We look for Kikkoman, Yamase, and any bottle that says "fermented" or "traditionally produced" and does not say "hydrolyzed" anywhere.

What diet would you recommend for vegetarians in order to get the proper amount of good fats?
Vegetarians can get all the healthy fats they need by including dairy and eggs in their diet, but it is particularly important for these to come from pastured animals.

I'm not a vegetarian, and I am fully committed to the Four Pillars. But I am just wondering what, if anything, can be adapted for my vegetarian family members.

Vegetarians can benefit from fermenting and sprouting foods, which is particularly important for non–meat eaters (who tend to get more carbohydrates than they need) because, as explained in Chapter 10, these processes reduce the empty carbohydrate content and generate new nutrients.

Are walnut and macadamia nut oils good for you?

If it tastes like walnut or macadamia nuts, then yes. The presence of a pleasant, identifiable flavor is one of the best indications of a good oil. Walnut is great for salads but not for cooking because it's very high in omega-3, while macadamia nut oil is high in saturated fats and great for both.

I eat Ezekiel 4:9 sprouted grain bread as toast in the morning. What is your take on this bread?

That's what we buy!

Is cold-pressed better than expeller-pressed?

It's the same thing, just a different term.

Is "high oleic" canola oil okay? I read about it and it seems to be more stable when cooking, equal to that of olive oil, but you never know.

Canola manufacturers try to emphasize the "high oleic" content of some canola oils as a selling point. But because canola has so much omega-3, unless the manufacturer avoids all the normal refining processes, much of that omega-3 will end up as distorted, harmful fats. This is true even for expeller-pressed oils. When it comes to factory-produced oils, as opposed to the artisanal (that tend to be much more expensive and will say unfiltered, unrefined), pressing is just the first step of many.

Does heat destroy the omega-3 fats and conjugated linoleic acid in grass-fed butter or is it more stable for some reason?

Heat also destroys the omega-3 and CLA in butter, so raw butter is superior. Keep in mind that cooking any butter at high heat (sizzling) starts to damage its special nutrients.

If people are supposed to burn body fat, why do we need any carbs?

Our fast-twitch muscle fibers use glycogen (a storage form of carb) to fuel bouts of intense exercise.

Beyond that, if we've optimized our fat-burning ability, then our bodies only need about two tablespoons (about thirty grams) of glucose per day to run cells lacking mitochondria, such as red blood cells. That amount is easily supplied by a gluconeogenesis, a process whereby the liver converts amino acids into glucose. Gluconeogenesis enables animals to manufacture glucose when their diet contains little to none.

I'd love to know your stance on prenatal vitamins versus receiving adequate nutrition through nourishing foods. I worry that if I am already eating grass-fed liver, bone broth, and varieties of nutrient-dense vegetables that I could be setting myself up for toxicity problems by adding a vitamin.

Toxicity is rare with naturally produced vitamins. However most pills are made using synthetic vitamins. These industrial products contain a mix of molecules we need and molecules that are close enough to the real thing to bind to receptors. But these almost-natural molecules will not function like the real thing and, because they grab up receptor real estate, their presence can actually block the real vitamin's ability to help you. This is why I recommend supplementing with no more than 100 percent of the RDA of a given vitamin, at least for the long term. A brand of vitamins called Standard Process sources the genuine vitamin from nature. However, their pills are really large and hard for some people to swallow.

Can *Deep Nutrition* save my children from braces?

Possibly, but there are many variables, including birth timing, genetics, and their current ages. As with everything else, optimal nutrition will have greater impact the earlier you start.

A quick story on braces. When I was six, my mouth was full of crooked teeth. By age nine they were perfectly straight. At the time my mom was making lots of chicken liver because it was cheap. We had no idea about good nutrition, so the liver went away once my dad started earning more money. When my wisdom teeth came in, there was not enough room and they were pulled. Of course, this personal anecdote is pretty weak support for the idea that *Deep Nutrition* can guarantee your child freedom from braces. But it does align nicely with the idea that optimal nutrition gives any child the best chance to develop as well as possible, an idea *Deep Nutrition* embraces with both arms.

Can vaccines cause autism?

Researchers have long since dismissed the idea that vaccines are the root cause of autism. However, there is an uncommon form of the disorder, associated with loss of aquired skills, called regressive autism—in contrast to other forms of autism—that can often be diagnosed between the ages of eighteen and thirty months. While it can occur in unvaccinated children, there is some possibility that the immune system stress of vaccines (or infections, or new foods being introduced) plays a contributing, but not primary, role in the disorder.

You say nutrient-dense foods are key to lasting health and giving birth to healthy babies, that wild over farmed is better, and that small family farms that have space for animals are best. But how are eight billion people supposed to get this stuff when, frankly, most people can't afford it?

To paraphrase William Money from the movie *Unforgiven*, "supposed to" has nothing to do with it. It's a great question, but it isn't a question of science. It's a political question best directed toward any policy-maker interested in encouraging a sustainable match between the human population and what remains of the natural environment we all depend upon to provide natural, nutrient-dense foods.

Is it okay to cook with ground flaxseed? I make a muffin with ground flaxseed and coconut flour but am not sure if the oil in the ground seed is being damaged by baking.

Whole flours, when freshly ground, still contain antioxidants that do protect the oils from oxidative damage during baking. The key is keeping your muffin moist.

Have you found any folks who, due to a lifetime of poor nutrition, etc., simply cannot optimize their fat digestion? What do you recommend in this case? Are more carbs "needed" by these people?

They don't need more carbs. They need to reactivate their fat-digestion enzymes (just as they need to revive fat-*burn* enzymes throughout the body). The body can do this but it takes patience. Start slow.

I cut my carbs and increased my healthy fats according to your suggestions. After twenty years of cramps, bloating, and horrible gas, I can now tolerate dairy. What explains this?

Eliminating the excess sugar (from starchy and sweet foods) that promotes pathogenic microbes and impedes the growth of beneficial ones, and eliminating pro-inflammatory fats, are two big factors that facilitate repair of the gastric and immune systems, allowing us to tolerate and digest a wider variety of foods, which would explain your renewed ability to enjoy dairy.

I'd like to buy sprouted breads but I notice they have added gluten. Can I buy it anyway or do I need to make my own?

Gluten is the protein in wheat that makes dough glue-y. It's added to Ezekiel brand bread because truly sprouted grain breads would be very crumbly without it. If you have a gluten allergy, Ezekiel is not a good choice. Otherwise, it's fine!

Of course, sourdough bread is another excellent option.

Weston Price didn't do any studies; his work was purely observational. What value is that?

Observational surveys such as the ones Price did on human populations are indeed a valuable research tool, and the now-famous Framingham Studies are largely observational surveys. Price also did extensive laboratory research. His book, *Nutrition and Physical Degeneration,* gives plenty of details on both.

How can I explain the fact that vegetable oil is unhealthy to my friends who don't like science?

Show them this list of foods nearly everyone agrees are not good for you: Doritos, Funions, McDonald's fries, Domino's Pizza, Frito-Lay potato chips, Hot Pockets, Oreos, Ring Dings, Twinkies, Krispy Kreme donuts, Goldfish crackers, Milky Way bars, Cheetos, Cool Whip, Easy Cheese (that spray cheese), Cinnabon. What is the one ingredient they all have in common? Vegetable oil. And lots of it.

Vegetable oils contain omega-6. Isn't that the reason they're bad for us?

No. The problem is the processing that distorts all the PUFA fatty acids, including both the omega-3 and the omega-6.

Would it be fair to conclude that all seed oils are bad and nut oils are good?

It's about the starting material as much as it's about the processing. You can get poor quality olive oil and high quality grapeseed. So I guess I could rephrase that: It's really about how much you are paying. If you have to pay more, it's probably because the manufacturer is doing it right.

You mentioned that when heating canola oil, it can actually increase the amount of trans fat. What kind of increase are we talking about?

The starting amount ranges from a low of 1.8 percent to a high of roughly 5 percent. After cooking, the content of trans fat depends entirely on details: time, temperature, acidity. I've read reports showing that it can increase to 25 percent during deep frying.

Our kids are allergic to dairy and won't eat very much collards, broccoli, or other calcium-rich vegetables or fish with bone. How can I get them enough calcium?

Calcium supplements are perfect for situations like yours. There are many arguments about which kind of calcium is the most bioavailable, but the differences are insignificant, so just get whatever is the easiest to swallow. I don't, however, advise coral calcium since destroying the coral reef to obtain calcium is incompatible with the core concept of the *Deep Nutrition* philosophy, that our genes depend on nature (and our ability to connect to it by way of the consumption of traditional food). And don't forget about bone broths! When made using standard aromatic vegetables (onion, celery, carrot) each cup has about 100 milligrams of calcium, about a third as much as milk.

What is the protein content of bone stock that gels nicely in the fridge?

The protein content of gelatin depends entirely upon details of your cooking process. As a guess I would say it is likely to be similar to the protein content of various prepared gelatins, which is about one gram per two to four ounces. The benefits of broth go beyond the amino acid counts, however.

I've considered fasting for extended periods based on the idea that our ancestors might go for weeks or more without eating when the hunt was bad or non-existent. Is that a good idea?

In general, our diets are less nutrient intense and more pro-inflammatory—both of these factors make us more fragile and less physiologically sound than our ancestors were. For these reasons, three or four days of fasting is probably the maximum amount of time that would benefit us before the downsides begin to outweigh the up.

Should I go for a lower-quality olive oil that is from a second press with a higher smoke point?

Although it's very useful to know that saturated fats have a higher smoke point than other natural oils, when it comes to processed oils smoke point can get a bit tricky, because highly processed oils, like saturated fat, can have a high smoke point as well. And that's a real problem, as it allows cooks to use, and reheat and reheat, oils that, although not smoking, are still undergoing massive chemical damage. The best chefs use saturated oils and fats rich in saturated fatty acids for high-heat cooking. Whenever using ingredients high in poly- or monounsaturated fats, they watch their dishes closely, stirring constantly and ensuring the more delicate fats, like olive oil, never smoke. So follow their lead: saturated fat for high heat. And use other quality, antioxidant-rich oils for moderate heat, but take care to keep these relatively delicate oils from smoking.

Is roasting a good way to cook meat?

Roasting generates more complex molecules that enhance flavor, but it can also generate unhealthy compounds. Adding antioxidants (fresh veggies, spices, and herbs) helps your body deal with those unhealthy compounds.

I don't like cold sauerkraut. If I heat it, am I destroying the probiotics?

If you heat it to steaming hot, there may not be many surviving bacteria. So I recommend warming it very gently, to something close to body temperature.

What is a good replacement for salad dressing oil if you don't like the taste of olive oil?

Try to match the flavor profiles of the salad with an oil that you like. For example, peanut and sesame for Asian themed salads, walnut with Mediterranean, avocado oil for a more citrusy flavor. Don't forget to use a vinegar that tastes good, for example, balsamic. A really good vinegar might even turn you into a fan of olive oil!

Is caffeine harmful?

Some people notice they feel bad from it, and if that's the case for you, then obviously you should avoid it. If not, I'm not sure it's a problem. For what it's worth, my dad has been drinking several quarts of coffee per day since I've known him, and he's still going strong!

I've read that Asians are genetically adapted to eating more starch. Is that true?

I've found that carbohydrates are an equal-opportunity metabolic offender. While I worked in Hawaii, folks who ate starchy foods regularly, whether Thai, Chinese, Korean, Japanese, Filipino, or what have you, developed diabetes as frequently as Caucasians, Hispanics, and African Americans who ate too many carbs. And no matter a person's race, blood sugars improve by cutting carbs.

What are your thoughts on microwaving?

Microwaves are good for heating liquids, melting cheese, and reheating previously cooked foods. Make sure to avoid microwaving in styrofoam and non-microwave-safe plastics.

Do you have any data to support the idea that microwaving food is unhealthy?

There is surprisingly little research on potential differences between microwaving food and conventional cooking. Most research supports the idea that any kind of cooking reduces nutritional content of foods, and the higher the temperature and longer the food is cooked, the more nutrition is lost. This makes sense to me.

In addition to the damage caused by heat, microwaves produce ionizing radiation. Of course they tell us that the wavelength of their microwaves specifically targets only water molecules. In my view, the radiation is unlikely to be 100 percent absorbed by water, and any escaping ionizing radiation could theoretically damage many molecules in ways that radiant heat does not. Supporting this idea is the fact that protein-rich foods often come out of the microwave rubbery—a sign of potentially harmful molecular polymerization.

Still, I don't feel it's necessary to toss your microwave. I would caution against using recipes that rely solely on microwaves for cooking, and be especially careful when reheating high-protein foods, like meat.

I had coronary bypass surgery three years ago. I started eating the Human Diet last year. My doctor wants me to stay on my cholesterol-lowering statin. How do I determine if I really need to be on statins or not?

The answer to whether statins will benefit you depends in part on your cholesterol numbers off the statin, but doing justice to this topic would require another book. It also depends on what you're putting into your body. For most people who have been following a *Deep Nutrition* diet for a full year, then, at this point, staying on target with the diet is going to do you far more good than any statin.

However, because doctors are so misinformed about the role of dietary fat in causing heart disease, we put way too much faith in statins. So if you are one of the millions of Americans on statins now learning about this topsy-turvy world of fats, you are probably finding yourself caught between your cardiologist and a hard place. The fact is, once you have undergone heart surgery, your doctor will consider it "proven" that you have dangerous amounts of atherosclerosis and is unlikely to seriously consider stopping your statin.

How do I talk to my doctor about ordering a test of my LDL particle size?

As I explain in Chapter 7, an overabundance of smaller size LDL particles can indicate a problem with your lipid cycle, most likely resulting from a dysfunctional (oxidized and/or glycated) protein coat. When your LDL particles are not working right, no matter whether your LDL cholesterol number is high or low, the particles are likely to precipitate out of circulation, land on your arterial walls, and promote plaque formation. But standard cholesterol testing won't provide LDL particle size information. To get the information on LDL (and HDL) particle size, ask your doctor for an advanced lipid panel.

There is only one company currently providing these kinds of tests: Lab-Corp NMR LipoProfile. They currently offer two tests that I find useful: the NMR profile and the Cardio IQ. Be aware you may need to foot the bill yourself, as insurance doesn't often pay for these more advanced tests. If your doctor refuses to order the test for you, there are several direct-to-consumer lab companies that can enable consumers in all but a few states to take charge of their own health and order tests without their doctors' help. (For the most up-to-date info on how to order, visit DrCate.com.)

I ordered my NMR LipoProfile. How do I interpret the results?

If you understand all the concepts in Chapter 7, you will be able to interpret the results yourself! If you need help, you can sign up for a consultation or join a group education class at DrCate.com.

What is your stance about vegetable juicing? I'm aware that it's not part of any traditional diet, but could it help to get more nutrients when you can't get enough veggies in one day?

Juicing wastes a good deal of the vegetable and ends up providing a lot of sugar. Blending into smoothies is much more nutritious.

I recommend using smoothie recipes that call for only one piece of fruit per serving at most. Otherwise you end up getting more sugar than you need. Some people don't do well with blended vegetables, though, because blender blades can completely homogenize the cells. That can expose the stomach and upper digestive tract to a load of nutrients to which we are unaccustomed, causing bloating or heartburn.

I buy pickles and sauerkraut. Can I do anything with the leftover juice?

I drink the leftover juice after workouts and splash some in my salad. We also use a few tablespoons of the juice as a starter culture when making our own sauerkraut.

I get that we should avoid sugar. What about other sweeteners like Nutrasweet, Splenda, and Stevia?

The sweetness receptors in your intestines—taste buds in your gut—react to all sweetness, whether from sugar, Stevia, or artificial sources, the same way. This "gut perception" of sweetness initiates insulin production, which can, in turn, promote the production of fat.

Even if artificial sweeteners were relatively safe, like Stevia, I'd still advise you to save your money for real food. These products desensitize your palate to the sweetness nature puts in almost everything.

If I'm not hungry in the morning, do I still need to eat breakfast?

No. If you're not hungry, don't eat. Just don't use the skipped breakfast as an excuse to eat junk food later on.

The research suggesting that people who skip breakfast gain more weight is flawed by, among other things, the fact that the surveys don't consider that people who say they skip breakfast typically eat something junky for a snack before lunch, like the sugar and trans fat coffee confections, muffins, danishes, and energy bars that most of my patients (the same ones who say they skip breakfast) with metabolic issues tell me they eat.

How much salt is too much?

The idea that most people need to watch their salt is a myth. If you have normal kidney and heart functions, then even on a high-sodium junk food diet, your body can deal with the sodium content. What your body can't deal with is—you guessed it—vegetable oils and sugars. The low-salt message is actually dangerous, not only because it confuses people into thinking that salt is the enemy when it's really these other toxins but also because, at least in my experience, more people get into trouble from not having enough salt in their diets than from having too much.

My friend who is into CrossFit is on a ketogenic diet. What is that?

A ketogenic diet brings about a state of nutritional ketosis, which maximizes your body's ability to burn stored body fat. It's a fat-burning diet taken to an extreme. Dr. Atkins discovered that it was so powerful at suppressing appetite, he almost never needed to use prescription appetite suppressants.

Unfortunately, depending on exactly how you do it and how active you are, a ketogenic diet may so deplete your body of carbohydrates that it forces it to convert protein into sugar to supply your body's carbohydrate needs.

Still, because ketogenic diets can optimize fat-burning, and fat-burning is a powerful tool to recalibrate your metabolism in a relatively short time, several researchers are studying ketogenic diets as a tool to help treat epilepsy, brain tumors, and breast cancer and as a way to optimize sports performance, with promising results.

Is the Human Diet a ketogenic diet?

The diet I describe in the previous chapter does not call for the kind of extreme carb restriction typical of a ketogenic diet. However, the principles outlined in this book are entirely compatible with a ketogenic diet. If you're already on a ketogenic diet, you'll find it easy to modify the plan to keep you in ketosis.

I'm weaning my toddler. How can I get him started eating the Human Diet?

Studies show that the foods mom eats during pregnancy have an influence on the taste preferences of the newborn. In my patients' experience, when a child is ready to accept foods, they'll accept whatever you give them—particularly if you're eating it, too. This even includes things like Brie cheese, egg yolks, chicken liver, and seaweed. Just be sure to give age-appropriate portions and blend or puree if needed as you would when introducing any food.

Shouldn't I supplement with omega-3?

Because omega-3 is so easily destroyed during extraction of the oil from the parent food, and because it degrades so quickly during storage, I recommend food as your go-to omega-3 source. If you don't eat grass-fed dairy or fish, you can still get plenty of omega-3 from raw or sprouted nuts and seeds. Your liver can elongate the short-chain omega-3 PUFAs into the longer DHA chain your brain requires, but only if your diet is free of vegetable oils (because they damage a key enzyme required for elongating PUFAs).

I'm too busy to make major changes. What are some simple things I can do instead of adapting the program wholesale that will still enable me to feel improvements?

Here are five ways to get started:

1. **Eat a big colorful salad four days per week with a non–vegetable oil dressing.** There should be four cups total salad volume, including a minimum of four kinds of vegetables. Fresh salads with a variety of vegetables are particularly important if you're not ready to go "deep" into *Deep Nutrition*. Because vegetable oil–free salad dressings are hard to find, you will need to make your own. But it doesn't have to take longer than one more minute: stock up on good quality oils and a couple of good vinegars, including a good balsamic, and learn to combine them in real time on your salads. I

have provided a few really quick ideas for combining these in the previous chapter.

2. Include some grass-fed dairy fat in your daily diet. This includes cheese, cream, cream cheese, butter, and full-fat cottage cheese and yogurt. Raw is better, where available.

3. Get bone stock. Not just for its health benefits but because it facilitates so many fast, healthy lunches (see the recipe for Drop-in Soup, in the previous chapter). Check your local Costco, a good source of discounted high-quality foods. And there are plenty of higher quality mail-order services popping up around the country (see Resources). If you like Asian food, trying buying *pho* (a Vietnamese soup; you have to ask if they make it with real bones) or fish head soup from a Filipino restaurant.

4. Eat organ meats at least once weekly. You can buy liver pate or liverwurst at most decent grocery stores and spread it on a vegetable oil–free cracker or sprouted grain toast. (US Wellness meats can mail you a liverwurst that is shockingly savory and delicious.) If that's not going to happen, then include seafood three times weekly, preferably raw at least once—raw oysters, *sashimi, ceviche,* pickled herring. If you hate seafood and fish or are allergic, then use pasture-raised eggs three times weekly instead, and be sure to cook only so long that the yolk stays runny. (I recommend this rule for anyone not including liver or other organ meats in their diet on a weekly basis.)

5. Eat probiotic-rich foods once a day. To keep your digestive and immune systems working smoothly, include probiotic-rich foods in your diet on a regular basis. The most popular probiotic-rich food in the United States is yogurt— buy plain and flavor it yourself—and real pickles and sauerkraut are also great sources of digestive-boosting organisms, and you only need a few bites to get some benefits if you use these to start your meal.

EPILOGUE: HEALTH WITHOUT HEALTHCARE

In *Selling Sickness,* authors Ray Moynihan and Alan Cassels explain that "there's a lot of money to be made telling healthy people they're sick." The prologue to their book, published in 2005, paraphrases a candid interview with Merck's former chief executive Henry Gadsen, originally published in *Fortune* more than thirty years ago. "Suggesting he'd rather Merck be more like chewing gum maker Wrigley's, Gadsen said it had long been his dream to make drugs for healthy people. Because then, Merck would be able to 'sell to everyone.'" The case that the healthcare industry does not exist for the betterment of our health has also been well-argued by a number of experts from respected institutions, including Harvard and the *New England Journal of Medicine,* and so for the most part I've resisted making grand indictments of the healthcare industry and attacking its failure to keep us well. But it's not just industry that's to blame. This kind of corporate thinking trickles down from the boardroom into your local clinic, contaminating individual doctors—like yours.

While I was building my practice, my boss explained to me that to be "successful" I would need more chronic patients in my panel. He explained that putting people on blood pressure and other medications, which would need periodic monitoring, was key to building a busy practice. I understood that from his perspective keeping my patients healthy—and medication free—was bad for business. This entrepreneurial mentality is endemic in today's healthcare model. But these days it's gone beyond populating one's own practice with as many unhealthy people as possible and doing little to improve their health. Now the name of the game is to push as many drugs as you can by whatever means you can get away with. When I interviewed with the Chief of Family Medicine at a large medical corporation on the West Coast, he explained that, since he was part of a team of people who arranged for pharmaceutical companies to issue cash grants, he was in a position to offer me a particularly enticing salary.

"What are the grants for?" I asked.

"We have a quality improvement program that tracks physician pre-scribing patterns. We call it 'quality' but it's really about money."

And that's all it's about. It works like this. In his organization, any pa-tient with LDL cholesterol over 100 is put on a cholesterol-lowering med-ication. Any person with a blood pressure higher than 140/90 is put on a blood pressure medication. Any person with "low bone density" is put on a bone-remodeling inhibitor. And so on. The doctors who prescribe the most get big bonuses. Those who prescribe the least get fired. With a hint of in-credulousness in his voice, he explained, "So far, every time we've asked for funding for our program, the drug companies give it to us." If this is where healthcare is headed, then these hybrid physicians-executives will instinc-tively turn their gaze to our children and invent more creative methods to bulldoze an entire generation into the bottomless pit of chronic disease.

Merck CEO Henry Gadsen's thirty-year-old dream was to make healthy people buy drugs they didn't really need. But he was dreaming small. What I now see happening is more sinister and more profitable, and promises to have longer-lasting repercussions than merely creating diagnoses that lead to unnecessary prescriptions. What I see is a massive campaign of nutri-tion-related misinformation that has reordered our relationship with food and reprogrammed our physiologies. Industry has moved past selling sick-ness and learned how to create it. Whether by intent or simply fortuitous coincidence, today's definition of a healthy diet enables corporations to sell us cheap, easily stored foods that will put more money in their pockets and more people in the hospital. By denying our bodies the foods of our an-cestors and severing ourselves from our culinary traditions, we are chang-ing our genes for the worse. Just as corporations have rewritten the genetic codes of fruit and vegetables to better suit their needs, they are now, in ef-fect, doing the same thing to us.

But there's one thing they've overlooked. Fruits and vegetables can't fight back. We can.

ACKNOWLEDGMENTS

To Dado and Steve for faith that truth has value and being the best in the business. To Whitney for talent and superhuman levels of hard work. To Kobe, Steve, Pau, and Dwight for taking the lead. To Gary Vitti and Tim DeFrancesco of the Lakers for introducing real nutrition to the world of professional sports. To dozens of physicians at UCLA and UCSF for interviews and opinions. To Dr. Stephen Marquardt for insights into his groundbreaking research. To Jo Robinson for her story of the discovery of omega-3 fatty acids. To the Price-Pottenger Nutrition Foundation for making the extensive works of Weston A. Price and Dr. Francis Pottenger publicly available. To my brother Dan Shanahan for cartoons. To Mark Sisson and Brad Kearns for fostering a vibrant and thoughtful community. And to all the scientists and researchers who still believe in the scientific method.

Resources

CARB COUNTING TOOL:
SIMPLY COUNTING CARBS

Milk Group

- 10 ounces of milk
- I cup of soy milk
- 10 ounces of buttermilk
- 16 ounces of plain whole milk yogurt

Carbs in Yogurt

- **Flavored yogurt** contains added sugars, averaging 35 grams per cup.
- **Plain yogurt** will contain fewer net carbs than what is listed here if it tastes very sour, indicating bacteria have fermented the sugar, and in so doing created more nutrition for you.

Starch Group (measured after cooking)

- I slice of bread (weighing I ounce)
- 1/4 large bagel or large muffin
- 1/2 hamburger bun, hotdog bun, pita bread, English muffin
- Rice, pasta millet, couscous (1/3 cup)
- Beans (pinto, kidney, garbanzo, lentils; 1/2 cup)
- Starchy vegetable (potato, corn, peas, sweet potato, yam; 1/2 cup)
- Tortilla, flour or corn (6-inch size)
- Crackers (6 saltine or 3 graham squares)
- Popcorn (3 cups)
- Oatmeal, kasha, grits, bulgur (1/2 cup)
- Boxed cereal (Cheerios, 3/4 cup; Raisin Bran, 1/2 cup)

Fruit Group

- I small apple, orange, peach, pear, or nectarine (1/2 if large fruit)
- I small banana (1/2 of average banana)
- 1/2 grapefruit
- 1/2 cup unsweetened applesauce
- 3/4 cup fresh pineapple chunks, blueberries, or blackberries
- 17 grapes
- 3 prunes
- I date
- 1¼ cups strawberries, or watermelon

- 1 cup cantaloupe, honeydew, or papaya
- 1 large kiwi
- 2 tablespoons raisins, dried and sweetened cranberries
- 1/2 cup orange juice, apple juice, or grapefruit juice

Sweets Group

- Cookie (2½-inch)
- Ice cream (1/2 cup)
- Chocolate or candy bar (1 ounce)

Non-Starchy Vegetables, Nuts, and Seeds

The following non-starchy vegetables contain about 5 grams of carbohydrate per 1/2 cup cooked or 1 cup raw:

Artichokes, asparagus, green beans, beets, broccoli, Brussels sprouts, cabbage, carrots, cauliflower, eggplant, greens, jicama, kohlrabi, leeks, okra, onions, pea pods, peppers, pumpkin, spinach, summer squash, tomato sauce, turnips, and zucchini.

Nuts and seeds contain about 5 grams of carbohydrate per ounce (handful).

Meats, Proteins, and Fats

The following meats, protein foods, and fats contain little or no carbohydrate:

meat	tuna	tofu
chicken	mayonnaise	eggs
butter	cheese	olives
fish	avocado	sour cream
liver/liverwurst	cottage cheese	oyster
marrow bones	cream cheese	shellfish
oil		

Free Foods

The following are insignificant sources of carbohydrate:

coffee	allspice	basil
tea (green, black, herbal)	tumeric	parsley
lettuce, salad greens	vanilla bean	thyme
broth	spices in general (dried and fresh)	oregano
salsa		tarragon
garlic	ginger	herbs in general (dried or fresh)
lemons/limes	mineral water	
cinnamon	sprouts	
nutmeg	radish	

PROTEIN-COUNTING TOOL:
SIMPLY COUNTING PROTEIN

Beef
- Hamburger patty, 4 ounces–28 grams of protein
- Steak, 6 ounces–42 grams of protein
- Most cuts of beef–7 grams of protein per ounce

Chicken
- Chicken breast, 3½ ounces–30 grams of protein
- Chicken thigh, average size–10 grams of protein
- Drumstick–11 grams of protein
- Wing–6 grams of protein
- Chicken meat, cooked, 4 ounces–35 grams of protein

Fish
- Most fish fillets or steaks are about 22 grams of protein for 3½ ounces (100 grams) of cooked fish, or 6 grams of protein per ounce
- Tuna, 6-ounce can–40 grams of protein

Pork
- Pork chop, average size–22 grams of protein
- Pork loin or tenderloin, 4 ounces–29 grams of protein
- Ham, 3-ounce serving–19 grams of protein
- Ground pork, 1 ounce raw–5 grams; 3 ounces cooked–22 grams of protein
- Bacon, 1 slice–3 grams of protein
- Canadian-style bacon (back bacon), 1 slice–5 to 6 grams of protein

Note: An ounce of meat or fish has about 7 grams of protein.

Eggs and Dairy
- Egg, large–6 grams of protein
- Milk, 1 cup–8 grams of protein
- Cottage Cheese, ½ cup–15 grams of protein
- Yogurt, 1 cup–usually 8 to 12 grams of protein; check label
- Soft cheeses (mozzarella, Brie, Camembert)–6 grams of protein per ounce
- Medium cheeses (cheddar, Swiss)–7 or 8 grams of protein per ounce
- Hard cheeses (Parmesan)–10 grams of protein per ounce

Beans (including soy)
- Tofu, ½ cup–20 grams of protein
- Tofu, 1 ounce–2.3 grams of protein
- Soy milk, 1 cup–6 to10 grams of protein
- Most beans (black, pinto, lentils, etc.), ½ cup cooked–about 7 to 10 grams of protein
- Soy beans, ½ cup cooked–14 grams of protein
- Split peas, ½ cup cooked–8 grams of protein

Nuts and Seeds
- Peanut butter, 2 tablespoons–8 grams of protein
- Almonds, ¼ cup–8 grams of protein
- Peanuts, ¼ cup–9 grams of protein
- Cashews, ¼ cup–5 grams of protein
- Pecans, ¼ cup–2.5 grams of protein
- Sunflower seeds, ¼ cup–6 grams of protein
- Pumpkin seeds, ¼ cup–8 grams of protein
- Flax seeds, ¼ cup–8 grams of protein

HELPFUL WEBSITES

When I'm consulting with clients across the country to optimize their diets, I refer people to the following websites to help folks secure the best locally sourced ingredients available in the area:

www.EatWild.com: Excellent information on where to buy pasture-raised meats and eggs. Organized by state.

www.RealMilk.com: Volunteer chapter leaders from the Weston A. Price foundation post sources of fresh dairy on this web site.

www.SlowFoodUSA.org: Supports consumption of good, clean, and fair food. Members join local convivia.

www.LocalHarvest.org: Interactive map for finding farmers markets, CSAs (Community Supported Agriculture), and events, including workshops for learning artesanal food production techniques.

RECOMMENDED BRANDS

■ LiveCulture Fermented Foods
Real pickles: Bubbies Whole Dill Pickles
Real saurkraut: Bubbies Saurkraut
Kombucha: GT Dave Synergy (lower in sugars than most other kombuchas)

■ Dairy
Yogurt: Wallaby, Soneyfield, Organic Valley, Kalona Supernatural
Cottage cheese: Kolona Supernatural, Organic Valley
Cream cheese: Organic Valley
Sour cream: Kolona Supernatural
Cream: Kolona Supernatural, Organic Valley Pasture Raised
Milk: Kolona Supernatural, Organic Valley Pasture Raised
Butter: Kerrygold, Kolona Supernatural, Organic Valley Pasture Butter
Cheese: Organic Valley, Dubliner (check Costco for great deals on Dubliner
    and other grass-fed or artisanal raw cheeses)

■ Fish and Meats
Liverwurst and bratwurst (surprisingly tasty): US Wellness Meats
    (exclusively online)
Beef jerky: Nick's Sticks Certified Paleo Grass-Fed Beef and Organ Meat
    (exclusively online)
100 percent grass-fed hotdogs: Applegate Naturals, Fork in the Road
Wild sardines in extra virgin olive oil: Crown Prince, Wild Planet, King Oscar
    (bone in, for bone-building minerals)
Kipper snacks, naturally smoked: Crown Prince
Smoked oysters in olive oil: Crown Prince
Grilled chicken strips: Applegate Naturals
Sausage: Applegate Naturals
Bacon: Applegate Naturals

■ Miscellaneous
Bone stock (chicken and beef, organic): Pacific Foods
Sprouted pumpkin and sunflower seeds: Go Raw, Living Intentions
    (usually found in the freezer section)
Sprouted almonds and flavored nuts: Living Intentions
Sprouted grain bread: Ezekiel 4:9, Alvarado Street Bakery
Mayo: Primal Kitchens (online and select stores)

DOCTORS IN YOUR AREA

Several webmasters maintain lists of doctors who are familiar with alternatives to the conventional USDA and ADA nutrition guidelines:

- Jimmy Moore's List of Low Carb Doctors www.lowcarbdoctors.blogspot.com/
- Robb Wolf's Paleo Physicians Network www.paleophysiciansnetwork.com/
- Chris Armstrong's Primal Docs www.primaldocs.com/members/

SUGGESTED READING

Abramson, John, *Overdosed America: The Broken Promise of American Medicine*, HarperCollins, 2004.

Baylock, Russel L., *Excitotoxins: The Taste That Kills*, Health Press, 1996.

Cohen, Mark Nathan, *Health and the Rise of Civilization*, Yale University Press, 1989.

Etcoff, Nancy, *Survival of the Prettiest: The Science of Beauty*, Anchor, 2000.

Fearnley-Whittingstall, Hugh, *The River Cottage Meat Book*, Ten Speed Press, 2007.

Furia, Thomas E., *Handbook of Food Additives*, The Chemical Rubber Company, 1968.

Gardeners and Farmers of Centre Vivante, *Preserving Food Without Freezing or Canning: Traditional Techniques Using Salt, Oil, Sugar, Alcohol, Vinegar, Drying, Cold Storage, and Lactic Fermentation*, Chelsea Green Publishing, 1999.

Hatfield, Elaine, *Mirror, Mirror . . . The Importance of Looks in Everyday Life*, State University of New York Press, 1986.

Hill, Annabella, *Mrs. Hill's New Cook Book: A Practical System for Private Families, In Town and Country*, Applewood Books (facsimile edition of the 1867 original).

Hurley, Don, *Natural Causes: Death, Lies and Politics in America's Vitamin and Herbal Supplement Industry*, Broadway, 2006.

Jablonka, Eva, and Marion J. Lamb, *Evolution in Four Dimensions: Genetic, Epigenetic, Behavioral, and Symbolic Variation in the History of Life*, MIT Press, 2006.

Kassirer, Jerome P., *On the Take: How Medicine's Complicity with Big Business Can Endanger Your Health*, Oxford University Press, 2004.

Katz, Ellix Sandor, *Wild Fermentation: The Flavor, Nutrition, and Craft of Live Culture Foods*, Chelsea Green Publishing, 2003.

Kipple, Kenneth F. and Kriemhild Conee Omelas (eds.), *The Cambridge World History of Food*, Cambridge University Press, 2000.

McWilliams, James E., *A Revolution in Eating: How the Quest for Food Shaped America*, Columbia University Press, 2005.

Moynihan, Ray, and Allan Cassels, *Selling Sickness: How the World's Biggest Pharmaceutical Companies are Turning Us All into Patients*, Nation Books, 2005.

Pollan, Michael, *In Defense of Food: An Eater's Manifesto*, Penguin, 2008.

Price, Weston Andrew, *Nutrition and Physical Degeneration*, Price-Pottenger Nutrition Foundation, 2008.

Ravnskov, Uffe, *The Cholesterol Myths: Exposing the Fallacy that Saturated Fat and Cholesterol Cause Heart Disease*, NewTrends, 2000.

Smith, Jeffrey M., *Seeds of Deception: Exposing Industry and Government Lies about the Safety of the Genetically Engineered Foods You're Eating*, Yes! Books, 2003.

NOTES

Author's Note

1. 1994 data shows annual U.S. per capita consumption of vegetable oil at 25.1 killograms per day, equating to 618 calories daily. Data from tables at USDA website shows 2014 consumption is 170 percent of 1995 consumption. Assuming 1994 and 1995 are about the same in terms of per capita consumption, then doing the math for 2014 per capita consumption, we get just over 1,000 calories per day from vegetable oils for the average American. The average calories consumed per day by Americans obviously ranges widely, but 2015 estimates put the average intake at 3,600, where thin people eat 1,700-3,000 depending on activity level. Estimates for health conscious consumers based on personal experience that most health conscious consumers cook at home more often and that reduces their exposure to all vegetable oils. Sources: 1995 data from Table 6 in the article: Polyunsaturated fatty acids in the food chain in the United States, Am J Clin Nutr, January, 2000, vol. 71, no. 1, pp. 179S-188. 2014 data from tables at www.ers.usda.gov/data-products/oil-crops-yearbook.aspx.

2. Protein lipoxidation: detection strategies and challenges, Giancarlo Aldini, Redox Biol, August 5, 2015, pp. 253–266.

3. Oral glycotoxins are a modifiable cause of dementia and the metabolic syndrome in mice and humans, Weijing Cai et al, PNAS, April 1, 2014, vol. 111, no. 13.

4. Changes in breast cancer incidence and mortality in middle-aged and elderly women in twenty-eight countries with Caucasian majority populations, C. Héry et al, Ann Oncol, 2008, 19 (5), pp. 1009–1018.

5. Source: Surveillance, epidemiology, and end results (SEER) program (www.seer.cancer.gov), SEER 9 area, Age 0-19, accessed online on April 2, 2016, via www.curesearch.org/Incidence-Rates-Over-Time

6. www.cdc.gov/heartdisease/facts.htm

7. Per Alzheimer's.net 2015 statistic on April 2, 2014, at http://www.Alzheimer's.net/resources/Alzheimer's-statistics/

Chapter I

8. Dr. Michael Dexter, Wellcome Trust.

9. Transposable elements: targets for early nutritional effects on epigenetic gene regulation, Waterland RA, Molecular and Cellular Biology, August 2003, vol. 23, no. 15, pp. 5293–5300.

10. *Nutrition and Physical Degeneration,* Price W, Price-Pottenger Foundation, 1945, p. 75.

11. Lifetime risk for diabetes mellitus in the United States, Venkat Narayan KM, JAMA, 2003, 290:1884-1890.

12. Guts and grease: the diet of native americans, Fallon S, Wise Traditions.

13. A mechanistic link between chick diet and December in seabirds? Proceedings of the Royal Society of Biological Sciences, vol. 273, no. 1585, February 22, 2006, pp. 445–550.

14. Maternal vitamin D status during pregnancy and childhood bone mass at age nine years: a longitudinal study, Javaid MK, Obstetrical and Gynecological Survey, 61(5):305-307, May 2006.

15. Epigenetic epidemiology of the developmental origins hypothesis, Waterland RA, Annual Review of Nutrition, vol. 27, August 2007, pp. 363-388.

16. See Chapter 11.

17. *The Paleo Diet: Lose Weight and Get Healthy By Eating the Food You Were Designed to Eat*, Loren Cordain, Wiley, 2002, p. 39.

18. *In Defense of Food: An Eater's Manifesto*, Michael Pollan, Penguin, 2008.

Chapter 2

19. We have between 10 and 100 trillion cells in our body, and each cell has two to three meters of DNA, totaling between 20 and 300 trillion meters. It's only 3,844,000,000 meters to the moon.

20. Pluripotency of mesenchymal stem cells derived from adult marrow, Jiang Y, Nature, July 2002, 4;418(6893):41-9, epub Jun 20, 2002.

21. Epigenetics, the science of change, Environ Health Perspect, March 2006, 114(3): A160–A167.

22. Environmental Health Perspectives, vol. 114, no. 3, March 2006.

23. Toxic optic neuropathy, Indian J Ophthalmol, Mar-Apr 2011, 59(2): 137–141.

24. Epigenetic differences arise during the lifetime of monozygotic , Fraga MF, PNAS, July 26, 2005, vol. 102, no. 30, pp. 10604–9.

25. Epigenetics: a new bridge between nutrition and health, Adv Nutr, November 2010, vol. 1: 8-16, 2010.

26. Osteoporosis: Diagnostic and Therapeutic Principles, Clifford J. Rosen, Humana Press, 1996, p. 51.

27. Genetics of osteoporosis, Peacock M, Endocrine Reviews 23 (3): 303-326.

28. The ghost in your genes, NOVA partial transcript accessed online at http://www.bbc.co.uk/sn/tvradio/programmes/horizon/ghostgenes.shtml

29. Accuracy of DNA methylation pattern preservation by the Dnmt1 methyltransferase, Rachna Goyal, Richard Reinhardt and Albert Jeltsch, Nucl Acids Res, 2006, 34 (4): 1182-1188 doi 10.1093/nar/gkl002.

30. Age-associated sperm DNA methylation alterations: possible implications in offspring disease susceptibility, Jenkins TG, Aston KI, Pflueger C, Cairns BR, Carrell DT, 2014, PLoS Genet, 10(7).

31. Effects of an increased paternal age on sperm quality, reproductive outcome and associated epigenetic risk to offspring, Rakesh Sharma et al, Reproductive Biology and Endocrinology, 2015, 13:35.

32. Age-associated sperm DNA methylation alterations: possible implications in offspring disease susceptibility, Jenkins TG, Aston KI, Pflueger C, Cairns BR, Carrell DT, 2014, PLoS Genet, 10(7).

33. Epigenetic programming by maternal nutrition: shaping future generations, Epigenomics, August 2010, 2(4):539-49.

34. Transposable elements: targets for early nutritional effects on epigenetic gene regulation, Waterland RA, Molecular and Cellular Biology, August 2003, pp. 5293-5300, vol. 23, no. 15.

35. Decreased birthweights in infants after maternal in utero exposure to the Dutch famine of 1944-1945, LH Lumey, Paediatr Perinat Ep, 6:240-53, 1992.

36. Pregnant smokers increases grandkids' asthma risk, Vince G, NewScientist.com news service, 22:00, April 11, 2005.

37. Rethinking the origin of chronic diseases, Mohammadali Shoja et al, BioScience, 62,5 (2012): 470–478.

38. Epigenetics: genome, meet your environment, Pray L, vol. 18, issue 13, 14, July 5, 2004.

39. Article accessed at www.bioinfo.mbb.yale.edu/mbb452a/projects/Dov-S-Greenbaum.html#_edn42

40. Ibid.

41. Influence of S-adenosylmethionine pool size on spontaneous mutation, dam methylation, and cell growth of escherichia coli, Posnick, LM, Journal of Bacteriology, November 1999, pp. 6756–6762, vol. 181, no. 21.

42. A unified genetic theory for sporadic and inherited autism, Proc Natl Acad Sci USA, July 31, 2007, 104(31): 12831–12836.

43. Whole-genome sequencing in autism identifies hot spots for de novo germline mutation, Jacob Michaelson et al, Cell, 151,7 (2012): 1431-1442.

44. Feature co-localization landscape of the human genome, Sci Rep, 2016, 6: 20650.

45. The effects of chromatin organization on variation in mutation rates in the genome, Nat Rev Genet, April 16, 2015, (4): 213–223.

46. Zipf's law states that, if one were to create a histogram containing the total amount of words in a language and their occurrence, the arrangement in rank order would be linear on a double logarithmic scale with a slope of -z. This is the case for all natural languages.

47. Hints of a language in junk DNA, Flam F, Science, 266:1320, 1994.

48. Power spectra of DNA sequences in phage and tumor suppressor genes (TSG), Eisei Takushi, Genome Informatics, 13: 412–413 (2002).

49. Mantegna RN et al, Physics Review Letters 73, 3169 (1994).

50. The relation of maternal vitamin A deficiency to microopthalmia in pigs, Hale F, Texas S J Med 33:228, 1937.

51. The modulation of DNA content: proximate causes and ultimate consequences, Gregory TR, Genome Research, vol. 9, issue 4, pp. 317-324, April 1999.

Chapter 3

52. Ancient precision stone cutting, Lee L, Ancient American: Archaeology of the Americas Before Columbus, February 1997.

53. *Nutrition and Physical Degeneration*, Weston A Price, Price-Pottenger Foundation, 1970, p. 279.

54. Ibid, p. 5.

55. Ibid.

56. Ibid, p. 1.

57. Ibid, p. 31.

58. This argument will be flushed out and supported with statistics in the next chapter.

59. Management of genetic syndromes, Suzanne B. Cassidy, Judith E. Allanson, Wiley, March 22, 2010.

60. *Nutrition and Physical Degeneration,* Price Pottenger Foundation, 1970, p. 12.

61. Effects of malocclusions and orthodontics on periodontal health: evidence from a systematic review, Journal of Dental Education, August 1, 2008, vol. 72, no. 8912-918.

62. *Nutrition and Physical Degeneration,* Weston A Price, Price Pottenger Foundation, 1945, p. 275.

63. Ibid., pp. 274-78.

64. Ibid.

65. Influence of vitamin B6 intake on the content of the vitamin in human milk, West KD, Am J Clin Nutr, September 29, 1976, (9):961-9.

66. *Nutrition and Physical Degeneration,* Weston A Price, Price Pottenger Foundation, 1945, p. 110.

67. Wise Traditions, vol. 8, no. 4, p. 24.

68. *Nutrition and Physical Degeneration,* Weston A Price, Price Pottenger Foundation, 1945, p. 402.

69. *The Ways of My Grandmothers,* Beverly Hungry Wolf, Quill, 1982, p. 186.

70. *Nutrition and Physical Degeneration,* Weston A Price, Price Pottenger Foundation, 1945, pp. 402–03.

71. Vitamins for fetal development: conception to birth, Masterjohn C, Wise Traditions, vol.8, no. 4, winter 2007.

72. *Nutrition and Physical Degeneration,* Weston A Price, Price Pottenger Foundation, 1945, p. 401.

73. Ibid., p. 402

74. Hiraoka, M, Nutritional status of vitamin A, E, C, B1, B2, B6, nicotinic acid, B12, folate, and beta-carotene in young women, J Nutr Sci Vitaminol, February 2001, 47(1):20-27.

75. Serum vitamin A concentrations in asthmatic children in Japan, Mizuno Y, Pediatrics International, vol. 48, issue 3, pp. 261–4.

76. Vitamin D inadequacy has been reported in up to 36 percent of otherwise healthy young adults, and up to 57 percent of general medicine inpatients in the United States, from High prevalence of vitamin D inadequacy and implications for health, Mayo Clin Proc, March 2006, 81(3):297-9.

77. Nutrient intakes of infants and toddlers, Devaney B, Journal of the American Dietetic Association, 104 (1), suppl 1, S14–S21 (2004).

78. Less than adequate vitamin E status observed in a group of preschool boys and girls living in the United States, J Nutr Biochem, February 2006, 17(2):132-8.

79. Vitamin K status of lactating mothers and their infants, Greer FR, Acta Paediatr Suppl, August 1999, 88(430):95-103.

80. Nutritional status of vitamin A, E, C, B1, B2, B6, nicotinic acid, B12, folate, and beta-carotene in young women, Hiraoka, M. J Nutr Sci Vitaminol, February 2001, 47(1):20-27.

81. Consumption of calcium among African American adolescent girls, Goolsby SL, Ethn Dis, spring 2006, 16(2):476-82.

Chapter 4

82. The body beautiful: the classical ideal in ancient greek art, New York Times Art and Design section, May 17, 2015, Alastair Macaulay.

83. The history of fitness, Lance C. Dalleck and Len Kravitz at www.unm.edu/~lkravitz/Article-percent20folder/history

84. The Spirit of Vitalism: Health, Beauty and Strength in Danish Art, 1890–1940, Gertrud Hvidberg-Hansen (editor), Gertrud Oelsner (editor), James Manley (translator), Museum Tusculanum Press, February 28, 2011.

85. National Ambulatory Medical Care Survey: 2012 State and National Summary Tables, table 16, accessed online on March 22, 2016 at: www.cdc.gov/nchs/data/ahcd/namcs_summary/2012_namcs_web_tables.pdf

86. Effects of pelvic skeletal asymmetry on trunk movement: three-dimensional analysis in healthy individuals versus patients with mechanical low back pain, spine, vol. 31(3), February 1, 2006.

87. Smiths recognizable patterns of human malformation, Jones KL, 6th ed, September 2005.

88. Evaluation of the palate dimensions of patients with perennial allergic rhinitis, DePreietas FCN, Int J Pediatric Dent, vol. 11, issue 5, p. 365, September 2001.

89. Dentofacial morphology of mouthbreathing children, Preto R, Braz Cent J, vol. 13, no. 2, 2002.

90. Cephalometric comparisons of craniofacial and upper airway structures in young children with obstructive sleep apnea syndrome, Kawashima S, Ear Nose and Throat Journal, July 2000.

91. Sleep apnea-related cognitive deficits and intelligence: an implication of cognitive reserve theory, Achantis M, J Sleep Res, Mar 2005, 12(1):69-75.

92. Central nervous malformations in presence of clefts reflect developmental interplay, Mueller AA, Int J Oral Maxillofac Surg, April 2007, 36(4):289-95, epub January 2007.

93. Body weight, waist-to-hip ratio, breasts and hips: role in judgments of female attractiveness and desirability for relationships, Singh D, Ethology and Sociobiology, 16, 1995, pp. 483–507.

94. Waist-to-hip ratio and body dissatisfaction among college women and men: the moderating role of depressed symptoms and gender, Joiner T, Int J Eating Disor, 16, 1994, pp. 199–203.

95. Appearance of symmetry, beauty and health in human faces, Zaidel DW, Brain and Cognition, 57, 2005, pp. 261–263.

96. Waist-to-hip ratio and body dissatisfaction among college women and men: the moderating role of depressed symptoms and gender, Joiner T, Int J Eating Disor, 16, 1994, pp. 199–203.

97. Physical attractiveness, dangerousness, and the Canadian criminal code 1, Esses V, Journal of Applied Social Psychology, 18 (12), pp. 1017–1031.

98. Cross-cultural implications of physical attractiveness stereotypes in personnel selection, Shahani-Denning C, Presentation at 27th Annual Conference on Personnel Assessment, available online at www.ipmaac.org/conf/03/shahani-denning.pdf

99. For more details on how the mask is constructed, visit Dr. Marquardt's website at www.Beautyanalysis.com

100. This four-part BBC series examines the science behind facial beauty, expression, and fame in an entertaining fashion. Learn more from IDMB: www.imdb.com/title/tt0280262/

101. Zeising, Adolf, 1854, Neue Lehre von den Proportionen des menschlichen Körpers aus einem bisher unerkannt gebliebenen, die ganze Natur und Kunst durchdringenden morphologischen Grundgesetze entwickelt und mit einer vollständigen historischen Uebersicht der bisherigen Systeme begleitet, Leipzig: Weigel.

102. Mathematical lives of plants: why plants grow in geometrically curious patterns, Julie J. Rehmeyer, July 21, 2007, www.mywire.com/pubs/ScienceNews/2007/07/21/4250760

103. Excerpted from the July 11, 1998 Sunday Telegraph, Simon Singh's review of Ian Stewart's book Nature's Numbers.

104. Chaotic climate dynamics, Selvan AM, Luniver Press, 2.

105. A superstring theory for fractal spacetime, chaos and quantumlike mechanics in atmospheric

flows, AM Selvan and Suvarna Fadnavis, published with modification in Chaos, Solitons, and Fractals, 10(8), pp. 1321-1334, 1999.

106. Language in context: emergent features of word, sentence, and narrative comprehension, Xu J, Neuroimage, April 15, 2005, 25(3):1002-15.

107. The effect of emergent features on judgments of quantity in configural and separable displays., Peebles D, J Exp Psychol Appl, Jun 14, 2008, (2):85-100.

108. Survival of the Prettiest: The Science of Beauty, Nancy Etcoff, Anchor, reprint edition July 11, 2000, p. 34.

109. Facial symmetry and judgments of apparent health support for a "good genes" explanation of the attractiveness–symmetry relationship, Jones BC, Evolution and Human Behavior, vol. 22, issue 6, November 2001, pp. 417–429.

110. An objective system for measuring facial attractiveness, Bashour M, Plast. Reconstr. Surg, 118: 757, 2006, Chapter 3, figure 8, "Checkerboard patterns trigger organized EEG waves," from: Lack of long-term cortical reorganization after macaque retinal lesions, Nature, vol. 435, May 2005, see figure 2 and text regarding cortical response to images lacking pattern. Attentive staring enables "optimization of sensory integration within the corticothalamic neural pathways," from Thalamic bursting in rats during different awake behavioral states, Proc Natl Acad Sci USA, 2001, 98:15330–15335. That our brains respond to pattern, from Spatial frequency modulates visual cortical response to temporal frequency variation of visual stimuli: an fMRI study, Physiol Meas, 28, pp. 547-554. That symmetrical objects trigger bloodflow to the pleasure centers, from: Sex, beauty, and the orbitofrontal cortex, International Journal of Psychophysiology, vol. 63, issue 2, February 2007, pp. 181-185. That infants prefer and learn symmetrical images faster than asymmetrical ones, from The effect of stimulus attractiveness on visual tracking in two- to six-month-old infants, Infant Behavior and Development, vol. 26, no. 2, April 2003, pp. 135–150(16).

111. Prevalence information from www.fitdeskjockey.com/female-body-types

112. Waist and hip circumferences and all-cause mortality: usefulness of the waist-to-hip ratio? Bigaard J, Nature Obesity, vol. 28(6), June 2004, pp. 741–747.

113. Waist circumference and body composition in relation to all-cause mortality in middle-aged men and women, Bigaard J, Int J Obes (London), July 2005, 29(7):778-84.

114. The shape of things to wear: scientists identify how women's figures have changed in fifty years, Helen McCormack, Independent UK, November 21, 2005.

115. Survival of the Prettiest: The Science of Beauty, Nancy Etcoff, Anchor, reprint edition July 2000, p. 12.

116. Anthropometric and biochemical characteristics of polycystic ovarian syndrome in South Indian women using aes-2006 criteria, Sujatha Thathapudi et al, Int J Endocrinol Metab, 5, 12(1), epub January 2014, 5.

117. Abdominal obesity and hip fracture: results from the Nurses' Health Study and the Health Professionals Follow-up Study, Haakon Meyer et al, Osteoporosis Intl, 27, 6 (2016):2127-36.

118. Comparison of anthropometric measures as predictors of cancer incidence: a pooled collaborative analysis of eleven Australian cohorts, Jessica Harding et al, Int J Cancer, 137, 7(2013), pp. 1699–708.

119. Apolipoprotein epsilon 4 allele modifies waist-to-hip ratio effects on cognition and brain structure, Daid Zade et al, J Stroke, Cerebrovasc Dis. 22, 2 (2013): 119-125.

120. Adiposity assessed by anthropometric measures has a similar or greater predictive ability than dual-energy X-ray absorptiometry measures for abdominal aortic calcification in community-dwelling older adults, Xianwen Shang et al, Int J Cardiovasc Imaging (2016), doi 10.1007/s10554-016-0920-2.

121. Waist circumference and body composition in relation to all-cause mortality in middle-aged men and women, Bigaard J, Int J Obes (London)., July 2005, 29(7):778-84.

Chapter 5

122. The impact of parity on course of labor in a contemporary population, Vahratian A, Hoffman MK, Troendle JF et al, Birth, March 2006, 33(1):12-7.

123. Nutritional supplements in pregnancy: commercial push or evidence based? Glennville M Curr, Opin Obstet Gynecol, Decemberember 2006, 18(6):642-7.

124. *The Contribution of Nutrition to Human and Animal Health,* Widdowson (editor), Cambridge University Press, p. 263.

125. Reduced brain DHA content after a single reproductive cycle in female rats fed a diet deficient in N-3 polyunsaturated fatty acids, Levant B, Biol Psychiatry, November 1, 2006, 60(9):987-90.

126. Maternal parity and diet (n-3) polyunsaturated fatty acid concentration influence accretion of brain phospholipid docosahexaenoic acid in developing rats, Levant B, J Nutr, January 2007, 137(1):125-9.

127. Change in brain size during and after pregnancy: study in healthy women and women with preeclampsia, American Journal of Neuroradiology, vol. 37, issue 3, pp. 19-26.

128. As we will learn in the coming chapters, vegetable oils and excess dietary sugar are major contributors to a state of metabolic imbalance called oxidative stress. Oxidative stress, in turn, impairs cell signaling function by disrupting the transmission of short-lived signaling molecules like nitric oxide and depleting the cell of antioxidants necessary for normal function, as well as direct free-radical mediated damage.

129. Effects of oxidative stress on embryonic development, Birth Defects, Res C Embryo Today, September 2007, 81(3):155-62.

130. Diabetes mellitus and birth defects, Correa A, Am J Obstet Gynecol, September 2008, 199(3):237.

131. Epigenetic regulation of metabolism in children born small for gestational age (review), Holness MJ, Curr Opin Clin Nutr Metab Care, July 2006, 9(4):4 82-8

132. Early-life family structure and microbially induced cancer risk, Blaser MJ, PLoS Med, January 2007, 4(1):e7.

133. The effect of birth order and parental age on the risk of type 1 and 2 diabetes among young adults, Lammi N, Diabetologia, Decemberember 2007, 50(12):2433-8, epub October 2007.

134. Associations of birth defects with adult intellectual performance, disability and mortality: population-based cohort study, Eide MG, Pediatr Res, June 2006, 59(6):848-53, epub April 2006.

135. Nutritional factors affecting the development of a functional ruminant—a historical perspective, Warner RG, pp. 1–12 in Proc Cornell Nutr Conf Feed Manuf, Syracuse, NY, Cornell University, Ithaca, NY, 1991.

136. The many faces and factors of orofacial clefts, Schutte B, Human Molecular Genetics, 1999, vol. 8, no. 10, pp. 1853–1859.

137. The effect of birth spacing on child and maternal health, Beverly Winikoff, Studies in Family Planning, vol 14, no 10, October 1983, pp. 231–245.

138. Does birth spacing affect maternal or child nutritional status? Matern Child Nutr, July 2007, 3(3):151-73, a systematic literature review.

139. Association between birth interval and cardiovascular outcomes at thirty years of age: a prospective cohort study from Brazil, Devakumar D et al, PLoS One, 2016; 11(2).

140. Developmental dysplasia of the hip, Am Fam Physician, October 15, 2006, 74(8):1310-1316, Stephen K. Storer.

141. A meta-analysis of common risk factors associated with the diagnosis of developmental dysplasia of the hip in newborns, Eur J Radiol, March 2012, 81(3):e344-51.

142. Idiopathic scoliosis: genetic and environmental aspects, Frances V. De George, J. Med Genet, 1967, pp. 4, 251.

143. Risk factors for deformational plagiocephaly at birth and at seven weeks of age: a prospective cohort study, Van Vlimmeren, LA Pediatrics, February 2007, 119(2):e408-18.

144. Asymmetry of the head and face in infants and in children, David Greene, Am J Dis Child, 1931.

145. A common form of facial asymmetry in the newborn infant; its etiology and orthodontic significance, Elena Boder, *American Journal of Orthodontics,* vol. 39, issue 12, December 1953, pp. 895–910.

146. On the current incidence of deformational plagiocephaly: an estimation based on prospective registration at a single center, Kevin M Kelly, Semin Pediatr Neurol, 11 :301-304, 2004, Elsevier.

147. Craniofacial deformity in patients with uncorrected congenital muscular torticollis: an assessment from three-dimensional computed tomography imaging, Yu C-C, Wong F-W, Lo L-J, et al, Plast Reconstr Surg, 2004, 113:24–33.

148. Intrauterine growth retardation (IUGR): epidemiology and etiology, Romo A, Pediatr Endocrinol Rev, February 2009, suppl 3:332-6.

149. Intrauterine growth retardation—small events, big consequences, Taimur Saleem, Ital J Pediatr, 2011, 37: 41.

150. Maternal and fetal indicators of oxidative stress during intrauterine growth retardation (IUGR), Ullas Kamath, Indian J Clin Biochem, March 2006, 21(1): 111–115.

151. Human conditions of insulin-like growth factor-I (IGF-I) deficiency, Juan E Puche, J Transl Med, 2012.

152. Unpublished communication with Ph.D. at UCLA Jonsson Comprehensive Cancer Center, October. 11, 2006.

153. Lillian Gelberg, UCLA Jonsson Comprehensive Cancer Center, unpublished communication, October 11, 2006.

154. Vitamin A and beta-carotene supply of women with gemini or short birth intervals: a pilot study, Schulz C, Eur J Nutr, November 10, 2006.

155. From Vitamin profile of 563 gravidas during trimesters of pregnancy, Baker H, J Am Coll Nutr, February 2002, 21(1):33-7.

156. High prevalence of vitamin D insufficiency in black and white pregnant women residing in the Northern United States and their neonates, Bodnar LM, J Nutr, February 2007, 137(2):447-52.

157. Maternal supplementation with very-long-chain in 3 fatty acids during pregnancy and lactation augments children's IQ at four years of age, Helland IB, Pediatrics, January 2003, 111(1):e39-44.

158. The fetal origins of memory: the role of dietary choline in optimal brain development, Zeises SH, J Pediatr, November 2006, 149(5 suppl):S131-6, review.

159. Choline: are our university students eating enough? Gossell-Williams M, West Indian Med J, June 2006, 55(3):197-9.

160. Fetal alcohol syndrome: historical perspectives, Neuroscience and Biobehavioral Reviews, vol. 31, issue 2, 2007, pp. 168–171; and Fetal alcohol syndrome: the origins of a moral panic alcohol and alcoholism, vol. 35, issue 3, May 1, 2000.

161. Prevention of neural tube defects: results of the Medical Research Council Vitamin Study, MRC Vitamin Study Research Group, Lancet, July 20, 1991, 338(8760):131-7.

162. Views: ergot and the salem witchcraft affair: an outbreak of a type of food poisoning known as convulsive ergotism may have led to the 1692 accusations of witchcraft, Mary K. Matossian, American Scientist, vol. 70, no. 4, July-August 1982, pp. 355–357.

163. Nutritional supplements in pregnancy: commercial push or evidence based? Glenville M, Current Opinion in Obstetrics and Gynecology, 2006, 18:642-647.

164. Beyond deficiency: new views on the function and health effects of vitamins, Annals of the New York Academy of Sciences, vol. 669, 1992, pp. 8–10.

165. Natural Causes: Death, Lies, and Politics in America's Vitamin and Herbal Supplement Industry, Dan Hurly, Broadway, 2006.

166. Changes in USDA food composition data for forty-three garden crops, 1950 to 1999, Donald R Davis, P. Journal of the American College of Nutrition, vol. 23, no. 6, 2004, pp. 669–682.

167. Comparison of tables in McCance and Widdowson, The chemical composition of foods versions from 1940 and 2002, published by His Majesty's Stationery Office, London.

168. Nutritional supplements in pregnancy: commercial push or evidence based? Glenville M, Current Opinion in Obstetrics and Gynecology, 2006, 18:642-647.

169. Traditional methods of birth control in Zaire, Waife RS, Pathfinder Papers No. 4, Chestnut Hill, MA, 1978.

170. "Le bebe en brousse": European women, African birth spacing and colonial intervention in the Belgian Congo, Hunt NR, International Journal of African Historical Studies, 21, 3 (1988), pp. 401–32.

171. Intimate colonialism: the imperial production of reproduction in Uganda, 1907-1925, Carol Summers, Signs, vol. 16, no. 4, Women, Family, State, and Economy in Africa, Summer 1991, pp. 787–807.

172. Nutrition and Physical Degeneration, Weston A Price, Price Pottenger Foundation, 1945, p. 398.

173. Mahatma Gandhi, quoted in Richard Frazer, Live as though you might die tomorrow and farm as though you might live forever, Christian faith and the welfare of the city, Johnston R. McKay (editor), Edinburgh: CTPI, 2008, p. 48.

174. Letter to all state governors on a uniform soil conservation law, February 26, 1937, Franklin D Roosevelt, pp. 1933–945.

175. Nutritional supplements in pregnancy: commercial push or evidence based? Glenville M, Current Opinion in Obstetrics and Gynecology, 2006, 18:642-647.

176. Changes in USDA food composition data for forty-three garden crops, 1950 to 1999, Donald R Davis, P. Journal of the American College of Nutrition, vol. 23, no. 6, 2004, pp. 669–682.

177. Comparison of tables in McCance and Widdowson, The chemical composition of foods versions from 1940 and 2002, published by His Majesty's Stationery Office, London.

178. Nutritional supplements in pregnancy: commercial push or evidence based? Glenville M, Current Opinion in Obstetrics and Gynecology, 2006, 18:642-647.

179. Lifetime risk for diabetes mellitus in the United States, Venkat Narayan, KM, JAMA, 2003, 290:1884-1890.

180. America's children in brief: key national indicators of well-being, 2008, Federal Interagency Forum on Child and Family Statistics.

181. Dairy products and physical stature: a systematic review and meta-analysis of controlled trials, Hans de Beer, Economics and Human Biology, 10,3 (2012), pp. 229–309.

182. Do variations in normal nutrition play a role in the development of myopia? Marion Edwards et al, Optometry and Vision Science, 73, 10 (1996), pp. 638–643.

183. There are several but one example is K Chen et al, Antioxidant vitamin status during pregnancy in relation to cognitive development in the first two years of life, Early Hum Dev, 85,7, 2009, pp. 421–27.

184. Maternal fatty acids in pregnancy, FADS polymorphisms, and child intelligence quotient at eight years of age, Colin Steer et al, Am J Clin Nutr, 98, 6, 2013, pp. 1575–582.

185. Dietary patterns in early childhood and child cognitive and psychomotor development: the Rhea mother-child cohort study in Crete, Vasiliki Levantakou et al, British Journal of Nutrition, 1, 8, 2016, pp. 1–7.

186. Recognition of a sequence: more growth before birth, longer telomeres at birth, more lean mass after birth, F de Zegher et al, Pediatric Obesity, doi 10.1111/ijpo.12137.

187. Muscularity and fatness of infants and young children born small- or large-for-gestational-age, Mary Hediger et al, Pediatrics, 102,5, 1998, E60.

188. The Potential Impact of Nutritional Factors on Immunological Responsiveness, in Nutrition and Immunity, M Eric Gershwin.

189. Early development of the gut microbiota and immune health, M. Pilar Franciino, Pathogens, 3,3, 2014, pp. 769–90.

190. Is dirt good for kids? Are parents keeping things too clean for their kids' good? Zamosky, Lisa, Medscape, www.webmd.com/parenting/d2n-stopping-germs-12/kids-and-dirt-germs

191. Early puberty: causes and effects, Maron, Dina Fine, Scientific American, Health, May 2, 2015, http://www.scientificamerican.com/article/early-puberty-causes-and-effects/

192. The regulation of reproductive neuroendocrine function by insulin and insulin-like growth factor-1 (IGF-1), Andrew Wolfe et al, Front Neuroendocrinol, 35,4(2014), pp. 558–72.

193. Anna Stainer-Knittel: portrait of a femme vitale, Kain E, Women's Art Journal, vol. 20, no. 2, pp. 13-71.

194. Mirror, Mirror . . . The Importance of Looks in Everyday Life, Hatfield E, SUNY Press, 1986.

195. Stature of early Europeans, Hormones, Hermanussen M, Athens, July-September 2003, 2(3):175-8.

196. New light on the "dark ages": the remarkably tall stature of Northern European men during the Medieval era, Steckel RH, Social Science History, 2004, 28(2), pp. 211–229.

197. The Cambridge World History of Food, Cambridge University Press, 2000.

198. Fighting the Food Giants, Paul A Stitt, Natural Press, 1981, pp. 61–66.

Chapter 6

199. Accessed online on July 27, 2008, at www.lostgirlsworld.blogspot.com/2006/12/becoming-maasai.html

200. Accessed online on September 4, 2008 at www.bluegecko.org/kenya/tribes/maasai/beliefs.htm

201. The emergence of Orwellian newspeak and the death of free speech, John W Whitehead, Commentary from the Rutherford Institute, June 29, 2015, accessed online on April 1, 2016, at www.rutherford.org/publications_resources/john_whiteheads_commentary/the_emergence_of_orwellian_newspeak_and_the_death_of_free_speech

202. Nutrition and Physical Degeneration, Weston A Price, Price WA, Price-Pottenger Foundation, 1945, p. 226.

203. Ibid., p. 10.

204. Ibid., p. 228.

205. Ibid., p. 248.

206. Archaeological Amerindian and Eskimo cranioskeletal size variation along coastal Western North America: relation to climate, the reconstructed diet high in marine animal foods, and demographic stress, Ivanhoe F, International Journal of Osteoarchaeology, vol. 8, issue 3, pp. 135–179.

207. Craniofacial variation and population continuity during the South African Holocene, Stynder DD, American Journal of Physical Anthropology, published online.

208. Craniofacial morphology in the Argentine center-West: consequences of the transition to food production, Marina L Sardi, American Journal of Physical Anthropology, vol. 130, issue 3, pp. 333–343.

209. *The Cambridge World History of Food*, Cambridge University Press, 2000, p. 1704.

210. Stone age economics, Sahlins M Aldine, Transaction, 1972, pp. 1–40.

211. Ibid.

212. The question of robusticity and the relationship between cranial size and shape in Homo sapiens, Lahr MM, Journal of Human Evolution, 1996, 31, pp. 157–191.

213. Dental caries in prehistoric South Africans, Dryer TF, Nature, 136:302, 1935, "The indication from this area . . . bears out the experience of European anthropologists that caries is a comparatively modern disease and that no skull showing this condition can be regarded as ancient."

214. Dental anthropology, Scott GR, Annual Review of Anthropology, vol. 17:99-126, October 1988, "Pronounced forms of malocclusion are a relatively recent development."

215. Bioarchaeology of Southeast Asia, Oxenham M, Cambridge University Press, 2006. "Hunter-gatherers typically have low frequencies of caries, calculus, malocclusion, and alveolar resorption, a high frequency of severe attrition [wear] and large jaw size. Agricultural populations typically have the opposite profile, low rates of severe attrition (except in cases where food contains abrasives), and high rates of caries, calculus, resorption, dental crowding, and malocclusion."

216. *Fannie Farmer 1896 Boston Cookbook*, Fannie Merritt Farmer, Boston Cooking School, Ottenheimer, commemorative edition, 1996, pp. 1–2.

217. *Nutrition and Physical Degeneration*, Price WA, Price-Pottenger Foundation, 1945, p. 279.

218. Ibid.

219. January 20, 2001, inaugural luncheon menu served at the U.S. State Capitol, accessed online on October 31, 2007, at: www.gwu.edu/percent7Eaction/inaulu.html

220. The content of bioactive compounds in rat experimental diets based on organic, low-input, and conventional plant materials, Leifert C, 3rd QLIF Congress, Honeheim, Germany, March 20-23, 2007, archived at www.orgprints.org/view/projects/int_conf_qlif2007.html

221. Nutritional comparison of fresh, frozen, and canned fruits and vegetables, vitamin A and carotenoids, vitamin E, minerals and fiber, Joy C Rickman, J Sci Food Agric.

222. The vitamin A, B, and C content of artificially versus naturally ripened tomatoes, House MC, Journal of Biological Chemistry, vol. LXXXI, no. 3, received for publication December 13, 1928.

223. Ibid.

224. Nutritional comparison of fresh, frozen and canned fruits and vegetables, Part 1, Vitamins C and B and phenolic compounds, Joy C Rickman, J Sci Food Agric, 87:930–944 (2007).

Chapter 7

225. Types of dietary fat and risk of coronary heart disease: a critical review, HU F, Journal of the American College of Nutrition, vol. 2, 1, 5-19, 2001.

226. *In Defense of Food: An Eater's Manifesto,* Michael Pollan, Penguin, 2009, p. 43.

227. *Eat Fat, Get Thin: Why the Fat We Eat Is the Key to Sustained Weight Loss and Vibrant Health,* Mark Hyman, Little, Brown, 2016.

228. *The Big Fat Surprise: Why Butter, Meat and Cheese Belong in a Healthy Diet,* Nina Teicholz, Simon and Schuster, reprint, 2015.

229. In food choices and coronary heart disease: a population based cohort study of rural Swedish men with twelve years of follow-up, Int J Environ Res Public Health 2009, 6, 2626-2638. The authors assert, "The diet-heart hypothesis from the 1950s stating that saturated fats lead to heart disease via blood lipid derangement is under re-evaluation." Barry Groves cites over 1,000 articles in his book, Trick and Treat: How Healthy Eating Is Making Us Ill, Hammersmith, 2008. Gary Taubes's 640-page book Good Calories, Bad Calories, Knopf, 2007, is similarly well-referenced.

230. In doing research for my own family's health I found out from my mom that she and her brother were both formula fed, as was the style of the well-educated women on the East Coast at the time. I asked my grandmother what convinced her to follow this trend, suspecting it was convenience or some idea that doing so would help her retain her figure. To my surprise she retold the story of a sales pitch given to her by a Nestle "milk nurse" after my uncle was born. My grandmother was advised that if she were to breastfeed she would need to use a number of supplements to best assure her baby's heath. But if she chose to use formula, which was "fortified," she would avoid the need to give the baby several supplements because the formulation devised was "more perfect than breastmilk."

231. *The Search* archive of the 1953 episode featuring Keys is available from University of Minnesota's www.epi.umn.edu/cvdepi/video/the-search-1953/

232. Health revolutionary: the life and work of Ancel Keys, accessed online at www.209.85.141.104/search?q=cache:PVHCLllMKzQJ:www.asph.org/movies/keys.pdf+percent22i'll+show+those+-guyspercent22+keys&hl=en&ct=clnk&cd=1&gl=us&client=firefox-a

233. Hydrogenated fats in the diet and lipids in the serum of man, Anderson JT, J Nutr, 75 (4):338, p. 1961.

234. Ibid.

235. Health revolutionary: the life and work of Ancel Keys, accessed online at www.209.85.141.104/search?q=cache:PVHCLllMKzQJ:www.asph.org/movies/keys.pdf+percent22i'll+show+those+-guyspercent22+keys&hl=en&ct=clnk&cd=1&gl=us&client=firefox-a

236. Tracing citations in consensus articles and other policy setting research statements leads us back to Keys and his junk science. Case in point, the 2004 National Cholesterol Education Program (NCEP) coordinating committee issued an update to the third Adult Treatment Panel (ATP III) Consensus panel statement.

237. *Time magazine,* March 26, 1984.

238. *Time magazine,* Jun 12, 2014.

239. Oxidation of linoleic acid in low-density lipoprotein: an important event in atherogenesis, Spiteller G, Angew Chem Int Ed Engl, February 2000, 39(3):585-589.

240. *Know Your Fats: The Complete Primer for Understanding the Nutrition of Fats, Oils, and Cholesterol,* Mary G Enig, Bethesda Press, 2000, p. 94.

241. *The Cholesterol Myths,* Uffe Ravnskov, New Trends Publishing, 2000, p. 30.

242. Myths and truths about beef, Fallon S, Wise Traditions in Food, Farming and the Healing

Arts, Spring 2000.

243. Trans fatty acids in the food supply: a comprehensive report covering sixty years of research, second edition, Enig Mary G, Enig Associates, Silver Spring, MD, 1995, pp. 4-8.

244. Heart disease and stroke statistics, 2003 update, American Heart Association.

245. The rise and fall of ischemic heart disease, Stallones RA, Sci Am, Nov 1980, 243(5):53-9.

246. Sex matters: secular and geographical trends in sex differences in coronary heart disease mortality, Lawlor DA, BMJ, September 8, 2001, 323:541-545.

247. The lowdown on oleo, Kapica C, Chicago Wellness Magazine, September-October 2007.

248. See Chapter 11.

249. The ABCs of vitamin E and ß-carotene absorption, Traber MG, American Journal of Clinical Nutrition, vol. 80, no. 1, July 3–4, 2004.

250. Absorption, metabolism, and transport of carotenoids, Parker RS, FASEB J, April 1996, 10(5):542-51.

251. Human plasma transport of vitamin D after its endogenous synthesis, Haddad JG, Matsuoka LY, Hollis BW, Hu YZ, Wortsman J.

252. Physicochemical and physiological mechanisms for the effects of food on drug absorption: the role of lipids and pH, Journal of Pharmaceutical Sciences, vol. 86, issue 3, pp. 269–282.

253. Plasma lipoproteins as carriers of phylloquinone (vitamin K1) in humans, Am J Clin Nutr, June 1998, 67(6):1226-31.

254. Vitamin E: absorption, plasma transport and cell uptake, Hacquebard M, Carpentier YA, Curr Opin Clin Nutr Metab Care, March 2005, 8(2):133-8.

255. PUFAs reduce the formation of post-prandial triglycerides that carry lipid soluble nutrients from your last meal.

256. ". . . It is now generally recognized that the replacement of saturated fats by vegetable oils containing high levels of polyunsaturated fatty acids (PUFAs) may also render individuals susceptible to cardiovascular lesions." In Vivo absorption, metabolism, and urinary excretion of alpha, beta-unsaturated aldehydes in experimental animals: relevance to the development of cardiovascular diseases by the dietary ingestion of thermally stressed polyunsaturate-rich culinary oils, Grootveld MJ, Clin Invest, vol. 101, no. 6, March 1998, pp. 1210–218.

257. Enig's report was published in the prestigious Food Chemical News and Nutrition Week, as well as other publications widely read by congressional members,The oiling of America, posted on January 1, 2000, by Sally Fallon and Mary G. Enig. See more at: www.westonaprice.org/know-your-fats/the-oiling-of-america/#sthash.xgjweoMn.dpuf

258. Dietary oxidized fatty acids: an atherogenic risk? Meera Penumetchaa M, Journal of Lipid Research, vol. 41, 1473-1480, September 2000.

259. Determination of total trans fats and oils by infrared spectroscopy for regulatory compliance, Mossoba M, Anal Bioanal Chem, 2007, 389:87–92.

260. Lipoxygenase-catalyzed oxygenation of storage lipids is implicated in lipid mobilization during germination, Feussner I, Proceedings of the National Academy of Sciences, vol. 92, 11849-11853.

261. Formation of modified fatty acids and oxyphytosterols during refining of low erucic acid rapeseed oil, aka canola oil, Lambelet PJ, Agric Food Chem, July 2003, 16;51(15):4284-90.

262. The effect of short-term canola oil ingestion on oxidative stress in the vasculature of stroke-prone spontaneously hypertensive rats, Lipids Health Dis, October 2011, 17;10:180.

263. Differential effects of dietary canola and soybean oil intake on oxidative stress in stroke-prone spontaneously hypertensive rats, Lipids Health Dis, June 2011, 13;10:98.

264. Formation of modified fatty acids and oxyphytosterols during refining of low erucic acid rapeseed oil, aka canola oil, Lambelet PJ, Agric Food Chem, July 2003, 16;51(15):4284-90.

265. Mastugo et al, Current medicinal chemistry, 1996, vol. 2, no. 4, Bentham Science Publishers, page 764, subheading The chemistry of free radicals and biological substrates, Table 1, Reaction rate constants of hydroxyl radical with organic compounds.

266. Familial hypercholesterolemia: risk stratifications in practice, ReachMD, program hosted by Alan J Brown podcast, accessible online at www.reachmd.com/programs/lipid-luminations/its-relative-screening-and-treating-familial-hypercholesterolemia/6421, Alan Brown's comment at 9 minutes.

267. Testosterone induces erythrocytosis via increased erythropoietin and suppressed hepcidin: evidence for a new erythropoietin/hemoglobin set point, Bachman EJ, Gerontol Biol Sci Med Sci, June 2014, 69(6):725-35, doi 10.1093/gerona/glt154, epub October 2013.

268. Lipid peroxidation in vivo evaluation and application of methods for measurement by Eva Södergren, comprehensive summaries of Uppsala Dissertations from the Faculty of Medicine, 949.

269. Antioxidant and inhibitory effects of aqueous extracts of Salvia officinalis leaves on pro-oxidant-induced lipid peroxidation in brain and liver in vitro, Oboh G, J Med Food, February 2009, 12(1):77-84.

270. Antioxidant and inhibitory effect of red ginger (Zingiber officinale var. Rubra) and white ginger (Zingiber officinale Roscoe) on Fe(2+) induced lipid peroxidation in rat brain in vitro, Oboh G, Exp Toxicol Pathol, January 2012, 64(1-2):31-6.

271. Autoxidation of human low density lipoprotein: loss of polyunsaturated fatty acids and vitamin E and generation of aldehydes, J Lipid Res, May 1987, 28(5):495-509, www.ncbi.nlm.nih.gov/pubmed/3598395

272. Impaired endothelial function following a meal rich in used cooking fat, Williams M, J Am Coll Cardiol, 1999, 33:1050-1055.

273. A local restaurant owner explained that one of the benefits of the new "reduced trans" cooking oils is that you can stretch their useful life from one week to two. By then, he said, the stuff turns so black and rancid, you've got no choice but to change it out. Bon appetit!

274. Two consecutive high-fat meals affect endothelial-dependent vasodilation, oxidative stress and cellular microparticles in healthy men, Tushuizen ME, J Thromb Haemost, May 2006, 4(5):1003-10.

275. Intake of calories and selected nutrients for the United States population, 1999-2000, published online and accessed on April 4, 2016, at: www.cdc.gov/nchs/data/nhanes/databriefs/calories.pdf.

276. A new role for apolipoprotein E: modulating transport of polyunsaturated phospholipid molecular species in synaptic plasma membranes, J Neurochem, January 2002, 80(2):255-61.

277. Oxidation of linoleic acid in low-density lipoprotein: an important event in atherogenesis, Angew, Chem Int Ed, 2000, 39, no. 3.

278. J Lipid Res, May 1987, 28(5):495-509, Autoxidation of human low density lipoprotein: loss of polyunsaturated fatty acids and vitamin E and generation of aldehydes, at: www.ncbi.nlm.nih.gov/pubmed/3598395

279. Oxidation of linoleic acid in low-density lipoprotein : an important event in atherogenesis, Angew, Chem Int Ed, 2000, 39, no. 3.

280. Non enzymatic glycation of apolipoprotein A-I: effects on its self-association and lipid binding properties, Calvo C, Biochem Biophys Res Commun, June 3, 1988, 153(3):1060-7.

281. Lipoprotein lipase mediates the uptake of glycated LDL in fibroblasts, endothelial cells, and macrophages, Robert Zimmermann.

282. Glycation of very low density lipoprotein from rat plasma impairs its catabolism, Mamo JC, Diabetologia, June 1990, 33(6):339-45.

283. Modification of low density lipoprotein by advanced glycation end products contributes to the dyslipidemia of diabetes and renal insufficiency, Bucala R, Proc Natl Acad Sci USA, September 27, 1994, 91(20):9441-5.

284. Glycation of very low density lipoprotein from rat plasma impairs its catabolism, Mamo JC, Diabetologia, June 1990, 33(6):339-45. The study concludes: "Glycation [sugar sticking to stuff] of VLDL appears to interfere with the lipolysis [the unloading] of its triglyceride. This may explain the delayed clearance of glycated VLDL triglyceride in vivo."

285. Stone NJ, et al, 2013 ACC/AHA blood cholesterol guideline, p. 1, 2013, ACC/AHA guideline on the treatment of blood cholesterol to reduce atherosclerotic cardiovascular risk in adults, a report of the American College of Cardiology/American Heart Association Task Force on Practice Guidelines.

286. Cholesterol and cancer: answers and new questions, Eric J Jacobs, Cancer Epidemiol Biomarkers Prev, November 2009, 18; 2805.

287. U. Ravnskov, High cholesterol may protect against infections and atherosclerosis, Q J Med, 2003, 96: 927-934.

288. Cholesterol quandaries relationship to depression and the suicidal experience, Randy A Sansone, Psychiatry (Edgmont), March 2008; 5(3): 22–34.

289. Editorial serum cholesterol concentration, depression, and anxiety, Mehmed YuÈcel AgÏarguÈn, Acta Psychiatr Scand, 2002: 105: 81±83.

290. Low cholesterol as a risk factor for primary intracerebral hemorrhage: a case-control study, Ashraf V. Valappil, Ann Indian Acad Neurol, January-March 2012; 15(1): 19–22.

291. Chronic kidney disease and its complications, Robert Thomas, Prim Care, Jun 2008, 35(2): 329–vii.

292. High density lipoprotein as a protective factor against coronary heart disease, Tavia Gordon et al, The Framingham Study, American Journal of Medicine, May 1977, vol. 62, pp. 707-714.

293. Accessible at: www.cvriskcalculator.com/

294. Oxidation of linoleic acid in low-density lipoprotein: an important event in atherogenesis, Spiteller D, Spiteller G. Angew, Chem Int Ed Engl, February 2000, 39(3):585-589.

295. Thermally oxidized dietary fats increase the susceptibility of rat LDL to lipid peroxidation but not their uptake by macrophages, Eder K, J Nutr, September 2003, 133(9):2830-7.

296. Myeloperoxidase and plaque vulnerability, Hazen SL, Arteriosclerosis, Thrombosis, and Vascular Biology, 2004, 24:1143.

297. Oxidation-reduction controls fetal hypoplastic lung growth, Fisher JC, J Surg Res, August 2002, 106(2):287-91.

298. Intake of high levels of vitamin A and polyunsaturated fatty acids during different developmental periods modifies the expression of morphogenesis genes in European sea bass (Dicentrarchus labrax), Villeneuve LA, Br J Nutr, April 2006, 95(4):677-87.

299. Neural tube defects and maternal biomarkers of folate, homocysteine, and glutathione metabolism, Zhao W, Birth Defects Res A Clin Mol Teratol, April 2006, 76(4):230-6.

300. Congenital heart defects and maternal biomarkers of oxidative stress, Hobbs CA, Am J Clin Nutr, September 2005, 82(3):598-604.

301. A reduction state potentiates the glucocorticoid response through receptor protein stabilization, Kitugawa H, Genes Cells, November 2007, 12(11):1281-7.

302. Trends in serum lipids and lipoproteins of adults, 1960-2002, Carrol MD, vol. 294, no. 14, October 12, 2005.

303. Application of new cholesterol guidelines to a population-based sample, Pencina MJ1, N Engl J Med, April 10, 2014, 370(15):1422-31, doi: 10.1056/NEJMoa1315665, epub March 2014.

304. *On the Take: How Medicine's Complicity with Big Business Can Endanger Your Health,* Jerome P. Kassirer, Oxford University Press, 2005.

305. *Overdosed America: The Broken Promise of American Medicine,* John Abramson, Harper Collins, 2004.

306. Adverse birth outcomes among mothers with low serum cholesterol, Edison RJ, Pediatrics, vol. 120, no. 4, October 2007, pp. 723-733.

Chapter 8

307. The stomach as a bioreactor: dietary lipid peroxidation in the gastric fluid and the effects of plant-derived antioxidants, Free Radical Biology and Medicine, vol. 31, issue 11, December 1, 2001, pp. 1388-1395.

308. Protective effect of oleic acid against acute gastric mucosal lesions induced by ischemia-reperfusion in rat, Saudi Journal of Gastroenterology, 2007, vol. 13, issue 1, p. 17.

309. Lipid peroxidation by "free" iron ions and myoglobin as affected by dietary antioxidants in simulated gastric fluids, J Agric Food Chem, May 4, 2005, 53(9):3383-90, www.ncbi.nlm.nih.gov/pubmed/15853376

310. Linoleic acid, a dietary n-6 polyunsaturated fatty acid, and the aetiology of ulcerative colitis: a nested case-control study within a European prospective cohort study, Gut, December 2009, 58(12):1606-11, doi 10.1136/gut.2008.169078, epub July 2009.

311. "Owing to the fact that DHA has a higher number of double bonds compared with AA, DHA is more susceptible to free radical-mediated oxidation," from page 34 of Omega-3 Fatty Acids in Brain and Neurological Health, edited by Ronald Ross Watson, Fabien De Meester, Academic Press, 2014, Elsevier.

312. Oxidation of marine omega-3 supplements and human health, Benjamin B Albert, 1, David Cameron-Smith, 1, Paul L Hofman, 1, 2, and Wayne S Cutfield, 1,2, BioMed Research International, vol. 2013, 2013, article ID 464921, 8 pages, www.dx.doi.org/10.1155/2013/464921

313. Formation of malondialdehyde (MDA), 4-hydroxy-2-hexenal (HHE) and 4-hydroxy-2-nonenal (HNE) in fish and fish oil during dynamic gastrointestinal in vitro digestion, Food Funct, February 17, 2016, 7(2):1176-87.

314. Association of proton pump inhibitors with risk of dementia, JAMA Neurol, published online February 15, 2016.

315. *Brain Maker: The Power of Gut Microbes to Heal and Protect Your Brain—For Life,* David Perlmutter, Little, Brown, April 28, 2015, from Gut: The Inside Story of Our Body's Most Underrated Organ, Graystone Books.

316. Obese-type gut microbiota induce neurobehavioral changes in the absence of obesity, Bruce-Keller AJ, Biol Psychiatry, April 1, 2015, 77(7):607-15.

317. Ibid.

318. Ibid.

319. Effect of intestinal microbial ecology on the developing brain, Douglas-Escobar M, JAMA Pediatr, April 2013, 167(4):374-9.

320. Aust N Z J Psychiatry, December 2011, 45(12):1023-5, Probiotics in the treatment of depression: science or science fiction? Dinan TG.

321. Intestinal microbiota, probiotics and mental health, from Metchnikoff to modern advances,

part III, Convergence toward clinical trials, Alison C Bested, Gut Pathog, 2013, 5: 4.

322. The role of gut microbiota in the gut-brain axis: current challenges and perspectives, Chen X, Protein Cell, June 2013, 4(6):403-14.

323. Obese-type gut microbiota induce neurobehavioral changes in the absence of obesity, Bruce-Keller AJ, Biol Psychiatry, April 1, 2015, 77(7):607-15.

324. Control Diet Ingredients, file:///Users/cateshanahan/Downloads/product_data_D12450B.pdf, High Fat Diet Ingredients: file:///Users/cateshanahan/Downloads/product_data_D12451.pdf.

325. Oxidation stability and fatty acid composition of selected storage and structural lipids: influence of different high fat diet compositions. The combination of sunflower oil and lard resulted in the highest amount of oxidation, compared to butter, lard, and partially hydrogenated oil, Nahrung, 1988, 32(4):365-74.

326. Mitochondrial formation of reactive oxygen species, Julyio F Turrens, Journal of Physiology, October 2003.

327. Chronic n-3 polyunsaturated fatty acid deficiency alters dopamine vesicle density in the rat frontal cortex, Luc Zimmer, Neuroscience Letters 284,1-2 (2000): 25-28.

328. Curr Neuropharmacol, March 2014, 12(2): 140–147, Oxidative stress and psychological disorders: "The brain with its extensive capacity to consume large amounts of oxygen and production of free radicals, is considered especially sensitive to oxidative stress." www.ncbi.nlm.nih.gov/pmc/articles/PMC3964745/

329. Curr Neuropharmacol, March 2009, 7(1): 65–74, Oxidative stress and neurodegenerative diseases: a review of upstream and downstream antioxidant therapeutic options.

330. Curr Neuropharmacol, March 2014, 12(2): 140–147, Oxidative stress and psychological disorders.

331. Toxicity of oxidized fats II: tissue levels of lipid peroxides in rats fed a thermally oxidized corn oil diet. Brain contains higher levels of lipid peroxides after a meal of repeatedly thermally oxidized oil.

332. Peroxyl radicals: inductors of neurodegenerative and other inflammatory diseases, their origin and how they transform cholesterol, phospholipids, plasmalogens, polyunsaturated fatty acids, sugars, and proteins into deleterious products, Spiteller G, Free Radic Biol Med, August 1, 2006, 41(3):362-87.

333. Triacylglycerol oxidation in pig lipoproteins after a diet rich in oxidized sunflower seed oil, Lipids, 40, 437–444, May 2005, "Studies suggest that oxidized dietary lipids increase the oxidation level of chylomicrons and VLDL. In addition to oxidized LDL, which has a central role in atherogenesis, oxidized chylomicrons and their remnants also seem to be potentially atherogenic. Oxidation of chylomicrons results in particles that may serve as a substrate for scavenger receptors. Chylomicrons and their remnants may associate with arterial tissue with even greater efficiency than LDL."

334. Effect of dietary oils on lipid peroxidation and on antioxidant parameters of rat plasma and lipoprotein fractions, C Scaccini, l. M. Nardini, M. D'Aquino, V. Gentili, M. Di Felice, and G. Tomassit, Istituto Nazionale della Nutrizione, Rome, Italy, and Universith della Tuscia, Viterbo, Italy, Journal of Lipid Research, vol. 33, 1992, 627-633, "The use of monounsaturated fats in the diet, rather than polyunsaturated fats, generates lipoprotein particles markedly resistant to oxidative modification. On the other hand, the dietary contribution of antioxidant compounds affects the overall resistance of lipoproteins to lipid peroxidation."

335. Associations between the antioxidant network and emotional intelligence: a preliminary study, Pesce, Mirko et al, Vladimir N Uversky (editor), PLoS ONE 9.7 (2014): e101247, PMC, Web, April 10, 2016.

336. Lipidomics and H218O labeling techniques reveal increased remodeling of DHA-containing membrane phospholipids associated with abnormal locomotor responses in α-tocopherol deficient zebrafish (danio rerio) embryos, Redox Biology, vol. 8, August 2016, pp. 165–174.

337. The adult brain makes new neurons, and effortful learning keeps them alive, Tracy J Shors, Current Directions in Psychological Science, October 2014, vol. 23, no. 5311-318.

338. Influence of dietary thermally oxidized soybean oil on the oxidative status of rats of different ages, Ann Nutr Metab, 1990, 34(4):221-31.

339. Biological studies on the protective role of artichoke and green pepper against potential toxic effect of thermally oxidized oil in mice, Arab J, Biotech, vol. 12, no. 1, January 2009, 27-40, http://www.acgssr.org/BioTechnology/Vol.12N1January2009_files/abstract/003.pdf

340. 2015 Gallup Poll (the largest poll conducted to date): One in five Americans include gluten-free foods in diet, accessed online on April 6, 2016, at www.gallup.com/poll/184307/one-five-americans-include-gluten-free-foods-diet.aspx

341. 2012 survey by the NPD Group, accessed online on April 6, 2016, at https://www.npd.com/wps/portal/npd/us/news/press-releases/percentage-of-us-adults-trying-to-cut-down-or-avoid-gluten-in-their-diets-reaches-new-high-in-2013-reports-npd/

342. The prevalence of celiac disease in average-risk and at-risk Western European populations: a systematic review, Dubé, C et al, Gastroenterology 128, suppl. 1, S57–S67 (2005).

343. Non-celiac gluten sensitivity: the new frontier of gluten related disorders, Carlo Catassi, Nutrients, October 2013, 5(10): 3839–3853.

344. Food allergy among U.S. children: trends in prevalence and hospitalizations, NCHS Data Brief No. 10, October 2008.

345. Effects of dietary oxidized frying oil on immune responses of spleen cells in rats, Reaeawh, W, Nutrition, 17, no. 4.

346. www.fmri.ucsd.edu/Research/whatisfmri.html

347. Ibid.

348. Role of nitric oxide and acetylcholine in neocortical hyperemia elicited by basal forebrain stimulation: evidence for an involvement of endothelial nitric oxide, 1995, Neuroscience 69, 1195–1204.

349. Ibid.

350. Endothelial nitric oxide: protector of a healthy mind, Zvonimir S. Katusic and Susan A. Austin, Eur Heart J, April 7, 2014, 35(14): 888–894, www-ncbi-nlm-nih-gov.prx.hml.org/pmc/articles/PMC3977136/

351. Essential role of endothelial nitric oxide synthase for mobilization of stem and progenitor cells, Aicher A, Heeschen C, Mildner-Rihm C, Urbich C, Ihling C, Technau-Ihling K, Leiher AM, Dimmeler S, Nat Med, 2003, 9:1370–1376.

352. Neurovascular regulation in the normal brain and in Alzheimer's disease, Iadecola C, Nat Rev Neurosci, May 2004, 5(5):347-60.

353. Endothelial nitric oxide: protector of a healthy mind, Zvonimir S Katusic and Susan A Austin, Eur Heart J, April 7, 2014, 35(14): 888–894, www,ncbi-nlm-nih-gov.prx.hml.org/pmc/articles/PMC3977136/

354. Tonic and phasic nitric oxide signals in hippocampal long-term potentiation, Hopper RA, Garthwaite J, J Neurosci, 20;26:11513–11521.

355. Endothelial function and oxidative stress in cardiovascular diseases, Circ J 2009; 73: 411–418.

356. Associations between the antioxidant network and emotional intelligence: a preliminary study, PLoS One, 2014; 9(7): e101247, www.ncbi.nlm.nih.gov/pmc/articles/PMC4077755/.

357. Cognitive cost as dynamic allocation of energetic resources, Front Neurosci, 2015, 9: 289, www.ncbi.nlm.nih.gov/pmc/articles/PMC4547044/

358. Impaired endothelial function following a meal rich in used cooking fat, Michael JA Williams, Journal of the American College of Cardiology, vol. 33, issue 4, March 15, 1999, pp. 1050–1055.

359. Effects of repeated heating of cooking oils on antioxidant content and endothelial function (review), Austin Journal of Pharmacology and Therapeutics, April 07, 2015.

360. Migraine, headache, and the risk of stroke in women: a prospective study, Kurth T, Slomke MA, Kase CS, et al, Neurology, 2005, 64:1020-6.

361. Migraine and ischaemic heart disease and stroke: potential mechanisms and treatment implications, Tietjen GE, Cephalalgia, 2007, 27:981–7.

362. Migraine aura pathophysiology: the role of blood vessels and microembolisation, Turgay Dalkara, Lancet Neurol, March 2010, 9(3): 309–317.

363. Arginine-nitric oxide pathway and cerebrovascular regulation in cortical spreading depression, Am J Physiol, July 1995, 269(1 pt. 2):H23-9.

364. Migraine aura without headache pathogenesis and pathophysiology,MedMerits.com, article section 6 of 14, Shih-Pin Chen, http://www.medmerits.com/index.php/article/migraineaurawithoutheadache/P5.

365. Arginine-nitric oxide pathway and cerebrovascular regulation in cortical spreading depression, Am J Physiol, July 1995, 269(1 pt. 2):H23-9.

366. Migraine aura without headache pathogenesis and pathophysiology,MedMerits.com, article section 6 of 14, Shih-Pin Chen, http://www.medmerits.com/index.php/article/migraineaurawithoutheadache/P5.

367. Perfusion-weighted imaging defects during spontaneous migrainous aura, Ann Neurol, January 1998, 43(1):25-31.

368. Migraine aura without headache pathogenesis and pathophysiology,MedMerits.com, article section 6 of 14, Shih-Pin Chen, http://www.medmerits.com/index.php/article/migraineaurawithoutheadache/P5.

369. Structural brain changes in migraine, JAMA, November 14, 2012; 308(18): 1889–1897, www.ncbi-nlm-nih-gov.prx.hml.org/pmc/articles/PMC3633206/

370. Ibid.

371. Oxidative stress and the aging brain: from theory to prevention, Gemma C, Vila J, Bachstetter A, et al, Riddle DR (editor); Brain Aging: Models, Methods, and Mechanisms, Chapter 15, Boca Raton, FL, CRC Press/Taylor and Francis, 2007, available from www.ncbi.nlm.nih.gov/books/NBK3869/

372. Peroxyl radicals: inductors of neurodegenerative and other inflammatory diseases, their origin and how they transform cholesterol, phospholipids, plasmalogens, polyunsaturated fatty acids, sugars, and proteins into deleterious products, Spiteller G, Free Radical Biology and Medicine, 41, 2006, pp. 362–387.

373. Linoleic acid peroxidation—the dominant lipid peroxidation process in low density lipoprotein—and its relationship to chronic diseases (review), Spiteller G, Chemistry and Physics of lipids, 95 (1998) pp. 105–162.

374. Concussions, and the NFL: how one doctor changed football forever, Laskas Jeanne Marie, Bennet Omalu, September 15, 2009, www.gq.com/story/nfl-players-brain-dementia-study-memory-concussions

375. Ibid.

376. Determination of lipid oxidation products in vegetable oils and marine omega-3 supplements, Food Nutr Res, 2011, 55: 10, www.ncbi-nlm-nih-gov.prx.hml.org/pmc/articles/PMC3118035/

377. Molecular aspects of medicine, vol. 24, issues 4–5, pp. 147-314, August–October 2003, 4 - Hydroxynonenal: a lipid degradation product provided with cell regulatory functions.

378. Involvement of microtubule integrity in memory impairment caused by colchicine, Pharmacology Biochemistry and Behavior, vol. 71, issues 1–2, January–February 2002, pp. 119-138.

379. 4-Hydroxy-2-nonenal, a reactive product of lipid peroxidation, and neurodegenerative diseases: a toxic combination illuminated by redox proteomics studies, Antioxid Redox Signal, December 1, 2012, 17(11): 1590–160.

380. Ibid.

381. Neuronal microtubules: when the MAP is the roadblock, Trends in Cell Biology, vol. 15, issue 4, April 2005, pp. 183-187.

382. 4-Hydroxy-2-nonenal, a reactive product of lipid peroxidation, and neurodegenerative diseases: a toxic combination illuminated by redox proteomics studies, Antioxid Redox Signal, December 1, 2012, 17(11): 1590–160.

383. MRI vs. clinical predictors of Alzheimer disease in mild cognitive impairment, Neurology, January 15, 2008, 70(3):191-9, vol. tric.

384. Neuron number and size in prefrontal cortex of children with autism, Courchesne E, Mouton PR, Calhoun ME, et al, JAMA, 2011, 306(18):2001-2010.

385. Local brain connectivity across development in autism spectrum disorder: a cross-sectional investigation, Autism Res, January 2016, 9(1):43-54, doi 10.1002/aur.1494, epub June 2015.

386. Dr. Anthony Bailey of the University of British Columbia presents Neurobiology of autism spectrum disorders, a care-ID web presentation, from Care ID YouTube Channel, accessed online on April 11, 2106, at www.youtube.com/watch?v=0IudE9OrIOE; minute 27:00 shows novel columns in the brainstem.

387. Using human pluripotent stem cells to model autism spectrum disorders, Carol Marchetto, YouTube video presentation online from the Salk Institute YouTube Channel, accessed online on April 11, 2016 at www.youtube.com/watch?v=eB9JonYy1xo, minute 13:00.

388. Patches of disorganization in the neocortex of children with autism, Stoner R, Chow ML, Boyle MP, Sunkin SM, Mouton PR, Roy S, Wynshaw-Boris A, Colamarino SA, Lein ES, Courchesne E. NEJM, March 27, 2014.

389. Non-verbal girl with autism speaks through her computer, 20/20 ABC News Story reported by John Stossel, accessible via STAR Center (Sensory Therapies and Research Center) YouTube Channel, accessed on April 11, 216 at www.youtube.com/watch?v=xMBzJleeOno.

390. Ibid.

391. Schizophrenic reaction, childhood type, DSM I, 1952, entry 000-x28, accessed online on March 5, 2016, at www.unstrange.com/dsm1.html

392. Diagnostic criteria for infantile autism, DSM III, 1980, accessed online on March 5, 2016, at www.unstrange.com/dsm1.html

393. Accessed online on March 5, 2016, www.cdc.gov/ncbddd/autism/addm.html

394. Combined vaccines are like a sudden onslaught to the body's immune system': parental concerns about vaccine 'overload' and 'immune-vulnerability, Hilton S, Petticrew M, Hunt K, Vaccine. 2006;24(20):4321–7.

395. Maternal smoking and autism spectrum disorder: a meta-analysis, Rosen BN, Lee BK, Lee NL, Yang Y, Burstyn I.

396. In utero exposure to selective serotonin reuptake inhibitors and risk for autism spectrum disorder, Gidaya NB, Lee BK, Burstyn I, Yudell M, Mortensen EL, Newschaffer CJ J, Autism Dev Disord, October 2014, 44(10):2558-67.

397. Reduced prefrontal dopaminergic activity in valproic acid-treated mouse autism model, Hara Y, Takuma K, Takano E, Katashiba K, Taruta A, Higashino K, Hashimoto H, Ago Y, Matsuda T, Behav Brain Res, August 1, 2015, 289:39-47.

398. Current research on methamphetamine-induced neurotoxicity: animal models of monoamine disruption (review), Kita T, Wagner GC, Nakashima T, J Pharmacol Sci, July 2003, 92(3):178-95

399. Prenatal exposure to a common organophosphate insecticide delays motor development in a mouse model of idiopathic autism, De Felice A, Scattoni ML, Ricceri L, Calamandrei G, PLoS One, Mar 24, 2015, 10(3):e0121663.

400. Neurodevelopmental disorders and prenatal residential proximity to agricultural pesticides: the CHARGE study, Shelton JF, Geraghty EM, Tancredi DJ, Delwiche LD, Schmidt RJ, Ritz B, Hansen RL, Hertz-Picciotto I, Environ Health Perspect, October 2014, 122(10):1103-9.

401. Early exposure to bisphenol A alters neuron and glia number in the rat prefrontal cortex of adult males, but not females, Neuroscience, October 24, 2014, 279:122-31, doi 10.1016/J Neuroscience, 2014.08.038, epub 2014.

402. Childhood autism and associated comorbidities, Brain and Development, June 2007, vol. 29, issue 5, pp. 257-272.

403. Mercury exposure and child development outcomes, Davidson PW, Myers GJ, Weiss B, Pediatrics, 2004, 113(4 suppl):1023-9.

404. Sleep spindles, mobile phones, lucid dreaming and sleep in Parkinson's disease and autism spectrum disorders, Dijk DJ, J Sleep Res, December 2012, 21(6):601-2.

405. Risk of autism spectrum disorders in children born after assisted conception: a population-based follow-up study, Hvidtjørn D, Grove J, Schendel D, Schieve LA, Sværke C, Ernst E, Thorsen P, J Epidemiol Community Health, June 2011, 65(6):497-502.

406. Perinatal factors and the development of autism: a population study, Arch Gen Psychiatry, June 2004, 61(6):618-27.

407. Out of time: a possible link between mirror neurons, autism and electromagnetic radiation, Thornton IM, Med Hypotheses, 2006, 67(2):378-82.

408. Polybrominated diphenyl ether (PBDE) flame retardants as potential autism risk factors (review), Messer A, Physiol Behav, June 1,2010, 100(3):245-9, doi 10.1016/j.physbeh.2010.01.011, epub January 2010.

409. Antenatal ultrasound and risk of autism spectrum disorders. Grether JK, Li SX, Yoshida CK, Croen LA. J Autism Dev Discord. Feb 2010;40(2):238-45.

410. Autism and attention-deficit/hyperactivity disorder among individuals with a family history of alcohol use disorders, Sundquist J, Sundquist K, Ji J, Elife, August 2014.

411. Med Hypotheses, August 2013, 81(2):251-2, doi 10.1016/j.mehy.2013.04.037, epub May 2013, May 21.Iatrogenic autism.Hahr JY1.

412. Influence of candidate polymorphisms on the dipeptidyl peptidase IV and μ-opioid receptor genes expression in aspect of the β-casomorphin-7 modulation functions in autism, Cieślińska A, Sienkiewicz, Szłapka E, Wasilewska J, Fiedorowicz E, Chwała B, Moszyńska-Dumara M, Cieśliński T, Bukało M, Kostyra E, Peptides, March 2015, pp. 6—11.

413. Soy infant formula may be associated with autistic behaviors, Westmark CJ, Autism Open Access, November 2013, 18;3, pp: 20727.

414. The relationship of autism and gluten, Buie T, Clin Ther, May 2013, 35(5):578-83.

415. A review of dietary interventions in autism, Annals of Clinical Psychiatry, 2009; 21(4):237-247.

416. Methods to create thermally oxidized lipids and comparison of analytical procedures to characterize peroxidation, J Anim Sci, July 2014, 92(7):2950-9, doi 10.2527/jas.2012-5708, epub May 2014.

417. 1994 data shows annual U.S. per capita consumption of vegetable oil at 25.1 killograms per day, equating to 618 calories daily. Data from tables at USDA website shows 2014 consumption is 170 percent of 1995 consumption. Assuming 1994 and 1995 are about the same in terms of per capita consumption, then doing the math for 2014 per capita consumption, we get just over 1,000 calories per day from vegetable oils for the average American. The average calories consumed per day by Americans obviously ranges widely, but 2015 estimates put the average intake at 3,600, where thin people eat 1,700-3,000, depending on activity level. Estimates for health conscious consumers based on personal experience that most health conscious consumers cook at home more often and that reduces their exposure to all vegetable oils. Sources: 1995 data from Table 6 in the article Polyunsaturated fatty acids in the food chain in the United States, Am J Clin Nutr, January 2000, vol. 71, no. 1, 179S-188, 2014 data from tables at www.ers.usda.gov/data-products/oil-crops-yearbook.aspx

418. Costs of autism spectrum disorders in the United Kingdom and the United States, Buescher AS, Cidav Z, Knapp M, Mandell DS, JAMA Pediatr, 2014, 168(8):721-728, doi10.1001/jamapediatrics.2014.210.

419. Chemistry and biology of DNA containing 1, N2-deoxyguanosine adducts of the α,β-unsaturated aldehydes acrolein, crotonaldehyde, and 4-hydroxynonenal, Chem Res Toxicol, May 18, 2009, 22(5): 759–778.

420. Mutational specificity of γ-radiation-induced g–thymine and thymine–guanine intrastrand cross-links in mammalian cells and translesion synthesis past the guanine–thymine lesion by human DNA polymerase, Biochemistry, August 5, 2008; 47(31): 8070–8079.

421. Rates of spontaneous mutation, Drake JW, Charlesworth B, Charlesworth D, Crow JF, Genetics, April 1998, 148 (4): 1667–86.

422. Mutagenic/recombinogenic effects of four lipid peroxidation products in Drosophila. Food Chem Toxicol, March 2013, 53:ch221-7, doi 10.1016/j.fct.2012.11.0,3, epub December 2012.

423. Dietary oxidized n-3 PUFA induce oxidative stress and inflammation: role of intestinal absorption of 4-HHE and reactivity in intestinal cells, J Lipid Res, October 2012, 53(10):2069-80, doi 10.1194/jlr.M026179, epub August 2012.

424. Role of glutathione in the radiation response of mammalian cells in vitro and in vivo, Bump EA, Brown JM, Pharmacol Ther, 1990, 47(1):117-36.

425. Glutathione modifies the oxidation products of 2'-deoxyguanosine by singlet molecular oxygen, Peres PS, Valerio A, Cadena SM, Winnischofer SM, Scalfo AC, Di Mascio P, Martinez GR, Arch Biochem Biophys, November 15, 2015, 586:33-44, doi 10.1016/j.abb.2015.09.020, epub September 2015.

426. Unequivocal demonstration that malondialdehyde is a mutagen, Carcinogenesis, 1983, 4(3):331-3.

427. Oxy radicals, lipid peroxidation and DNA damage, Toxicology, December 27, 2002, 181-182:219-22.

428. Ibid.

429. Malondialdehyde, a major endogenous lipid peroxidation product, sensitizes human cells to UV- and BPDE-induced killing and mutagenesis through inhibition of nucleotide excision repair, Mutat Res, October 10, 2006, 601(1-2):125-36, epub July 2006.

430. Trans-4-hydroxy-2-nonenal inhibits nucleotide excision repair in human cells: a possible mechanism for lipid peroxidation-induced carcinogenesis, Proc Natl Acad Sci USA, June 2004, 8;101(23):8598-602.

431. Global increases in both common and rare copy number load associated with autism, Hum Mol Genet, July 15, 2013, 22(14): 2870–2880.

432. Global increases in both common and rare copy number load associated with autism, Hum Mol Genet, July 15, 2013, 22(14): 2870–2880. The article discusses primarily the category of mutation called copy number load, meaning long portions of DNA are present in either abnormally high amount or a copy of the gene is absent. This study found a 7.7-fold increase in duplications and a 2.3-fold increase in deletions.

433. Global increases in both common and rare copy number load associated with autism, Hum Mol Genet, July 15, 2013, 22(14): 2870–2880.413, MMWR CDC Surveill Summ, December 1990, 39(4):19-23, Temporal trends in the prevalence of congenital malformations at birth based on the birth defects monitoring program, Edmonds LD, United States, 1979–1987.

434. Global increases in both common and rare copy number load associated with autism, Hum Mol Genet, July 15, 2013, 22(14): 2870–2880.

435. Global increases in both common and rare copy number load associated with autism, Hum Mol Genet, July 15, 2013, 22(14): 2870–2880.

436. The association between congenital anomalies and autism spectrum disorders in a Finnish national birth cohort, Dev Med Child Neurol, January 2015, 57(1): 75–80.

437. Minor malformations and physical measurements in autism: data from Nova Scotia, Teratology, 55:319–325 (1997).

438. MMWR CDC Surveill Summ. 1990 Dec;39(4):19-23). Temporal trends in the prevalence of congenital malformations at birth based on the birthdefects monitoring program, United States, 1979-1987. Edmonds LD (Yes this is the most recent report, apparently the CDC didn't find these statistics disturbing enough to see if the trend was continuing.)

439. Prevalence of autism spectrum disorder among children aged eight years—autism and developmental disabilities monitoring network, eleven sites, United States, 2010, Surveillance Summaries, March 28, 2014/63(SS02);1-21.

440. Advancing paternal age and risk of autism: new evidence from a population-based study and a meta-analysis of epidemiological studies, Mol Psychiatry, December 2011, (12):1203-12.

Chapter 9

441. Cane sugar: 160 pounds per capita per year; high fructose corn syrup: 44 pounds per capita per year.

442. Maternal obesity and risk for birth defects, Watkins ML, Pediatrics, vol. 111, no. 5, May 2003, pp. 1152-1158.

443. Fasting glucose in acute myocardial infarction, incremental value for long-term mortality and relationship with left ventricular systolic function, Aronson D, Diabetes Care, 30:960-966, 2007.

444. IGT and IFG, time for revision? K. Borch-Johnsen, Diabetic Medicine. vol. 19, issue 9, September 2002, pp. 707—707.

445. The modern nutritional diseases, Ottoboni F, 2002: "Epidemiologic studies among human populations showed that atherosclerotic cardiovascular diseases occurred at higher rates in affluent societies and among the higher socioeconomic classes. These studies associated the high disease rates with 'luxurious food' consumption, excessive caloric intake, sweets, sedentary lifestyle, and stress."

446. America's eating habits: changes and consequences, Frazao E (editor), Agriculture Information Bulletin No. (AIB750) 484, May 1999, Chapter 7: Trends in the US. food supply: 1970–97.

447. Insulin and glucagon modulate hepatic 3-hydroxy-3-methylglutaryl-coenzyme a reductase activity by affecting immunoreactive protein levels, G Ness, Journal of Biological Chemistry, 18 November 1994, 29168-72.

448. Restricted daily consumption of a highly palatable food (chocolate Ensure) alters striatal enkephalin gene expression, Kelley AE, European Journal of Neuroscience, 18 (9), pp. 2592–2598. The authors conclude that "repeated consumption of a highly rewarding, energy-dense food induces neuroadaptations in cognitive-motivational circuits." Numerous other similar studies exist to support the idea that animals addicted to sugar have the same chemical changes in their brains as if they were addicted to opiates.

449. Routine sucrose analgesia, during the first week of life in neonates younger than thirty-one weeks' postconceptional age, Johnston CC, Pediatrics, vol. 110, no. 3, September 2002, pp. 523-528.

450. Ibid.

451. Ibid.

452. Central insulin resistance as a trigger for sporadic Alzheimer-like pathology: an experimental approachreview, Salkovic-Petrisic M, Hoyer S, J Neural Transm Suppl, 2007, (72):217-33.

453. Aging of the brain (review), Mech Aging Dev, Anderton BH, April 2002, 123(7):811-7.

454. Taste preference for sweetness in urban and rural populations in Iraq, Jamel HA, J Dent Res, 75(11): 1879-1884, November 1996.

455. Pediasure brand nutritional supplement label information, accessed online on August 22, 2007 from www.pediasure.com/pedia_info.a.px

456. Observations on the economic adulteration of high value food products, Fairchild GF, Journal of Food Distribution Research, vol. 32, no. 2, July 2003, pp. 38–45.

457. From the ingredients listed on a box of Kellogg's Raisin Bran Crunch.

458. Fructose and non-fructose sugar intakes in the US population and their associations with indicators of metabolic syndrome, Sam Sun et al, Food and Chemical Toxicology, 49,11 (2011): 2874-2882.

459. Dietary fructose consumption among US children and adults: the third national health and nutrition examination survey, Miriam Vos et al, Medscape J Med, 10,7 (2008) 160.

Chapter 10

460. The Cambridge World History of Food, Cambridge University Press, 2000, p. 1210.

461. Ibid.

462. Dietary advanced glycation endproducts (AGEs) and their health effects—PRO, Sebeková K, Mol Nutr Food Res, September 2007, 51(9):1079-84.

463. Methylglyoxal in food and living organisms (review), Nemet I, Mol Nutr Food Res, December 2006, 50(12):1105-17.

464. Multidimensional scaling of ferrous sulfate and basic tastes, Stevens D, Physiology and Behavior, 2006, vol. 87, no. 2, pp. 272–279.

465. Neural circuits for taste: excitation, inhibition, and synaptic plasticity in the rostral gustatory zone of the nucleus of the solitary tract, Bradley RM, Annals of the New York Academy of Sciences, 855 (1), 467–474.

466. Excitotoxins: the taste that kills, Russel Blaylock, Health Press, 1996.

467. Body composition of white tailed deer, Robbins C, J, Anim Sci, 1974, 38:871-876.

468. University of New Hampshire Cooperative Extension, accessed online on August 19, 2008, at: www.extension.unh.edu/news/feedeer.htm

469. *The Journals of Samuel Hearne,* S Hearne, 1768, "On the twenty-second of July, we met several strangers, whom we joined in pursuit of the caribou, which were at this time so plentiful that we got everyday a sufficient number for our support, and indeed too frequently killed several merely for the tongues, marrow and fat."

470. *The Narrative of Cabeza De Vaca,* Cabeza de Vaca, Álvar Núñez, translation of La Relacion by Rolena Adorno and Patrick Charles Pautz, University of Nebraska Press, 2003.

471. CD36 involvement in orosensory detection of dietary lipids, spontaneous fat preference, and digestive secretions, Laugusterette FJ, Clin Invest, 115:3177-3184, 2005.

472. Evidence for human orosensory (taste) sensitivity to free fatty acids, Chale-Rush A, Chem Senses, June 1, 2007, 32(5): 423--431.

473. Multiple routes of chemosensitivity to free fatty acids in humans, Chale-Rush A, Am J Physiol Gastrointest Liver Physiol, 292: G1206-G1212, 2007.

474. Seeds of deception, exposing industry and government lies about the safety of the genetically engineered foods you're eating, Smith J, Yes Books, 2003, pp. 77-105.

475. Nutraceuticals as therapeutic agents in osteoarthritis: the role of glucosamine, chondroitin sulfate, and collagen hydrolysate, Deal CL, Rheumatic Disease Clinics of North America, vol. 25, issue 2, May 1, 1999, pp. 379-395.

476. Ibid.

477. The heparin-binding (fibroblast) growth factor family of proteins, Burgess W, Annual Review of Biochemistry, vol. 58: 575-602, July 1989.

478. As posted on the Stone Foundation for Arthritis Help and Research website, accessed on October 10, 2007, at: www.stoneclinic.com/jJanuaryews.htm

479. Determinants and implications of bone grease rendering: a Pacific Northwest example, Prince P, North American Archaeologist, vol. 28, no.1, 2007.

480. A new approach to identifying bone marrow and grease exploitation: why the "indeterminate" fragments should not be ignored, Outram AK, Journal of Archaeological Science, 2001, 28, pp. 401–410.

481. The Ladies New Book Of Cookery: A Practical System for Private Families in Town and Country; With Directions for Carving and Arranging the Table for Parties, Etc., Also Preparations of Food for Invalids and for Children, Sara Hosepha Hale, New York, H Long and Brother, 1852, p. 93.

482. Freezing for two weeks at -4 degrees F. will kill parasites.

483. *Let's Cook It Right,* Adelle Davis, Signet, 1970, p. 87.

484. USDA Agricultural Resource Service Nutrient Data Library, accessed online on December 23, 2005, at www.nal.usda.gov/fnic/foodcomp/search/

485. Paraphrased by HE Jacob in Six Thousand Years of Bread: It's Holy and Unholy History, Skyhorse, 2007, p. 26.

486. *The Cambridge World History of Food,* Cambridge Unviersity Press, 2000, p. 1474.

487. *Wind, Water, Work: Ancient and Medieval Milling Technology,* Adam Lucas, Brill Academic Publishers, 2005.

488. The gut flora as a forgotten organ, Shanahan F, EMBO reports 7, 7, 688–693, 2006.

489. Nutrition and colonic health: the critical role of the microbiota, O'keefe SJ, Curr Opin Gastroenterol, January 2008, 24(1):51-58.

490. Serum or plasma cartilage oligomeric matrix protein concentration as a diagnostic marker in pseudoachondroplasia: differential diagnosis of a family, A Cevik Tufan et al, Eur J Hum Genet, 15: 1023-1028.

491. *The Cambridge World History of Food,* Cambridge Unviersity Press, 2000, p. 1473.

492. Effects of soy protein and soybean isoflavones on thyroid function in healthy adults and hypothyroid patients: a review of the relevant literature, Messina M, Thyroid, March 2006, 16(3):249-58.

493. Infant feeding with soy formula milk: effects on puberty progression, reproductive function and testicular cell numbers in marmoset monkeys in adulthood, Tan KA, Hum Reprod, April 2006, (4):896-904.

494. *Food Values Of Portions Commonly Used,* Pennington J, Harper, 1989.

495. Quorum sensing: cell-to-cell communication in bacteria, Waters CM, Bassler BL, Annu Rev Cell Dev Biol, 21:319-346, 2005.

496. The gut flora as a forgotten organ, Shanahan F, EMBO reports 7, 7, 688–693, 2006.

497. Probiotics in human disease (review), Isolauri E, Am J Clin Nutr, June 2001, 73(6):1142S-1146S.

498. Commensal bacteria (normal microflora), mucosal immunity and chronic inflammatory and auto-immune diseases (review), Sokol D, Immunol Lett, May 15, 2004, 93(2-3):97-108.

499. Probiotics and their fermented food products are beneficial for health (review), Parvez S, J Appl Microbiol, Jun 2006, 100(6):1171-85.

500. Nutritional comparison of fresh, frozen, and canned fruits and vegetables, Executive Summary of the Department of Food Science and Technology, University of California Davis, Davis, CA, Rickman J, accessed online at: www.mealtime.org/uploadedFiles/Mealtime/Content/ucdavisstudyexecutivesummary.pdf

501. Whole wheat and white wheat flour—the mycobiota and potential mycotoxins, Weidenbörner M, Food Microbiology, vol. 17, issue 1, February 2000, pp. 103–107.

502. The impact of processing on the nutritional quality of food proteins, Meade S, Journal of AOAC International, 2005, vol. 88, no. 3, pp. 904–922.

503. Let's Have Healthy Children, Adelle Davis, Signet, 1972, p. 95.

504. Bioavailability and bioconversion of carotenoids, Castenmiller JJM, Annual Review of Nutrition, vol. 18: 19-38, July 1998.

505. *Mrs. Hill's Southern Practical Cookery and Receipt Book,* AP Hill, Damon Lee Fowler, University of South Carolina Press, 1872.

506. The apparent incidence of hip fracture in Europe: a study of national register sources, Johnel O, Ostoporosis International, vol. 2, no. 6, November 1992.

507. *The Last Hours of Ancient Sunlight: The Fate of the World and What We Can Do Before It's Too Late,* revised and updated, Thom Hartman, Broadway, 2004.

508. *The Milk Book: The Milk of Human Kindness Is Not Pasteurized,* William Campbell Douglass II, Rhino Publishing, 2005.

509. Continuous thermal processing of foods: pasteurization and Uht, Heppell NJ, Springer 2000, p. 194.

510. Dr. North and the Kansas City Newspaper war: public health advocacy collides with main street respectability, Kovarik B, paper presented at the Annual Meeting of the Association for Education in Journalism and Mass Communication (72nd, Washington, D.C., August 10-13, 1989,

accessed online on December 27, 2007, at: www.radford.edu/wkovarik/papers/aej98.html

511. *The Milk Book: The Milk of Human Kindness Is Not Pasteurized,* William Campbell Douglass II, Rhino Publishing, 2005.

512. Ibid., p. 11.

513. Modifications in milk proteins induced by heat treatment and homogenization and their influence on susceptibility to proteolysis, Garcia-Risco MR, International Dairy Journal, 12 (2002) pp. 679–688.

514. Soluble, dialyzable and ionic calcium in raw and processed skim milk, whole milk and spinach, Reykdal O, Journal of Food Science, 56 3, pp. 864–866, 1991.

515. Calcium bioavailability in human milk, cow milk and infant formulas—comparison between dialysis and solubility methods, Roig MJ, Food Chemistry, vol. 65, issue 3, pp. 353-357.

516. Carbonylation of milk powder proteins as a consequence of processing conditions, François Fenaille, Proteomics, vol. 5, issue 12, pp. 3097-3104.

517. Modifications in milk proteins induced by heat treatment and homogenization and their influence on susceptibility to proteolysis, Garcia-Risco MR, International Dairy Journal, 12 (2002) pp. 679–688.

518. *Chemistry and Safety of Acrylamide in Food,* Friedman M, p. 141, Springer, 2005.

519. Lancet, May 8, 1937, p. 1142.

520. Nutrition abstracts and reviews, Fischr RA and Bartlett S, October 1931, vol. 1, p. 224.

521. Dietary fat requirements in health and development, Thomas H Applewhite, American Oil Chemists Society, 1988, p. 30.

Chapter 11

522. Jaenisch, R, Epigenetic regulation of gene expression: how the genome integrates intrinsic and environmental signals, Nature Genetics, 33, 245-254 (2003).

523. Orexins in the brain-gut axis, Kirchgessner AL, Endocrine Reviews, 23 (1): 1-15.

524. Adipose tissue as an endocrine organ, Prins JB, Best Practice and Research Clinical Endocrinology and Metabolism, 2002, vol. 16, no. 4, pp. 639-651.

525. Reduction in adiposity affects the extent of afferent projections to growth hormone-releasing hormone and somatostatin neurons and the degree of colocalization of neuropeptides in growth hormone-releasing hormone and somatostatin cells of the ovine hypothalamus, Javed Iqbal J, Endocrinology, vol. 146, no. 11, pp. 4776-4785.

526. Peroxisome proliferator-activated receptor {gamma} and adipose tissue—understanding obesity-related changes in regulation of lipid and glucose metabolism, Sharma AM, Journal of Clinical Endocrinology and Metabolism, vol. 92, no. 2, pp. 386-395.

527. Leptin-induced growth stimulation of breast cancer cells involves recruitment of histone acetyltransferases and mediator complex to CYCLEN D1 promoter via activation of stat 3, Saxena NK, J. Biol Chem, vol. 282, issue 18, pp. 13316-13325, May 4, 2007.

528. Effect of dietary trans fatty acids on the delta 5, delta 6 and delta 9 desaturases of rat liver microsomes in vivo, Mahfouz M, Acta Biol Med Ger, 1981, 40(12):1699-1705. "This study shows that the dietary trans fatty acids are differentially incorporated into the liver microsomal lipids and act as inhibitors for delta 9 and delta 6 desaturases. The delta 6 desaturase is considered as the key enzyme in the conversion of the essential fatty acids to arachidonic acid and prostaglandins. This indicates that the presence of trans fatty acids in the diet may induce some effects on the EFA metabolism through their action on the desaturases."

529. A defect in the activity of delta 6 and delta 5 desaturases may be a factor predisposing to the development of insulin resistance syndrome, Das UN, Prostaglandins, Leukotrienes and Essential Fatty Acids, vol. 72, issue 5, May 2005, pp. 343–350.

530. Regulation of stearoyl-CoA desaturase by polyunsaturated fatty acids and cholesterol, M Ntambi, September 1999, Journal of Lipid Research, 40, pp. 1549–1558.

531. Role of stearoyl-CoA desaturases in obesity and the metabolic syndrome, H E Popeijus, International Journal of Obesity, 32, 1076–1082, doi 10.1038/ijo.2008.55, published online April 22, 2008.

532. Interruption of triacylglycerol synthesis in the endoplasmic reticulum is the initiating event for saturated fatty acid-induced lipotoxicity in liver cells, Mantzaris, February 2011, 278(3):519–30, doi 10.1111/j.1742-4658.2010.07972.x.

533. The significance of differences in fatty acid metabolism between obese and non-obese patients with non-alcoholic fatty liver disease, Nakamuta M, Int J Mol Med, November 2008, 22(5):663-7.

534. Liver mitochondrial dysfunction and oxidative stress in the pathogenesis of experimental nonalcoholic fatty liver disease, Oliveira CP, Braz J Med Biol Res, February 2006, 39(2):189-94, epub February 2006.

535. Insulin resistance, inflammation, and non-alcoholic fatty liver disease, Tilg H, Trends Endocrinol Metab, October 15, 2008, epub prior to print.

536. Apoptosis in skeletal muscle myotubes is induced by ceramide and is positively related to insulin resistance,Turpin SM, Am J Physiol Endocrinol Metab, 291: E1341–E1350, 2006.

537. Weapons of lean body mass destruction: the role of ectopic lipids in the metabolic syndrome (review), Unger RH, Endocrinology, December 2003, 144(12):5159-65.

538. Prostaglandins, Chuck S. Bronson, Nova Publishers, 2006. p. 51.

539. Dietary fat intake and risk of type 2 diabetes in women, Salmeron J, American Journal of Clinical Nutrition, vol. 73, no. 6, pp. 1019-1026, June 2001.

540. Sex differences in lipid and glucose kinetics after ingestion of an acute oral fructose load, Tran C, Jacot Descombes D, Lecoultre V, Fielding BA, Carrel G, Le KA, Schneiter P, Bortolotti M, Frayn KN, Tappy L, Br J Nutr, 2010, 104:1139–1147.

541. Regulation of adipose cell number in man, Prins JB, Clin Sci, London, 1997, 92: 3-11.

542. Neural Innervation of White Adipose Tissue and the Control of Lipolysis, Bartness, Timothy J. et al, Frontiers in Neuroendocrinology, 35.4 (2014): 473–493.PMC, web, April 15, 2016.

543. The cellular plasticity of human adipocytes, Tholpady SS, Annals of Plastic Surgery, vol. 54, no. 6, June 2005, pp. 651–6.

544. Transdifferentiation potential of human mesenchymal stem cells derived from bone marrow, Song L, FASEB Journal, vol. 18, June 2004, pp. 980–82.

545. Reversible transdifferentiation of secretory epithelial cells into adipocytes in the mammary gland, Morron M, PNAS, November 30, 2004, vol. 101, no. 48, pp. 16801–16806.

546. Identification of cartilage progenitor cells in the adult ear perichondrium: utilization for cartilage reconstruction, Togo T, Laboratory Investigation, 2006, 86, pp. 445–457.

547. The cellular plasticity of human adipocytes, Tholpady SS, Annals of Plastic Surgery, vol. 54, no. 6, June 2005, pp. 651–56.

548. The Health Report, ABC Radio International transcript, July 9, 2007, presented by Norman Swain.

549. Insulin-resistant subjects have normal angiogenic response to aerobic exercise training in skeletal muscle, but not in adipose tissue, Walton RG, Physiol Rep, June 2015, 3(6), pii, e12415, doi 10.14814/phy2.12415.

550. Transdifferentiation potential of human mesenchymal stem cells derived from bone marrow,

Song L, FASEB, vol. 18, June 2004, pp. 980–82.

551. Adipose cell apoptosis: death in the energy depot, A Sorisky, International Journal of Obesity, 2000, 24, suppl. 4, S3±S7.

552. In vivo dedifferentiation of adult adipose cells, Liao, Yunjun et al, Guillermo López Lluch (editor), PLoS ONE 10.4 (2015): e0125254, PMC, web, April 15, 2016. "Adipocytes can highly express embryonic stem cell markers, such as October 4, Sox2, c-Myc, and Nanog, after dedifferentiating [34]. Thus, they may represent a reservoir of pluripotent cells in dynamic equilibrium with organ-specific cellular components and be capable of phenotypic transformation."

553. Changes in nerve cells of the nucleus basalis of Meynert in Alzheimer's disease and their relationship to ageing and to the accumulation of lipofuscin pigment, Mann DM, Mech Ageing Dev, April-May 1984, 25(1-2):189-204.

554. Mechanisms of disease: is osteoporosis the obesity of bone? Rosen CJ, Nature Clinical Practice Rheumatology, 2006, 2, pp. 35–43.

555. Endocrinology of adipose tissue – an update, Fischer-Pozovsky P, Hormone Metabolism Research, May 2007, 36(5):314-21.

556. Exercise and the treatment of clinical depression in adults: recent findings and future directions, Brosse A, Sports Medicine, 32(12):741-760, 2002.

557. Beta-endorphin decreases fatigue and increases glucose uptake independently in normal and dystrophic mice, Kahn S, Muscle Nerve, April 2005, 31(4):481-6.

558. The differential contribution of tumour necrosis factor to thermal and mechanical hyperalgesia during chronic inflammation, Inglis JJ, Arthritis Res Ther, 2005, 7(4):R807-16, epub April 2005.

559. TNF-related weak inducer of apoptosis (TWEAK) is a potent skeletal muscle-wasting cytokine, Faseb J, June 2007, 21(8):1857-69.

560. Aerobic exercise training increases brain volume in aging humans, Colcombe J, Journals of Gerontology Series A: Biological Sciences and Medical Sciences, 2006, 61:1166-1170.

561. Running increases cell proliferation and neurogenesis in the adult mouse dentate gyrus, Gage FH, Nat Neurosci, Mar 1999, 2(3):266-70.

562. Six sessions of sprint interval training increases muscle oxidative potential and cycle endurance capacity in humans, Burgomaster KA, J Appl Physiol, 98: 1985-1990, 2005.

563. Ibid.

564. Plasma ghrelin is altered after maximal exercise in elite male rowers, Jürimäe J, Exp Biol Med, Maywood, July 2007, 232(7):904-9.

Chapter 12

565. Update on food allergy, Sampson, H, Journal of Allergy and Clinical Immunology , vol. 113, issue 5, pp. 805–819.

566. Food allergy among U.S. children: trends in prevalence and hospitalizations, NCHS Data Brief No. 10, October 2008, Amy M. Branum, M.S.P.H. Figure 4, accessible online at http://www.cdc.gov/nchs/products/databriefs/db10.htm

567. The relationship between lower extremity alighment charactheristics and anterior knee joint laxity, Shultz SJ, Sports Health 1, 1 (2009) 53-100.

568. Update on food allergy, Sampson H, Journal of Allergy and Clinical Immunology, vol. 113, issue 5, pp. 805-819.

569. Food allergy among U.S. children: trends in prevalence and hospitalizations, NCHS Data

Brief No. 10, October 2008, Amy M. Branum, M.S.P.H. Figure 4, accessible online at http://www.cdc.gov/nchs/products/databriefs/db10.htm

570. Facial soft tissue reconstruction: Thomas procedures in facial plastic surgery Gregory H, Branham Pmph USA, November 30, 2011, p. 17.

571. Glycation stress and photo-aging in skin, Masamitsu Ichihashi, Anti-Aging Medicine, 2011, vol. 8, no. 3, pp. 23-29.

572. Ageing and zonal variation in post-translational modification of collagen in normal human articular cartilage: the age-related increase in non-enzymatic glycation affects bio-mechanical properties of cartilage.

573. Ruud A. Bank, Biochemical Journal, February 15, 1998,330(1)345-351.

574. Diabetes, advanced glycation endproducts and vascular disease, Jean-Luc Wautier, Vasc Med, May 1998, vol. 3, no. 2, pp. 131-137.

575. Role of advanced glycation end products in aging collagen, Gerontology, 1998, 44(4):187-9.

576. See how AGEs cross-link collagen in Chapter 10, Beyond Calories.

577. Session 3: Joint Nutrition Society and Irish Nutrition and Dietetic Institute Symposium on 'Nutrition and auto-immune disease' PUFA, inflammatory processes and rheumatoid arthritis, Proc Nutr Soc, November 2008, 67(4):409-18.

578. Facial plastic surgery, scar management: prevention and treatment strategies, Chen, Margaret, Current Opinion in Otolaryngology and Head and Neck Surgery, August 2005, vol. 13, issue 4, pp. 242–247.

579. Metabolic fate of exogenous chondroitin sulfate in the experimental animal, Palmieri L, Arzneimittelforschung, March 1990, 40(3):319–23.

580. Proteoglycans and glycosaminoglycans, Silbert JE, in Biochemistry and Physiology of the Skin, Goldsmith LA (editor), Oxford University Press, 1983, pp. 448–461.

581. Anti-inflammatory activity of chondroitin sulfate, Ronca F, Osteoarthritis Cartilage, May 6, 1998, suppl. A:14-21.

582. Nutraceuticals as therapeutic agents in osteoarthritis: the role of glucosamine, chondroitin sulfate, and collagen hydrolysate, Deal CL, Rheumatic Disease Clinics of North America, vol. 25, issue 2, May 1, 1999.

583. The effect of concentrated bone broth as a dietary supplementation on bone healing in rabbits, Mahmood A, Aljumaily Department of Surgery, College of Medicine, University of Mosul, Ann Coll Med Mosul, 2011; 37 [1 and 2]: 42-47).

584. Cell death in cartilage, K. Kühn, Osteoarthritis and Cartilage, vol. 12, issue 1, January 2004, pp. 1–16.

585. The effect of hyaluronic acid on IL-1β-induced chondrocyte apoptosis in a rat model of osteoarthritis, Pang-Hu Zhou, Journal of Orthopaedic Research, December 2008, vol. 26, issue 12, pp. 1643–1648.

586. Cellulite and its treatment, Rawlings A, International Journal of Cosmetic Science, 2006, 28, pp. 175–190.

587. Mediators of Inflammation, vol. 2010 (2010), article ID 858176, 6 pages, Lipid mediators in acne, Monica Ottaviani.

588. Antioxidant activity, lipid peroxidation and skin diseases, what's new, S Briganti, Journal of the European Academy of Dermatology and Venereology, vol. 17, issue 6, pp. 663–669, November 2003.

589. Inflammatory lipid mediators in common skin diseases, Kutlubay Z, Skinmed, February 1, 2016, 1;14(1):23-7, eCollection 2016.

590. Inflammation in acne vulgaris, Guy F Webster, Journal of the American Academy of Dermatology, vol. 33, issue 2, part 1, August 1995, pp. 247–253.

591. Antioxidant activity, lipid peroxidation and skin diseases, what's new, S Briganti, Journal of the European Academy of Dermatology and Venereology, vol. 17, issue 6, pp. 663–669, November 2003.

592. Inflammatory lipid mediators in common skin diseases, Kutlubay Z, Skinmed, February 1, 2016, 1;14(1):23-7, eCollection 2016.

593. Dietary glycemic factors, insulin resistance, and adiponectin levels in acne vulgaris, Çerman AA, J Am Acad Dermatol, Apr 6, 2016, pii: S0190-9622(16)01485-7.

594. Glycemic index, glycemic load: new evidence for a link with acne, Berra B J, Am Coll Nutr, August 2009, 28 suppl., 450S-454S.

595. Modern acne treatment, Zouboilis C, Aktuelle Dermatologie, 2003, vol. 29, no. 1-2, pp. 49–57.

596. Diet and acne redux, Valori Treloar, CNS Arch Dermatol, 2003, 139(7):941.

597. Flesh eating bacteria: a legacy of war and call for peace, Shanahan C, Pacific Journal, vol. 1, issue 1, 2007.

598. Kinetics of UV light–induced cyclobutane pyrimidine dimers in human skin in vivo: an immunohistochemical analysis of both epidermis and dermis, Katiyar S, Photochemistry and Photobiology, vol. 72, issue 6, pp. 788–793.

599. Ultraviolet irradiation increases matrix metalloproteinase-8 protein in human skin in vivo, GJ Fisher, Journal of Investigative Dermatology, vol. 117, issue 2, August 2001, pp. 219–226.

600. Vitamin D deficiency: a worldwide problem with health consequences, Michael F Holick, Am J Clin Nutr, April 2008, vol. 87, no. 4, 1080S-1086S.

601. The vitamin D content of fortified milk and infant formula, Holick MF, NEJM, vol. 326:1178-1181, April 30, 1992.

602. Vitamin D intoxication associated with an over-the-counter supplement, Koutikia P, N Engl J Med, July 5, 2001, 345(1):66-7.

603. Vitamin D: the underappreciated D-lightful hormone that is important for skeletal and cellular health, Holick M, Current Opinion in Endocrinology and Diabetes, February 2002, 9(1):87-98.

604. The evolution of human skin coloration, Jablonski, Nina G, and George Chaplin, Journal of Human Evolution, 39: 57-106, 2000. With the exception of Northern American Native peoples. The exception may be due to the fact that they only migrated far north recently, or that they ate so much vitamin D rich animal tissue their skin never needed to lose the melanin to enable UV to penetrate enough to make their own.

605. The protective role of melanin against UV damage in human skin, Michaela Brenner, Photochem Photobiol, 2008, 84(3): 539–549.

606. Ibid.

607. Ultraviolet radiation accelerates BRAF-driven melanomagenesis by targeting TP53, Viros, A, et al, Nature, 2014, 511(7510): pp. 478-82.

608. Skin aging induced by ultraviolet exposure and tobacco smoking: evidence from epidemiological and molecular studies, Lei Y, Photodermatol Photoimmunol Photomed, 2001, 17: 178–183.

609. Molecular basis of sun-induced premature skin ageing and retinoid antagonism, Fisher GJ, Nature, vol. 379(6563), January 25, 1996, pp. 335-339.

610. Eicosapentaenoic acid inhibits UV-induced MMP-1expression in human dermal fibroblasts, Hyeon HK, Journal of Lipid Research, vol. 46, 2005, pp. 1712-20.

611. Influence of glucosamine on matrix metalloproteinase expression and activity in lipopoly-saccharide-stimulated equine chondrocytes, Byron CR, American Journal of Veterinary Research, June 2003, vol. 64, no. 6, pp. 666-671.

612. The structures of elastins and their function, Debelle L and Alix AJ, Biochimie 81, 1999, pp. 981-994.

613. *The Lung: Development, Aging and the Environment,* Plopper C (editor), Elsevier Publishing, 2003, p. 259.

614. Anti-oxidation and anti-wrinkling effects of jeju horse leg bone hydrolysates, Dongwook Kim, Korean J Food Sci Anim Resour, 2014, 34(6): 844–851.

615. Collagen hydrolysate intake increases skin collagen expression and suppresses matrix metal-loproteinase 2 activity, Zague V, J Med Food, June 2011, 14(6):618-24, doi 10.1089/jmf.2010.0085, pub April 2011.

Chapter 13

616. Gallup Poll 2012, accessible online at: www.gallup.com/poll/156116/Nearly-Half-Ameri-cans-Drink-Soda-Daily.aspx?utm_source=google&utm_medium=rss&utm_campaign=syndication

617. Dietary and physical activity behaviors among adults successful at weight loss maintenance, Judy Kruger, International Journal of Behavioral Nutrition and Physical Activity, December 2006, 3:17.

618. Body mass index and neurocognitive functioning across the adult lifespan, Stanek KM, Neu-ropsychology, March 2013, (2):141-51.

619. Altered executive function in obesity; exploration of the role of affective states on cognitive abilities, Appetite, vol. 52, issue 2, April 2009, pp. 535–539.

620. Opinion of the panel on food additives, flavourings, processing aids and food contact ma-terials (AFC), EFSA Journal, 2008, 754, 1-34 © European Food Safety Authority, 2007 Scientific (question nos. EFSA-Q-2006-168 and EFSA-Q-2008-254, adopted on May 22, 2008.

621. Opinion of the panel on food additives, flavourings, processing aids and food contact ma-terials (AFC), EFSA Journal, 2008, 754, 1-34 © European Food Safety Authority, 2007 Scientific (question nos. EFSA-Q-2006-168 and EFSA-Q-2008-254, adopted on May 22, 2008.

622. www.webmd.com/parenting/baby/baby-food-nutrition-9/baby-food-answers

623. www.caringforkids.cps.ca/handouts/feeding_your_baby_in_the_first_year

Chapter 14

624. The risk of lead contamination in bone broth diets, Medical Hypotheses, vol. 80, issue 4, April 2013, pp. 389–390.

625. Evaluation of lead content of kale (brassica oleraceae) commercially available in Buncombe County, North Carolina, Journal of the North Carolina Academy of Science, 124(1), 2008, pp. 23–25.

626. Mercury, arsenic, lead and cadmium in fish and shellfish from the Adriatic Sea, Food Addit Contam, March 2003, 20(3):241-6.

627. WebMD Report: Protein drinks have unhealthy metals, Kathleen Doheny, reviewed by Lau-ra J. Martin on June 3, 2010. Consumer Reports study finds worrisome levels of lead, cadmi-um, and other metals, accessed online on March 8, 2015 at: http://www.webmd.com/food-reci-pes/20100603/report-protein-drinks-have-unhealthy-metals

628. Lead in New York City community garden chicken eggs: influential factors and health impli-cations, Environ Geochem Health, August 2014, 36(4):633-49, doi 10.1007/s10653-013-9586-z, epub November 2013.

629. Cadmium and lead levels in milk, milk-cereal and cereal formulas for infants and children up to three years of age, Rocz Panstw Zakl Hig, 1991, 42(2):131-8.

630. Arsenic, cadmium, lead and mercury in canned sardines commercially available in eastern Kentucky, USA, Mar Pollut Bull, January 2011, 62(1).

631. Mercury, arsenic, lead and cadmium in fish and shellfish from the Adriatic Sea, Food Addit Contam, March 2003, 20(3):241-6.

632. Biochemical characterization of cyanobacterial extracellular polymers (EPS) from modern marine stromatolites (Bahamas), Alan Decho, Prep Biochem and Biotechnol, 30(4), 321-330 (2000).

633. Antioxidant and antiinflammatory activities of ventol, a phlorotannin-rich natural agent derived from Ecklonia cava, and its effect on proteoglycan degradation in cartilage explant culture, Kang K, Res Commun Mol Pathol Pharmacol, 2004, 115-116:77-95.

634. www.ionsource.com/Card/protein/beta_casein.htm

635. Comparative effects of A1 versus A2 beta-casein on gastrointestinal measures: a blinded randomised cross-over pilot study, European Journal of Clinical Nutrition, 2014, 68, 994–1000.

636. CDC tool available at cdc.gov/foodbornoutbreaks/. Accessed March 9 2016, data collection period 1998-2014 (all available) states: all 50.

637. www.westonaprice.org/press/government-data-proves-raw-milk-safe/. This is based on data available in the 2010 census.

638. Estimated based on reports that 60 percent of U.S. adults do not drink milk and from data on children from this website: www.agriview.com/news/dairy/americans-drinking-less-milk-can-the-tide-be-turned/article_14ed2c88-d9bd-11e2-a7b9-0019bb2963f4.html

639. www.realmilk.com/press/wisconsin-campylobacter-outbreak-falsely-blamed-on-raw-milk/

640. Eating in restaurants: a risk factor for foodborne disease? Oxford Journals Medicine and Health Clinical Infectious Diseases, vol. 43, issue 10, pp. 1324-1328.

641. The ten riskiest foods regulated by the US food and drug administration, accessed online on March 9, 2016, at www.cspinet.org/new/pdf/cspi_top_10_fda.pdf626. High intakes of milk, but not meat, increase s-insulin and insulin resistance in eight-year-old boys, C Hoppe, European Journal of Clinical Nutrition, 2005, 59, 393–398.

642. European Journal of Clinical Nutrition (2005) 59, 393-398. High intakes of milk, but not meat, increase s-insulin and insulin resistance in 8-year-old boys. C Hoppe.

643. High intake of milk, but not meat decreasses bone turnover in prepubertal boys after seven days, Eur J Clin Nutr, August 2007, 61(8):957-62, epub January 2007.

644. Animal protein intake, serum insulin-like growth factor I, and growth in healthy 2.5-year-old Danish children, Am J Clin Nutr, August 2004, 80(2):447-52. "An increase in milk intake from 200 to 600 mL/d corresponded to a 30 percent increase in circulating IGF-I. This suggests that milk compounds have a stimulating effect on sIGF-I concentrations and, thereby, on growth."

645. Role of the enteric microbiota in intestinal homeostasis and inflammation, Free Radic Biol Med, Mar 2014, 0: 122–133.

646. Mechanisms of disease: the role of intestinal barrier function in the pathogenesis of gastrointestinal auto-immune diseases, Alessio Fasano and Terez Shea Donohue, Nature Clinical Practice Gastroenterology and Hepatology, September 2005, vol. 2, no. 9, pp. 416–422.

647. Surprises from celiac disease, Scientific American, August 2009, pp. 32-39.

648. Gliadin, zonulin, and gut permeability: effects on celiac and non-celiac intestinal mucosa and intestinal cell lines, Alessio Fasano, Scandinavian Journal of Gastroenterology, 2006; 41: 408-419.

649. Zonulin and its regulation of intestinal barrier function: the biological door to inflammation,

autoimmunity, and cancer, Physiological Reviews, January 1, 2011, vol. 91, no. 1, pp. 151-175.

650. Non-celiac gluten sensitivity: the new frontier of gluten related disorders, Nutrients, October 2013, 5(10): 3839–3853.

651. Epidemiology of food allergy, Scott H. Sicherer, March 2011, vol. 127, issue 3, pp. 594–602.

652. Toxic metal distribution in rural and urban soil samples affected by industry and traffic, Polish J of Environ Stud, vol. 18, no. 6 (2009), 1141-1150.

653. The elephant in the playground: confronting lead-contaminated soils as an important source of lead burdens to urban populations, Filippelli GM and Laidlaw MAS, 2010, Perspectives in Biology and Medicine 53, 31-45.

654. The role of immune dysfunction in the pathophysiology of autism, Brain Behav Immun, author manuscript available in PMC, March 1, 2013, Brain Behav Immun, March 2012, 26(3) pp. 383–392.

655. Is a subtype of autism an allergy of the brain? Clin Ther, May 2013, 35(5):584-91, doi 10.1016/j.clinthera.2013.04.009.

656. Focal brain inflammation and autism, J Neuroinflammation, 2013, 10: 46.

657. Sugar-sweetened carbonated beverage consumption and coronary artery calcification in asymptomatic men and women, Chun S, Choi Y, Chang Y, et al, Am Heart J, 2016; doi 10.1016/j.ahj.2016.03.018.

658. Added sugar intake and cardiovascular diseases mortality among US adults, Yang Q, Zhang Z, Gregg EW, et al, JAMA Intern Med, 2014, doi 10.1001/jamainternmed.2013.13563.

ILLUSTRATION CREDITS

Page ii, *Blending Cultures, Blending Time,* Flickr Creative Commons, Mark Byzewski

Page 2, *What Do the Toughest Men in History All Have in Common?* Klitschko: Sven Teschke; Samuelson: Frankie Fouganthin; Kahn: Fanghong; all other images in public domain

Page 41, *Old-Fashioned Breakfast,* courtesy Imam MP Heijboer

Page 43, *Profiles in Genetic Wealth,* Thai woman: courtesy David Miller, Flickr Creative Commons; Danish barmaid: ©Bill Bachman

Page 54, *Eight Historical Studies of Human Anatomy,* Le-Courbusier: Wasily Wikimedia Commons; all other images in public domain

Page 59, *The Golden Rectangle,* Cate Shanahan

Page 60, *Beauty Emerges From Math,* ©2001 Stephen R. Marquardt

Page 61, *Blueprint for Beauty, Stephen Marquardt, Marquardt Beauty Analsysis,* courtesy of Dr. Marquardt, www.beautyanalysis.com

Page 62, *Price Meets Marquardt,* photos © Price Pottenger Nutrition Foundation, www. PPNE.org; Marquardt Mask © Stephen Marquardt, www.beautyanalysis.com

Pages 66-67, *Why Attractive People Entrance Us,* Cate Shanahan

Page 71, *An Average Face,* Cate Shanahan

Page 75, *Number One Son—Why So Lucky? Matt Dillon:* Wikimedia Commons, Festival International de Cine en Guadalajara; Kevin Dillon: Flickr Creative Commons, Allistair McMannis

Page 78, *Different Geometry,* Paris Hilton: Pad Schafermeier; Nicky Hiton: Eduardo Sciämmarello Page 81, *Biradial Symmetry Can Be a Pain in the Neck,* courtesy of Dan Shanahan

Page 87, *Fetal Alcohol Syndrome,* Modern Pharmacology, vol. 6, 1977.

Page 90, *Under-Developed Jaw Impacting Airway,* courtesy of Alexander V. Antipov, D.D.S.

Page 94, *The Reason Men Should Take Preparation for Pregnancy as Seriously as Women,* courtesy of Arielle Shanahan

Page 98, *Skeletal Responses to Diet Change,* Cate Shanahan

Page 114, *Changing Our Diet May Change Us,* Cate Shanahan

Page 124, *How Keys Faked It,* Cate Shanahan

Page 130, *Partial Hydrogenation Squashes Fats Flat,* Cate Shanahan

Page 136, *Why Vegetable Oils Are Prone to Oxidation,* Cate Shanahan

Page 140, *French-Fried Heart,* Cate Shanahan

Page 141, *How Free Radicals Damage Membranes,* Cate Shanahan

Page 147, *Lipoproteins: Superheroes of Lipid Circulation,* Cate Shanahan

Page 152, *How Dysfunctional Lipoproteins Cause Arteriosclerosis,* Cate Shanahan

Page 226, *High-Sugar Diets May Lead to Dementia* © 2006 National Academy of Sciences, U.S.A.

Page 245, *Hydrolytic Cleavage,* Cate Shanahan

Page 256, *Organ Meats Versus Fruits and Vegetables,* Cate Shanahan

Page 271, *African Petroglyph,* courtesy of Andras Zboray, Fliegel Jerniczy Expeditions. Gourd portion of petroglyph was digitally modified for better viewing in black and white.

Page 287, *Pro-Inflammatory Fats Prevent Weight Loss,* Cate Shanahan

Page 291, *The Right Signals Can Turn Fat Cells Into Muscle, Bone, or Nerve,* Cate Shanahan

Page 307, *Feeding Your Skin With Beauty Cream,* courtesy of Reza Kafi, M.D.

Page 308, *Anatomy of Skin,* Blausen.com staff, "Blausen Gallery 2014," Wikiversity Journal of Medicine.

Page 309, *A Classic Sign of Weak Collagen,* Cate Shanahan

Page 312, *Cellulite Fat Lacks Adequate Collagen Support,* Cate Shanahan

Page 316, *A Scar Is Born,* Cate Shanahan

Page 319, *How the Sun Causes Wrinkling,* Cate Shanahan

Page 320, *Battle of the Diets,* Ornish: courtesy of Pierre Omidyar; Maasai man by Ninara

Page 322, *Test for Premature Wrinkling,* Cate Shanahan

Page 323, *Brains Like It Smooth,* public domain images by Alfred Yarbus

Page 340, *Macronutrient Breakdown,* left image: Average patient files; right image: Health, United States, 2015, with special feature on Racial and Ethnic Health Disparities, page 207

INDEX